Working
with Immigrant
Women

Working with Immigrant Women

Issues and Strategies for Mental Health Professionals

Edited by
Sepali Guruge, RN, BScN, MSc, PhD
Enid Collins, RN, MS, MEd, EdD

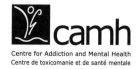

Centre for Addiction and Mental Health
Centre de toxicomanie et de santé mentale

Library and Archives Canada Cataloguing in Publication

Working with immigrant women : issues and strategies for mental health professionals / executive editors: Sepali Guruge and Enid Collins.

ISBN: 978-0-88868-535-3 (PRINT)
ISBN: 978-0-88868-728-9 (PDF)
ISBN: 978-0-88868-729-6 (HTML)

1. Women immigrants—Canada—Services for. 2. Women immigrants—Canada—Mental health. 3. Mental health services—Canada. I. Guruge, Sepali, 1967– II. Collins, Enid M. (Enid Monica), 1936–

HQ1453.W67 2008   305.48'8'00971   C2008-900959-2

Printed in Canada
Copyright © 2008 Centre for Addiction and Mental Health

This publication may be available in other formats. For information about alternate formats or other CAMH publications, or to place an order, please contact Sales and Distribution:

Toll free: 1 800 661-1111
Toronto: 416 595-6059
E-mail: publications@camh.net
Website: www.camh.net

This book was produced by:
Development: Julia Greenbaum, CAMH
Editorial: Martha Ayim, Diana Ballon, Jacquelyn Waller-Vintar, CAMH
Design: Eva Katz, Mara Korkola, CAMH
Typesetting: Laura Brady, Brady Typesetting and Design
Print production: Christine Harris, CAMH

2862/ 03-08 / PG124

*To women dealing with mental illness in the
post-migration context in Canada*

*To health care professionals working
to improve care to immigrant women*

Acknowledgments

This book is a product of both individual and collective efforts of many people. We wish to thank all the authors who have contributed their expertise and devoted numerous hours of their time to writing and revising their chapters. This effort is a testament to the authors' commitment to making life better for the many women who have arrived in Canada from countries around the world, and who struggle with a mental health system that is not adequately equipped to address their concerns and needs.

Our deepest gratitude to the many expert reviewers who generously offered their time to provide thoughtful feedback on draft chapters of this book: Branka Agic, Sheila Banerjee, Saleha Bismilla, Catherine Chan, Ena Chandha, Isolde Daiski, Marlinda Freire, Kathy Gates, Usha George, Axelle Janczur, Yasmin Jiwani, Mahboubeh Katirai, Anu Lala, Basanti Majumdar, Grazyna Mancewicz, Notisha Massaquoi, Ishwar Persad, Gloria Roberts-Fiati, Cheryl Rolin Gilman, Nalini Pandalangat, Laura Simich, Farah Shroff, Jacqueline Silvera, Taryn Tang, Debbie Thompson, Wilfreda Thurston, Colleen Varcoe, Bilkis Vissandjée, Janice Waddell, Charmaine Williams, Josephine Wong, Nargess Zahraei and Sajedeh Zahraei.

We are also very grateful to Martha Ayim, who so conscientiously yet gently provided editorial support to all the authors; to Diana Ballon, who worked tenaciously and diligently to help us with the final stretch of editorial work; and to Eva Katz for the page layout and cover design. And we thank the Centre for Addiction and Mental Health, which recognized the need for this kind of publication, and enabled it to be produced.

Finally, we are deeply indebted to Julia Greenbaum, our publishing developer and project manager, who proposed the idea of this book several years ago and worked patiently with us to ensure its completion.

Contents

Part 1: Understanding the Context of Immigrant Women's Lives

Part 2: Theoretical Perspectives

Part 3: Current Realities for Immigrant Women and New Paradigms for Mental Health Practice

Part 4: Working with Specific Groups

Part 5: Highlighting Critical Mental Health Concerns

Part 6: Conclusion

Preface

SEPALI GURUGE AND ENID COLLINS

Working with Immigrant Women: Issues and Strategies for Mental Health Professionals focuses on women's mental health and illness following migration and through the process of resettlement. The vision for creating this book came from conversations about a perceived dissonance between the needs of newcomer women and established structures and practices in Canada's mental health care system. Many of the contributors have immigrated to Canada themselves, and presently work in various health care positions: as nurses, counsellors, social workers, psychologists, social scientists, researchers and educators. They combine their knowledge gleaned through practice, education and research to bring forward perspectives that portray the complexity and diversity of immigrant women's experiences.

Most of the chapters critically interrogate existing literature and current research on the mental health and illness concerns of immigrant women. With an interest in changing paradigms in mental health practice, the authors have used critical frameworks to analyze a range of issues affecting women's mental health and illnesses in the context of post-migration and resettlement. Issues explored throughout the book point to women's concerns at the individual level, within the community and in the larger society.

A key goal of the book is to move the experiences of women immigrants to Canada from the margins to the centre. While aiming to highlight the intersecting oppressions experienced by women, the authors also emphasize the strengths and resiliencies of women, demonstrating how they are active participants in shaping their mental health and in responding to mental illness. Another major goal is to highlight the critical needs of newcomer women who are consumers of mental health services, so that the health care professionals can respond to their concerns more effectively. Each chapter includes strategies that mental health professionals can draw from if they wish to critically examine their practice, incorporate innovative approaches or build on those already established to create equitable, relevant and comprehensive care to the growing numbers of immigrant women in Canada who use mental health services. Where authors identify gaps in knowledge, these are indicated, along with recommendations for ongoing research. Some chapters examine systemic, social and structural issues and identify barriers that interfere with women receiving optimum mental health care.

While the book covers a number of key issues and a wide range of perspectives, some important issues such as homelessness and substance use among immigrant women are not included because there is not much research or practice-based evidence to sufficiently address the topics and make recommendations for practice.

Much work still needs to be done in moving mental health practice forward to meet the needs of all women.

The book is intended primarily, though not exclusively, as a resource for health care professionals working in the mental health field and for students entering the field. We hope the book will also be a valuable resource for administrators, educators, researchers and policy-makers in the mental health field.

A Note on Language

In this book—including in its title—we have used the term "immigrants" to refer to anyone born outside of Canada. However, where someone's experience differs because of their status in Canada, we have identified them according to this status. For instance, three of the chapter titles include the word refugee because the authors are writing specifically about how being a refugee has a direct effect on mental health that is different from the experience of someone who has arrived in Canada as a landed immigrant.

There is considerable literature on the topic of what is variously called acculturation, adaptation and integration, and on the stages an individual might undergo in the process of settling in a new country. These terms refer to a dynamic process of retaining previously held social, cultural and religious values and beliefs while choosing to embrace certain new values and beliefs in the context of settlement or resettlement. We use the term *resettlement* to apply to the act, process or context of starting a life in a new country in the first 10 years after arriving. The term *post-migration* (as in "after" migration) refers to the happenings any time following migration. Depending on the context, in this book, the authors have used one or the other or both terms.

Introduction

SEPALI GURUGE AND ENID COLLINS

While immigrant women face common issues that can influence their health, how they respond to and deal with these challenges is unique to each woman's situation. In this book, we explore how multiple identities—such as age, race, gender and class—among other social identities—intersect to influence immigrant women's mental health. By bringing together various theoretical, research and clinical perspectives, we have attempted to capture the complexity and diversity of immigrant women's experiences.

We recognize that immigrant women's experiences of mental health and mental illness are integrally related to the totality of their life experiences. However, women also claim unique experiences that are shaped by the economic, cultural, social and historical contexts in which they currently live. To effectively care for immigrant women as clients in the mental health care system, professionals need to move beyond the singular focus on culture to understand their individual experiences. They need to explore the varied and complex ways women experience migration and resettlement, and how this affects their mental health.

PART 1: UNDERSTANDING THE CONTEXT OF IMMIGRANT WOMEN'S LIVES

In **CHAPTER 1**, Guruge and Collins describe emerging trends in Canadian immigration and challenges for newcomers. They provide statistics around the growing numbers of immigrants coming to Canada. The authors also describe the many challenges immigrant women confront as they resettle in Canada, and the impact that these challenges have on their mental health.

PART 2: THEORETICAL PERSPECTIVES

In this section, the authors examine various theoretical perspectives and conceptual frameworks surrounding the intersection of gender, race and class with variables such as age, citizenship status, culture and sexual orientation in order to understand women immigrants' mental health and illness concerns.

In **CHAPTER 2**, Collins and Guruge provide a summary of a number of key theoretical perspectives—including transcultural nursing, anti-racism strategies and postcolonial feminist perspectives—with a critical view to understanding how each framework might guide mental health practitioners' work toward effective and quality mental health care to women of all backgrounds and cultures. The authors invite readers to question whose interests are being served when mental health professionals incorporate into their practice particular ways of thinking, understanding and acting in relation to social differences.

In **CHAPTER 3,** Gustafson discusses both explicit and hidden assumptions in two key theoretical approaches—namely, the cultural competence approach and the critical cultural approach—to working with newcomer women with mental illnesses. Using examples, the author invites the reader to reflect on the strengths and limitations of each approach and to examine how each approach can be used in health care professionals' practices. She encourages professionals to move beyond the notion of cultural sensitivity to focus on advocating for change in institutional practices and processes that create and sustain power dynamics that affect the everyday life of newcomer women and the mental health professionals who care for them.

PART 3: CURRENT REALITIES FOR IMMIGRANT WOMEN AND NEW PARADIGMS FOR MENTAL HEALTH PRACTICE

This section looks at the current realities of immigrant women's experiences and explores their implications for clinical practice. Among these realities is the fact that women who immigrate to Canada experience racism, sexism, classism and heterosexism, and cope with other challenges to resettlement that increase their vulnerability to mental illness. They are also confronted by a mental health care system that does not address the social determinants of mental health; that fails to recognize what is integral to their health and well-being (such as spirituality); and that presents barriers to accessing care (such as lack of trained interpreters).

In **CHAPTER 4,** Mawani examines social determinants of depression among women immigrants and refugees. While depression may be a universal phenomenon, there is variation in its prevalence and clinical presentation between countries around the world, between communities within each country, and between women and men. While women are more likely to experience depression than men, this phenomenon remains poorly understood, with research failing to emphasize the totality of women's life experiences. The chapter includes a review of the empirical literature on intersecting social determinants that influence women's depression, such as gender, socio-economic status, discrimination, social support, and violence and trauma. It concludes with evidence-based practice strategies to address these determinants.

Women give and receive social support when they connect with other women. The meanings, expressions and practices of spirituality can link women with each other, and bring extended families and community together. When separated from familiar culture and community, women lose these connections and the ability to take part in rituals, which can create challenges, stresses and resulting ill health. In **CHAPTER 5,** Collins examines the important role of spirituality in addressing mental health and illness concerns of women. Using a synthesis of concepts from critical feminism, feminist spirituality and anti-racism, the author suggests that when immigrant women become recipients of health care, they experience a disconnect between their lived experience and approaches used in "mainstream" mental health services. The meaning and expression of mental illness, help-seeking and spirituality are often interrelated, and can be incorporated in mental health care. The author presents holistic strategies that mental health practitioners can use in their practice.

In **CHAPTER 6,** Abraham and Rahman examine the intricacies of addressing the language and cultural interpretation needs of women seeking mental health services. The consequences of not having an interpreter to bridge the communication barriers, and the debates and controversies surrounding language versus cultural interpretation are also discussed. In addition, the authors highlight such issues as: lack of funding; challenges faced by health care institutions in setting up professional interpretation services; the implications of inadequate interpretation services on clients receiving mental health care; and approaches to address these concerns. They provide guidelines for working with interpreters and suggest the need for public policy that recognizes the right of all people to access the care and services they need.

Demonstrating the link between immigration, settlement and mental health in **CHAPTER 7,** Collins, Shakya, Guruge and Santos address the importance of settlement services and other resources that address social determinants of health. Key features of various programs and services at the societal, community, neighbourhood and familial levels are discussed. The authors note that despite the existence of many programs and services, some newcomer women encounter barriers in accessing them. They highlight three agencies that address the mental health and illness needs of immigrant women—one at the national level and two in the Greater Toronto Area.

PART 4: WORKING WITH SPECIFIC GROUPS

In this section, the authors address particular issues and concerns related to working with specific groups: newcomer girls, Sudanese women, Caribbean women and their children, lesbian and bisexual women of colour, women refugees and older women. While there are commonalities among the mental health care concerns of women, in general, the socioeconomic, ethnocultural, political and historical location of women in society affect their vulnerability to illness and influence their ability to access care and treatment.

In **CHAPTER 8,** Berman and Jiwani discuss critical issues facing racialized newcomer girls and young women in Canada. The authors contest the narrow notion of "the newcomer girl" —recognizing that girls are not defined solely by their newcomer status, but also by the multiple and intersecting realities of their everyday lives. Based on a review of the literature, the authors address a number of complexities surrounding this group, including how they develop and negotiate identities within the context of family, peer, community and society at large. While newcomer girls use a number of strategies when trying to fit in with Canadian born peers and the Canadian culture, the authors propose that such practices could be interpreted as a response to racism and discrimination in the larger context of society. Programs and policies that fail to consider gender are of particular concern for newcomer girls. The chapter concludes with recommendations for mental health professionals working with this group to address systemic racism, sexism and other forms of oppression, and to foster a more equitable and just society.

Drawing from a number of theoretical frameworks, in **CHAPTER 9,** Baya, Simich and Bukhari discuss the varied and complex influences of resettlement experiences on the mental health of Sudanese women in Southern Ontario. The chapter draws substantively—but not exclusively—from the first major study in Canada on the settlement and integration experiences of recent Sudanese immigrants from a protracted conflict zone. In spite of diversity within this community in Ontario, the women share commonalities in their struggle to adapt, settle and integrate into Canadian society. The many ways they experience oppression within Canada's stratified and racialized social system interact to negatively affect their mental health. Family issues that were once a communal responsibility become the sole burden of the couple—and particularly the woman—as they struggle to cope with issues such as role reversal and increased work for women. Based on their research and practice within this community, the authors provide guidelines and strategies for working with Sudanese women that incorporate a broader, holistic, anti-racist paradigm of mental health.

Incorporating Bowlby's theory of attachment, in **CHAPTER 10,** Campbell and Flaman discuss the importance of maternal-child attachment in the context of separation and reunification of Caribbean women and their children in Canada. The chapter emphasizes the diverse roles that many Caribbean women, as heads of families, undertake to improve their lives and that of their children, which includes seeking better employment opportunities in other countries such as Canada. The authors address the physical, social and emotional challenges both the mothers and their children face when reunited after a period of separation. Some of the factors addressed include the impact of length of separation, financial concerns and familial factors (such as other significant attachments the child forms while separated from the mother). The authors offer strategies for health care providers to respond to families' needs and suggest areas for future research, including the influence of fathers on the outcome of reunification and the need to learn from successful reunions the variables that contribute to their success.

Based on their psychotherapy practice grounded in an anti-oppression framework, in **CHAPTER 11,** Doctor and Bazet explore the complexities of counselling lesbian and bisexual women of colour in the context of racism and heterosexism. The authors address the cultural, social and emotional losses experienced by clients and the importance of community connections. Lesbian and bisexual women of colour face multiple challenges in their lives. The authors examine the factors that contribute to clients' complex identities, including being bicultural, bilingual or multiracial. They also discuss the impact of these identities on clients' daily life, and some strategies they use to survive an often hostile environment. Clinical cases are used to illustrate themes of assimilation and integration into "mainstream" Canadian society as well as "mainstream" lesbian and bisexual communities. The authors address issues of racism within clients' intimate relationships. They also explore power dynamics inherent in therapeutic relationships and how racism and heterosexism are expressed within these relationships.

In **CHAPTER 12**, Ortiz addresses a number of clinical and ethical issues encountered in his work with refugee claimants receiving mental health care. He notes that refugee women are confronted with complex social issues including poverty, distrust, limited language skills, devalued qualifications and social isolation—all of which can have a negative impact on their mental health. The chapter reviews some of the difficulties women face in negotiating the complexities of the immigration system—including filing and successfully obtaining refugee status (and later, permanent residency) in Canada. Case examples describe people who are pressured to go "underground" with no legal status, who have no health coverage, and who are without a work permit (thus are unable to find paid employment nor garner an income) and the influence of these factors on seeking and receiving care. Of special concern are women fleeing domestic violence, sexual abuse and/or discrimination due to their sexual orientation. Ortiz discusses ethical issues mental health professionals face in caring for women refugee claimants when their role involves supporting—or not supporting—the client's immigration application (and process).

Drawing on their community-based settlement work in Canada and research within the Sri Lankan Tamil community, in **CHAPTER 13**, Guruge, Kanthasamy and Santos discuss the often neglected topic of older immigrant women's mental health needs. Their review of health sciences literature on the topic—and their work with the Sri Lankan Tamil community in the Greater Toronto Area—highlight common health and settlement concerns among older immigrant women. Focusing on the intersection of gender, race, ethnicity and culture, the authors examine critical issues for this group of women, and highlight how their concerns are linked to both the pre-migration context in war-torn Sri Lanka as well as the influence on mental health of changing family dynamics, social isolation, altered social status and increased vulnerability to abuse in the post-migration context. The authors discuss gaps in services for older immigrant women, and provide recommendations for health and settlement workers to more effectively address the needs of this group.

PART 5: HIGHLIGHTING CRITICAL MENTAL HEALTH CONCERNS

Most women seeking refugee status in Canada flee their countries for reasons related to violence and traumatic events. Some have survived wars or conditions similar to war, experienced torture, kidnapping, rape and/or witnessed murder of loved ones. Some women might have fled such situations with the help of people demanding high prices to smuggle them out of their country. However, we know little about the plight of women who experience such situations and how their mental health is affected. Similarly, little attention has been paid to the topic of postpartum depression, which—until recently—was considered a concern unique to women in western countries. In this section, authors explore these critical mental health concerns.

In **CHAPTER 14**, Saphir locates women's trauma and suffering within their socio-cultural context, and emphasizes the strong values placed on women's roles within the family and the conflicts they experience when they are separated from family. She bases her writing on her experience of working with Latin American women dealing with multiple forms of trauma. Saphir notes that the traumatic experience dealt with in the therapy is not based on a single event but, rather, reflects a lifetime of upheaval. Dealing with trauma often entails reopening old wounds before dealing with and receiving care for the mental (and physical) health consequences of trauma and violence. The author proposes that therapeutic approaches must entail a holistic approach to healing that incorporates the physical, emotional and cognitive aspects of the woman's experience.

Highlighting a number of gaps in Canadian health sciences literature on intimate partner violence (IPV), in **CHAPTER 15**, Hyman and Mason identify the need for more in-depth research into factors that influence the choices women make when facing new and unique barriers in Canada. Using the available literature, they address: the prevalence and etiology of IPV; its risk and protective factors; its health impacts; and legal, contextual and cultural barriers to help-seeking. Implications for mental health professionals are discussed in terms of documentation, risk assessment, safety planning, mandatory reporting and referral. The authors highlight the importance of developing primary prevention strategies at the individual, couple, community and societal level.

In **CHAPTER 16**, Ardiles, Dennis and Ross use a health promotion framework, together with a broader social determinants of health approach, to critically review the literature to-date on postpartum depression (PPD) among immigrant women. Based on the findings of Canadian and cross-cultural studies, the authors address prevalence rates of PPD, limitations in its measurements, barriers to assessment, potential risk factors (including acculturation, acculturative stress, and social isolation and loss of support), gaps in intervention and culturally appropriate preventive care and treatment approaches. The authors discuss the role various social and cultural practices and rituals might play in reinforcing social bonds and protecting women from PPD. Strategies for multidisciplinary teams to facilitate continuity of care for women experiencing PPD in the post-migration context are proposed.

PART 6: CONCLUSION

Despite the fact that Canada's foreign-born population is increasing at a rate that is four times higher than the Canadian-born population, the needs of immigrants and refugees are not adequately addressed nor understood. Accordingly, much work remains to be done in order to adequately address the mental health concerns, care needs and treatment of mental illnesses among this group. Using the information, insights and speculations presented by the book's contributors as a jumping off ground, Collins and Guruge offer ways of moving forward in **CHAPTER 17**: they make recommendations for education, practice and policy, and suggest areas for future research.

Part 1

Understanding the Context of Immigrant Women's Lives

Chapter 1

Emerging Trends in Canadian Immigration and Challenges for Newcomers

SEPALI GURUGE AND ENID COLLINS

Immigration Trends

Canada is dependent on continued immigration for its economic and population growth. Since the mid-1980s, the numbers of immigrants to Canada have steadily increased. Since the 1990s, more than 200,000 immigrants and refugees come to Canada every year (Statistics Canada, 2001). In the last two decades, most immigrants to Canada have come from Asia, Africa, the Caribbean, Central and South America, and the Middle East. Immigrants from Asia account for the largest proportion (63 per cent in 2001 compared to 10 per cent in 1966) while the proportion of European immigrants has fallen (from over 80 per cent prior to 1967 to 47 per cent in 1996, and 17 per cent by 2001). Most newcomers are settling in major cities such as Toronto, Vancouver, Montreal, Ottawa and Edmonton, thereby significantly transforming their demographic make-up. According to 2001 census data, immigrants accounted for 44 per cent of the population in Metropolitan Toronto. Further, immigrant arrivals accounted for two-thirds of the population growth of Toronto between 1986 and 2001 (Statistics Canada, 2001).

The term *immigrant* refers to those who were not born in Canada who have come to Canada under the broad immigration categories of business, skilled-worker or family class.[1]

1. However, as noted in Guruge (2007) we recognize the problematic use of the term "immigrant" in everyday discourse as including any woman who is "seen" by others as an immigrant because of her skin colour, language, dress and/or socioeconomic status, even if they were born in Canada.

(Provinces may also nominate immigrants who enter under separate agreements, such as the program run by Quebec.) Business class immigrants are admitted as investors, entrepreneurs or self-employed. Skilled or professional workers arrive in Canada after being assessed on a point system that strongly considers the applicants' proficiency in English or French as well as on Canada's job market. Those included under the family class are sponsored by family members in Canada. In 2004, the business and skilled-worker classes comprised 57 per cent of immigrants, while the family class formed only 26 per cent of the total immigration.

The number of women entering Canada as "economic immigrants" (that is those arriving under the business or skilled worker categories) compared to "family class" immigrants or refugees is slowly increasing. This is partly due to the increase in the number of women who are immigrating to Canada as skilled or professional workers, such as nurses. Under the present immigration laws, professional women who migrate with their spouses are often admitted as family class immigrants, even when both women and their husbands hold equal qualifications. The implication is that they are dependent on their spouses, rather than being counted as economic class immigrants, which perpetuates the idea that women are dependent on their husbands or fathers. In reality, professional women may be the sole or higher income earners for their family during resettlement. However, under the present legislation, their classification as family class immigrants fails to acknowledge their potential for economic contribution.

FIGURE 1-1
Permanent Residents by Category, Canada 1980–2006

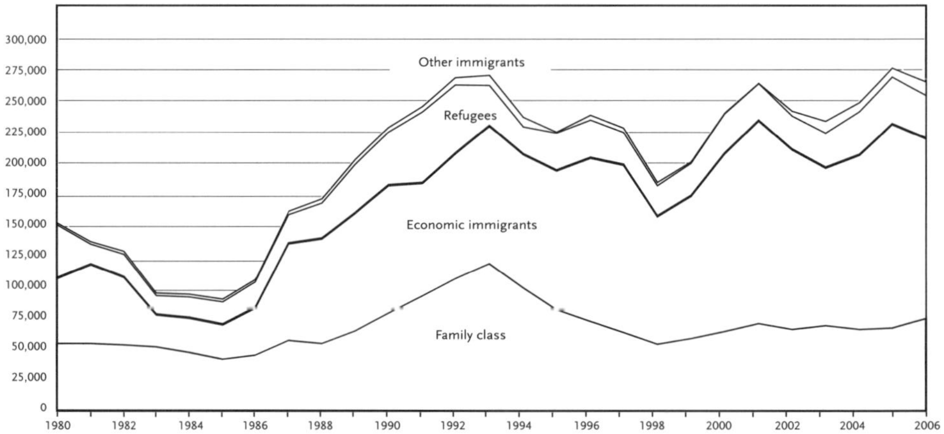

Source: Citizenship and Immigration Canada, 2006. www.cic.gc.ca/english/resources/statistics/facts2006/permanent/01.asp. Reproduced with the permission of the Minister of Public Works and Government Services, 2008.

While immigrants often arrive in a country voluntarily, **refugees** are forced to flee their home countries. According to the United Nations Convention, refugees have been persecuted, or fear persecution due to race, religion, nationality or because of their affiliation with "a particular social group or political opinion." In 1993, the Immigration and Refugee Board expanded this definition to recognize that women refugees also need protection based on "gender persecution"—from experiences of beatings, rape, torture and other types of violence, which are sometimes carried out by family members (Boyd, 2002).

The term *refugee* refers to those who were born outside of Canada and who have claimed refugee status either within or outside of the country and who belong to one of the following three classes identified by Citizenship and Immigration Canada: the convention refugee abroad class, the country of asylum class and the source country class. In addition, under the Canada–Quebec Accord, Quebec selects refugees who will live in that province. With growing political, economic and social upheaval in many countries around the world over this last decade, Canada has received a large number of refugees. According to data from the Canadian Council for Refugees, the number of refugees who settled in Canada in 2001 included 8,693 government-assisted refugees and 3,570 privately sponsored refugees. In the same year, another 211 refugees arrived under the urgent protection program (Canadian Council for Refugees, 2002). More recently, Canada has granted refugee status to approximately 20,000 to 30,000 people annually. However, the number of people applying for refugee status in Canada far exceeds this. For example, at the end of 2003, approximately 46,000 claimants were awaiting hearings from the Canadian Immigration and Refugee Board.

(We refer the reader to Table 1-1 and Table 1-2 on page 6 and Figure 1-1 on page 4 for an overview of the categories under which immigrants have successfully obtained permanent residency from 1993 to 2006 and the differences in these categories for men and women.)

Not only have the numbers of **women immigrants and refugees** increased over the years; the percentage of women settling in Canada as immigrant (and refugees whose claims have been approved to become permanent residents) usually exceeds that of men by two to seven per cent. While the difference seems small from year to year, this number becomes significant when assessed cumulatively. For example, between 1996 and 2005, Canada received 48,800 more women immigrants than men (CIC, 2006).

Because **fluency in one of Canada's official languages** is a major factor in the point system upon which acceptance to Canada is based, many immigrants to Canada are fluent in English. However, the number of immigrants who speak or do not speak English or French as their primary language and those who do not speak either of these languages fluently generally varies between the immigration classes. For example, in 2004, only 18 per cent of the principal applicants for permanent residency in Canada spoke neither English nor French; however, this number was 39 per cent among the family class immigrants, 51 per cent for spouses or dependants and 81 per cent for refugees (CIC, 2004).

A considerable number of women do not speak fluently in either of Canada's official languages. For example, between 1996 and 2005, 71,842 women arriving in the Census Metropolitan Area alone spoke neither English nor French. Among this group, most spoke Mandarin, Cantonese, Urdu or Punjabi as their primary language. Not only do many adult women who arrive as dependants or as sponsored family members not speak English upon arrival, but many are still unable to speak it during subsequent census enumerations (noted in Kilbride et al., 2007).

TABLE 1-1
Canada—Male Permanent Residents by Category, 1993 to 2006

Category	1993	1994	1995	1996	1997	1998	1999	2000	2001	2002	2003	2004	2005	2006
						Percentage distribution								
Family Class	39.5	37.9	31.7	25.5	22.7	23.4	23.1	20.7	21.1	21.5	23.4	20.8	19.6	23.3
Economic immigrants	42.6	47.9	52.7	58.4	62.9	60.5	62.2	64.7	66.8	65.3	60.0	61.4	63.3	58.9
Refugees	14.7	10.7	15.1	14.0	12.7	14.5	14.2	14.4	12.1	11.7	12.9	14.9	14.5	13.7
Other immigrants	3.2	3.5	0.5	2.1	1.8	1.6	0.6	0.2	0.1	1.4	3.7	3.0	2.6	4.1
Category not stated	0.0	0.0	0.0	0.0	0.0	0.0	0.0	0.0	0.0	0.0	0.0	0.0	0.0	0.0
	100.0	100.0	100.0	100.0	100.0	100.0	100.0	100.0	100.0	100.0	100.0	100.0	100.0	100.0

Source: Citizenship and Immigration Canada, 2006. www.cic.gc.ca/english/resources/statistics/facts2006/permanent/01.asp.
Reproduced with the permission of the Minister of Public Works and Government Services, 2008.

TABLE 1-2
Canada—Female Permanent Residents by Category, 1993 to 2006

	1993	1994	1995	1996	1997	1998	1999	2000	2001	2002	2003	2004	2005	2006
						Percentage distribution								
Family Class	47.7	45.6	40.7	34.8	32.7	34.7	34.9	32.4	32.1	32.7	35.0	31.7	28.5	32.4
Economic immigrants	39.9	43.5	47.7	52.6	56.1	52.1	53.1	55.3	57.6	55.2	49.7	52.3	56.1	51.2
Refugees	9.5	7.7	11.4	11.3	9.9	11.8	11.6	12.1	10.2	10.2	10.6	12.9	12.8	12.2
Other immigrants	2.8	3.2	0.3	1.3	1.4	1.3	0.5	0.2	0.1	1.9	4.6	3.1	2.6	4.1
Category not stated	0.0	0.0	0.0	0.0	0.0	0.0	0.0	0.0	0.0	0.0	0.0	0.0	0.0	0.0
	100.0	100.0	100.0	100.0	100.0	100.0	100.0	100.0	100.0	100.0	100.0	100.0	100.0	100.0

Source: Citizenship and Immigration Canada, 2006. www.cic.gc.ca/english/resources/statistics/facts2006/permanent/01.asp.
Reproduced with the permission of the Minister of Public Works and Government Services, 2008.

However, the lack of proficiency in English or French does not equate with poor education; it simply means that their education may not have included learning English or French. In fact, the **level of education** is higher for both women and men immigrants to Canada than it is for their Canadian-born counterparts. For example, 35.7 per cent of recent immigrants held a university degree compared to 13.8 per cent of the Canadian-born population. The table on page 7 provides a comparison of women and men immigrants' education. It shows that, over the last 10 years, among those who obtained permanent residency in Canada, the percentage of women and men who had a bachelor's or master's degree or a doctorate has increased. Furthermore, the percentage of women with a master's or doctorate is higher than that of men immigrants.

TABLE 1-3
Canada—New Workers 15 Years of Age or Older
by Gender and Level of Education

Level of education	1997	1998	1999	2000	2001	2002	2003	2004	2005	2006
				Percentage distribution						
Males	**100.0**	**100.0**	**100.0**	**100.0**	**100.0**	**100.0**	**100.0**	**100.0**	**100.0**	**100.0**
0 to 9 years of schooling	14.4	14.1	13.6	14.4	12.8	13.8	13.3	13.1	12.3	14.2
10 to 12 years of schooling	30.5	26.3	23.3	22.0	20.9	20.6	19.0	18.8	18.8	20.2
13 or more years of schooling	11.6	11.1	11.1	12.4	12.2	12.4	12.9	11.5	11.1	10.0
Trade certificate	11.0	10.4	9.7	7.5	6.3	5.7	5.4	6.3	6.0	5.9
Non-university diploma	10.5	13.1	12.9	11.7	13.9	13.7	14.9	16.2	16.7	16.6
Bachelor's degree	18.3	21.1	25.1	26.9	28.7	28.3	28.8	28.0	28.0	26.2
Master's degree	3.0	3.2	3.8	4.7	4.7	5.0	5.1	5.4	6.1	6.1
Doctorate	0.7	0.6	0.6	0.4	0.4	0.4	0.6	0.8	0.8	0.9
Females	**100.0**	**100.0**	**100.0**	**100.0**	**100.0**	**100.0**	**100.0**	**100.0**	**100.0**	**100.0**
0 to 9 years of schooling	15.8	15.5	15.0	15.8	14.4	15.9	15.3	13.7	12.9	14.7
10 to 12 years of schooling	31.3	28.2	25.7	25.3	23.6	22.9	21.5	21.1	20.2	21.2
13 or more years of schooling	11.6	11.2	11.2	12.1	11.8	11.9	12.1	11.1	10.7	9.8
Trade certificate	11.1	10.6	9.6	7.5	6.7	6.0	5.8	6.9	6.4	6.4
Non-university diploma	9.2	11.3	11.2	10.1	12.0	11.8	12.9	14.4	14.9	14.9
Bachelor's degree	17.3	19.3	22.7	24.1	26.2	25.9	26.5	26.2	27.0	25.1
Master's degree	3.0	3.1	3.8	4.5	4.6	5.0	5.2	5.6	6.6	6.6
Doctorate	0.7	0.8	0.7	0.6	0.6	0.7	0.8	1.1	1.3	1.4

Source: Citizenship and Immigration Canada, 2006. www.cic.gc.ca/english/resources/statistics/facts2006/permanent/31.asp.
Reproduced with the permission of the Minister of Public Works and Government Services, 2008.

Women tend to migrate for various reasons, including to gain economic mobility; to be reunited with family; to have more educational opportunities; to escape gender-based and/or political violence; and to gain more social independence (DeLaet, 1999). For example, Canadian immigration statistics show that more newcomers to the country are women. Half of the refugees are women, and both single and married women comprise a significant proportion of illegal immigrants. However, because of the assumption that women merely follow immigrant men as their wives or daughters, much less is known about **women's migratory process** (Delaet; Gastaldo et al., 2004). Further, conceptualization of them as followers "can and does play important roles in shaping immigration policies and regulations" (Guruge, 2007). The policies and regulations, in turn, shape immigration flows, which, consequently, influence expectations of family roles in the settlement countries (United Nations, 1993). Furthermore, the assumption that women are mere followers of men reinforces the myth that they are without skills and are financially dependent on their husbands. As Shamsuddin (1999) and Mojab (1999), among others, have noted, the repercussions of this myth are sexist immigration policies that can result in a labour market where women's skills and qualifications are not recognized or matched for the Canadian labour market.

The **circumstances of immigration** influence women's mental health not only in terms of whether or not they had control over relocating (which can differ for immigrants and refugees) but also whether they have been separated from their family or community, if they have been uprooted due to violence, and if they suffered exploitation on their journey to Canada and once in the country. Immigrants come to North America for a variety of reasons, the most important of which is the hope of securing a better future for themselves and, especially, for their children. The message about North America that is promoted across the world through various forms of media implies that anyone who arrives there can enjoy economic prosperity, freedom, rights and equality (Jiwani, 2001). While there are many benefits of immigrating to Canada, the reality is that life in Canada is also mired in hardships. When immigrants arrive in Canada the realities of navigating social systems, government bureaucracy, new cultures and unfamiliar languages can be daunting. Further, the processes associated with immigration and resettlement can be dehumanizing (Sandys, 1996). Besides having to establish themselves, meeting the basic necessities of life such as employment, housing, food and shelter can present enormous challenges. Even after the initial resettlement period women continue to encounter various challenges in their adopted country.

Resettlement in Canada: Common Challenges

Immigrants coming to Canada generally are in better health than the average Canadian (Chen et al., 1996a; 1996b; Parakulum et al., 1992). Several factors related to immigration selection criteria (such as rigorous health screening) and the immigration process itself (i.e., healthier people are more likely to travel and/or immigrate than those with a poor health status) have been associated with this **healthy-immigrant effect**. However, the health advantage is lost after being in Canada for 10 years, when long-term immigrants appear to be in poorer health than their Canadian-born counterparts and are more likely to experience a number of chronic health conditions (Chen et al., 1996a; 1996b; Hyman, 2001). Factors identified as contributing to both declining mental and physical health of the long-term immigrants include multiple responsibilities, financial and employment constraints, and difficulties obtaining services in a timely manner due to language differences (Chen et al., 1996a; 1996b; Hyman, 2001).[2]

Woven throughout this book are **common challenges** that immigrant women face regardless of the circumstances within which they left their home countries to settle in Canada: social isolation, social exclusion, language barriers, unemployment and under-employment, poverty, discrimination, intergenerational struggles, as well as trauma

---

2. Another explanation often noted in the literature alludes to exposure to the physical, social, cultural and environment influences in Canada that sets in motion a process in which morbidity and mortality patterns among immigrants change to resemble (or often become worse than) the health status and norms in Canada.

and violence. These are all aspects of immigrant women's experiences that influence their mental health.

Social isolation is a significant reality for immigrant women. Many women who arrive in Canada come from societies where extended family is a critical part of their support system. Despite comprising about 20 per cent of the Canadian population, they are often without their extended family and community. Even when present, family members might be too busy or geographically distant, leaving many women without instrumental, informational and psychological support. Uprooting from familiar culture, family and community can leave a social vacuum in women's relationships that can have a negative impact on women's mental health. The losses and their effects are even more paramount when we consider specific life stages, such as adolescence and life as an older adult.

Immigrant women who did not have opportunities to learn English prior to migration or those who had no reason to learn English in their country of origin often experience many barriers during resettlement in Canada. Without ways to deal with the **language barrier**, women are denied economic and social mobility (Kenise et al., 2007) and face other challenges to their accessing and using mental health care. Refugee women, in particular, might face additional barriers if unable to communicate with their lawyers and be fully informed of their immigration cases and procedures. Their fears and concerns may be misrepresented or misinterpreted in a way that might lead to their deportation. Even those who speak English encounter discrimination in the educational, employment and health institutions if they have an accent that is different than that of Canadian-born English speakers. Thus, issues related to language expression are integrally related to and have a significant impact on women's mental health and well-being.

Not only will these barriers prevent women from accessing mental health services; even when they do access care, they may get the wrong treatments, limited follow-up care and/or limited referral to specialists due to a lack of interpreters. While many institutions are aware of the need for and the pivotal role of interpreters, especially in mental health care and counselling, appropriate and adequate **interpreter services** are not available in most settings. In addition, many health care professionals have not received adequate training to work with interpreters, nor have students in health disciplines. Language differences can create particular challenges for women who are dealing with intimate partner violence.

Discriminatory actions toward individuals, and at an institutional or societal level create barriers to women achieving successful resettlement and realizing their full potential. Both subtle and overt discrimination interacts with other social determinants such as social isolation to hinder immigrant women from achieving social inclusion in Canada (Mulvihill et al., 2001; Omidvar & Richmond, 2003). **Social inclusion** refers to the notion that immigrants are able to participate fully and equally in all facets of life in their new country, including in social, economic and political areas (Omidvar & Richmond, 2003).

Mounting research evidence demonstrates that **race and gender discrimination** are major deterrents to racialized immigrants being able to achieve economic and social inclusion. In their analysis of factors that contribute to barriers to immigrants achieving social inclusion, Omidvar and Richmond cite research studies that substantiate that immigrants arriving in Canada since the 1980s and 1990s are experiencing increased difficulty in establishing an economic base in Canada. They experience high rates of under- and unemployment, consequently chronic individual and family poverty. Some of the research cited are studies by Devoretz (1995), Harvey and Siu (2001), Orenstein (2000), Pendakur (2000), Shields (2002) and Reitz (1998). Evidence indicates that racialized minority immigrants experience wage discrimination in the labour market. Immigrant women are further disadvantaged by gender discrimination. Newcomer women are forced into low wage jobs, in service sector and manufacturing. These women are further disadvantaged because they are burdened with the bulk of responsibility for domestic and family responsibilities.

Recent immigrants often are unable to find employment that is commensurate with their education and/or training. Employers who use racist and discriminatory practices fail to recognize the skills, knowledge and education obtained by immigrants from most other countries in the world, and do not provide job training and skills development opportunities (Mojab, 1999; Schaafsma & Sweetman, 1999). Immigrants and refugees, particularly those who are newcomers and those from racialized communities, are disproportionately over-represented in the low-income categories, and in substandard housing in under-serviced neighbourhoods.

Even though (as noted earlier) immigrants are more educated than the Canadian born population, the average annual **income** for immigrants tends to be significantly lower, particularly for recent immigrants from racialized communities and women. For example, from 1995 to 2000, the employment rate for university-educated, Canadian-born men was 94 per cent, in comparison to the rate of 81 per cent for immigrant men and 66 per cent for immigrant women at a similar educational level (Statistics Canada, 2004).

According to CIC (2001), the average annual income for immigrant men in Toronto from 1996 to 1999 was $27,790 (compared to the city average of $51,090 for annual income of Canadian-born men). The average annual income for women immigrants to Toronto during this same period was only $16,490 on average (compared to a city average of $41,130 for annual income for Canadian-born women). In fact, immigrant and refugee women's incomes were approximately 40 per cent of the income of their Canadian counterparts for the same job or position, due to a legacy of subordination and colonial practices. The proportion of immigrants whose family or individual income during this period was below one-half of the median income was nearly 30 per cent, which was more than twice the proportion among the Canadian-born. The proportion of immigrants with income below the median was approximately 70 per cent. While for the Canadian-born women and men and earlier immigrants, the highest proportion of incomes that were below the median were among the seniors, among the immigrants from 1996 to 1999, the proportion with income below the median was higher among younger age groups.

Recent immigrants, in general, cannot afford to be unemployed or depend on welfare, as this situation would jeopardize their plans for sponsoring and reuniting with their family members. (Someone sponsoring a family member has to show a minimum annual income of $15,000 to $20,000, which is difficult to do if one is paid close to minimum wage.) Many are forced to hold several jobs, to work long hours, and/or to work six to seven days a week to make the bare minimum. **Un/underemployment** is often associated with Canada's failure to have professional qualifications recognized in a quick and efficient manner as well as the racial inequities prevalent in the job market, especially in higher status and professional jobs.

Immigrant women are more likely to take on low-status jobs (albeit paid employment outside the home) to meet the basic necessities for their families and gain satisfaction by being able to financially contribute to their family. Especially for the women who did not hold paid employment prior to immigration, this new situation might give them more status and authority within the household. However, the change can also threaten men's previously held status and authority within the family and the community, creating frustration, shame and stress for men. This, in turn, can lead to conflicts at home: Bui's 2003 IPV study in the Vietnamese community in the United States, for instance, found that women's economic contributions did not reduce their husbands' dominant positions and use of violence at home, but that economic hardships prevented the women from leaving an abusive relationship. Furthermore, experiences of and perceptions of racial discrimination prevented the women from relying on the formal social support systems to cope with abuse (Bui, 2003).

Skills that immigrant women hold when they arrive in Canada are devalued or underutilized through **de-skilling**, a process whereby newly arrived immigrants who are educated and possess professional knowledge and skills have difficulty entering the Canadian labour market. They often remain unemployed or are pressured into non-skilled jobs, mostly manual labour. (De-skilling is discussed by Mojab [1999]). Obtaining professional accreditation poses formidable barriers, including going through lengthy and costly periods of re-training in order to gain accreditation for specific occupations. Most newly arrived women lack the financial resources to cover transportation, child care and additional courses or training. For some women who find employment, working situations might lead to disruptions in family life, especially if they are raising children as single parents and have no social networks and supports in Canada. Many women are caught in a dead-end employment cycle, and are unable to upgrade skills that would enable them to seek upward mobility in the labour market.

Findings from numerous studies (such as Krulfeld, 1994; Kulig, 1994) suggest that the process of immigrating to a new country may offer women possibilities that had not been previously available to them or that had been difficult to negotiate before relocating. However, other studies (e.g., Bui & Morash, 1999; Fernandez, 1997; Jiwani, 2001) suggest that women are not so advantaged by coming to North America. Paid labour, which may be a necessity for the family's basic survival, does not necessarily lead to a change in women's status relative to men at home or within the community. In fact, the women may be facing more discriminatory experiences in the post-migration context. According to a Canadian study on stress management by Majumdar, Ellis and Dye (1999)—involving 67 focus group participants consisting of immigrant, refugee and minority women in the workforce— "racial, cultural, linguistic, social and sexual areas were most frequently cited types of discrimination" (p. 159). An increase in occupational and financial difficulties without adequate child care and social support has been noted in various studies as contributing to ill health (Baker et al., 1994; Beiser, 1988a; 1988b; Sundquist, 1995; Vissandjee et al., 2001). Based on a number of previous studies, Majumdar, Ellis and Dye (1999) observed that, "As the number of women in the workforce increases, so does their exposure to these unique stressors (Gurber & Bjorn), which include open racial/sexual harassment; isolation/loneliness; and noisy, unclean, dangerous working environments" (p. 154). Health care professionals generally recognize that **social determinants of health** increase immigrant women's vulnerability to depression.

Dealing with both subtle and overt racism can be even a bigger challenge for newcomer girls who have to deal with peer group pressures to fit into Canadian culture, as well as respond to cultural expectations of their family and community. Concerns about sexual orientation also add another layer of struggle for newcomer girls who are in the process of developing their own identity. While identity formation is part of all adolescents' development, for **newcomer girls**, identity formation is also shaped by multiple and intersecting identities such as race, culture and language. Newcomer girls must also navigate new family and societal contexts. Based on their research, Khanlou et al. (2002) noted that newcomer youth face challenges and tensions related to their familial, cultural and social roles and responsibilities and expectations based on their age and gender. In the context of Canadian society, cultural differences and discrimination may also lead to social isolation and present challenges to their potential opportunities for higher education and employment.

In addition to discrimination based on race, gender, culture and language, newcomer girls and women who are lesbian, bisexual or transgendered may also face **heterosexism**. Girls and young women may experience pressures from within their families (who subscribe to dominant heterosexual orientation) to marry and reproduce. They face taboos that originate in male dominant power structures from within their ethnocultural communities as well as Canadian society.

Violence against women can take many forms, including emotional, psychological, verbal and physical abuse and, in extreme cases, rape as an act of war. The most common form of violence is carried out by male intimate partners. For girls and women, the impact of **intimate partner violence** (IPV) results in both short-term and long-term mental and physical health problems, which require urgent and comprehensive attention at all levels of community, economic, legal and health care systems. Existing literature attempts to explain causes of IPV through various theoretical approaches, including psychological theories and sociological theories, such as feminist analysis and status inconsistency theory. However, some theories do not account for the multiple sites of oppression both men and women experience in the post-migration and settlement context and do not account for the day-to-day struggles of resettlement. The current literature contains other gaps in knowledge of IPV among immigrant and refugee women: this is particularly evident in Canadian health sciences literature (Guruge, 2007).

While there has been increased interest in the role of the "wife" in the post-migration context, not much attention has been devoted to the **role of the mother**. Some beginning work is available on the topic of women who have had to leave their children behind and the impact of the loss on women. In some cases, **reunification** occurs incrementally, with children from the same family being reunited with their mothers at different times. Such **separation** creates difficulties in women managing their lives in a new country; it can also disrupt the women's perception of their ability to fulfill socially defined family responsibilities, creating intense feelings of guilt, shame and anxiety that may, over time, affect their mental health. Parenting teens—a challenge for all parents—can be particularly difficult for parents who have been separated from their children for significant periods, especially if the children had felt abandoned by their parents. Newcomer girls may clash with their parents over the degree to which they want to preserve or retain beliefs and values from their home country versus assimilate into a new culture, augmenting the familial stress. Grandparents and other older adults may have their own struggles, such as experiencing social, cultural and spiritual isolation. In general, current educational and health care systems do not adequately deal with the broader **long-term effects of family dispersal**.

Despite the challenges, barriers and difficulties that immigrant women face in Canada, the fact that most women eventually lead successful lives is a testament to their strengths and resilience.

References

Baker, C., Arseneault, A.M. & Gallant, G. (1994). Resettlement with the support of an ethnocultural community. *Journal of Advanced Nursing, 20* (6), 1064–1072.

Beiser, M. (1988a). Influences of time, ethnicity, and attachments on depression in Southeast Asian refugees. *American Journal of Psychiatry, 145* (1), 46–51.

Beiser, M. (1988b). The mental health of immigrants and refugees in Canada. *Sante Culture Health, 5*, 197–213.

Boyd, M. (1994, Spring). Canada's refugee flows: Gender inequality. *Canadian Social Trends*, no. 32.

Bui, H.N. (2003). Help seeking behaviours among abused immigrant women: A case of Vietnamese American women. *Violence Against Women, 9* (2), 207–239.

Bui, H.N. & Morash, M. (1999). Domestic violence in the Vietnamese Immigrant community: An exploratory study. *Violence Against Women, 5* (7), 769–795.

Canadian Council for Refugees. (2002, November). State of Refugees in Canada. Author.

Chen, J., Ng, E. & Wilkins, R. (1996a). The health of Canada's immigrants in 1994–1995. *Health Reports, 7* (4), 33–45.

Chen, J., Ng, E. & Wilkins, R. (1996b). Health expectancy by immigrant status. *Health Reports, 8* (3), 29–37.

Citizenship and Immigration Canada (2001). Recent immigrants in metropolitan areas: Toronto—A comparative profile based on the 2001 census. Available: www.cic.gc.ca/english/resources/research/census 2001/toronto/parte.asp. Accessed February 28, 2008.

Citizen and Immigration Canada. (2004). *Facts and Figures 2004. Immigration Overview: Permanent Residents*.

Citizen and Immigration Canada. (2006). *Facts and Figures 2006. Immigration Overview: Permanent Residents*. Available: www.cic.gc.ca/english/resources/statistics/facts2006/permanent/31.asp. Accessed December 31, 2007.

DeLaet, D.L. (1999). Introduction: Invisibility of women in scholarship on international migration. In G.A. Kelson & D.L. DeLaet (Eds.). *Gender and Immigration* (pp. 1–17). New York: New York University Press.

DeVoretz, D.J. (Ed.). (1995). *Diminishing Returns: The economics of Canada's recent immigration policy*. Toronto: C.D. Howe Institute.

Fernandez, M. (1997). Domestic violence by extended family members in India: Interplay of gender and generation. *Journal of Interpersonal Violence, 12* (3), 433–455.

Gastaldo, D., Gooden, A. & Massaquoi, N. (2004). *Transnational health promotion: Social well being across borders and immigrant women's subjectivities*. Unpublished report.

Guruge, S. (2007). *The Influence of Gender, Racial, Social, and Economic Inequalities on the Production of and Responses to Intimate Partner Violence in the Post-Migration Context*. Unpublished doctoral dissertation, University of Toronto, Toronto, Canada.

Harvey, E.B. & Siu, B. (2001). Immigrants' socioeconomic situation compared, 1991–1996. INSCAN 15, no. 2 (Fall).

Hyman, I. (2001). *Immigration and health* (Working Paper 01-05, Health Policy Working Paper Series). Ottawa, Ontario, Canada: Health Canada.

Jiwani, Y. (2001). *Intersecting inequalities: Immigrant women of colour, violence, and healthcare*. Vancouver, British Columbia, Canada: Feminist Research, Education, Development, and Action (FREDA) Centre.

Khanlou. N., Beiser, M., Friere, M., Hyman, I. & Cole, M. (2002). Mental Health Promotion Among Newcomer Female Youth: Post-Migration Experiences and self-esteem. Ottawa: Status of Women. Available: www.swc-cfc.gc.ca/pubs/pubsprc/0662320840/200206_0662320840_12_e.html. Accessed June 15, 2007.

Kilbride, K.M., Tyyska, V., Berman, R., Ali, M., Woungang, I., Guruge, S. et al. (2007). Reclaiming Voice: Challenges and Opportunities for Immigrant Women Learning English. Report submitted to Canadian Council on Learning, Ottawa, Ontario, Canada. Available: http://ceris.metropolis.net/Virtual%20LibraryEResources/kilbride_et_al2007.pdf. Accessed February 18, 2008.

Krulfeld, R.M. (1994). Changing concepts of gender roles and identities in refugee communities. In L.A. Camino & R.M. Krufiled (Eds.). *Reconstructing lives, recapturing memory: refugee identity, gender and culture change*. Washington, DC: Gordon and Breach Publishers.

Kulig, J. (1994). Old traditional in a new world: Changing gender relations among Cambodian refugees. In L.A. Camino & R.M. Krulfeld (Eds.), *Reconstructing lives, recapturing memory: refugee identity, gender and culture change*. Washington, DC: Gordon and Breach Publishers.

Majumdar, B., Ellis, S. & Dye, P. (1999). Stress indicators and management for immigrant, refugee, and minority women. In M. Denton, M. Hadjukowski-Ahmed, M. O'Conner, & I.U. Zeytinoglu (Eds.), *Women's voices in health promotion* (pp. 152–163). Toronto, Ontario, Canada: Canadian Scholars Press.

Mojab, S. (1999). De-skilling immigrant women. *Canadian Woman Studies/Les Cahiers De La Femme, 19* (3), 123–127.

Mulvihill, M., Mailloux, L. & Atkin, W. (2001). Advancing policy and research responses to immigrant and refugee women's health in Canada. Prepared for the Centres of Excellence in Women's Health. Canadian Women's Health Network. Available: www.cewf-cesf.ca/en/resources/im=ref_health/immigration.html. Accessed February 7, 2008.

Omidvar, R. & Richmond, T. (2003). Perspectives on social inclusion: Immigrant settlement and social inclusion in Canada. Working Paper Series. Toronto: The Laidlaw Foundation. Available: www.maytree.com/PDF_Files/OmidvarRichmond.pdf. Accessed February 7, 2008.

Orenstein, M. (2000). Ethno-racial inequality in the City of Toronto: An analysis of the 1996 census. Toronto: City of Toronto.

Parakulam, G., Krishnan, V. & Odynak, D. (1992). Health status of Canadian-born and foreign-born residents. *Canadian Journal of Public Health, 83*, 311–314.

Pendakur, R. (2000). Immigrants and the labour force: Policy, regulation and impact. Montreal: McGill-Queen's University Press.

Reitz, J. G. (1998). Warmth of the welcome: the social causes of economic success for immigrants in different nations and cities. Boulder, CO: Westview Press.

Sandys, J. (1996) Immigration and Settlement Issues for Ethno-racial People with Disabilities: An Exploratory Study. Available: http://ceris.metropolis.net/Virtual%20Library/RFPReports/Sandys1996.pdf. Accessed February 7, 2008.

Schaafsma, J. & Sweetman, A. (1999). Immigrant earnings: Age at immigration matters. Research on Immigration and Integration in the Metropolis, Working Paper Series #99-04. Vancouver, BC.

Shamsuddin, A.F.M. (1999). The double-negative effect on the earnings of foreign-born females in Canada (Research on Immigration and Integration in the Metropolis Working Paper Series # 99-04). Vancouver, BC.

Shields, J. (2002, June). No safe haven: markets, welfare and migrants. Paper presented to the Canadian Sociology and Anthropology Association, 2002, Congress of the Social Sciences and Humanities, Toronto.

Statistics Canada (2004). Study: Immigrants in Canada's urban centres. *The Daily*, Wednesday, August 18, 2004. Available: www.statcan.ca/Daily/English/040818/d040818b.htm. Accessed February 7, 2008.

Statistics Canada. (2001). *Census of Canada 2001.* Available: http://www12.statcan.ca/english/census01/home/index.cfm. Accessed February 7, 2008.

Sundquist, J. (1995). Ethnicity, social class, and health. A population-based study on the influence of social factors on self-reported illness in 223 Latin American refugees, 333 Finnish, and 126 South European labour migrants and 841 Swedish controls. *Social Science & Medicine, 40*, 777–787.

United Nations. (1993). Declaration on the elimination of violence against women. *Canada-USA Women's Health Forum, New York,* p.6.

Vissandjee, B., Desmeules, M., Cao, Z. & Abdool, S. (2004, August). Integrating ethnicity and migration as determinants of Canadian Women's Health. *BMC Women's Health* 1472–6872, S1, S32.

Vissandjee, B., Weinfeld, M., Dupere, S. & Abdool, S. (2001). Sex, gender, ethnicity, and access to health care services: Research and policy challenges for immigrant women in Canada. *Journal of International Migration and Integration, 2* (1), 55–75.

Part 2

Theoretical Perspectives

Chapter 2

Theoretical Perspectives and Conceptual Frameworks

ENID COLLINS AND SEPALI GURUGE

Critical theories include a wide range of perspectives that are concerned with power and oppression, and with how social inequalities are created and maintained through societal structures and processes. The critical perspective "is part of a cluster of theories which analyze all aspects of social life from an explicitly political perspective. This political perspective intertwines theory and practice in order to produce knowledge aimed at both interpreting the world and changing it" (Baines, 1998, p. 5). According to Leonard (1993 as noted in George & Tsang, 1999, p.59), the three requirements of critical theory are that it must: a) locate the sources of domination and oppression; b) present an alternative vision of life without such domination and oppression; and c) communicate these ideas and findings in a format that is accessible to those who are oppressed by this domination.

The emergence of critical theories can be traced back to some of the early thinkers who advocated for transforming societal structures that create and maintain various forms of oppression. For example, Karl Marx (1818–1893) attributed peasants' oppression to the exploitation of their labour by ruling classes who owned economic resources, means of production and control of knowledge. Based on his work with peasants in South America, Friere (1989) posited that every human being, with the right tools, can develop critical awareness of their reality, become empowered to resist oppression, and take action to bring about transformation of social structures to change their situation.

Critical theoretical perspectives depart from "traditional" concepts and theories that focus on explaining and predicting social situations as they exist. In other words, critical theories go beyond the obvious to raise such questions as: How can the status quo be changed? How can oppressions be removed, and social justice and equity achieved for all members of society? The ultimate goal of approaching situations from a critical theoretical standpoint is to engage in political action that leads to the unravelling of multiple intersecting oppressions (such as racism, classism, sexism, homophobia and subjugation of knowledge) to achieve social change, social justice and equity in society.

Over the years, there has been a move toward critical inquiry in health and a greater emphasis in social work, psychology and nursing, in particular, on engaging in reflective practice. With this change has come an interest in recognizing diversity and addressing the inequalities among women—and between groups of women— caused by racism, colonialism, ethnocentrism, heterosexism, ageism and able-bodiedism. As a result, health care professionals are incorporating various theoretical perspectives and conceptual frameworks that help to recognize and respond to the issues of power, oppression and privilege.

In this chapter, we outline key elements of a number of approaches that respond to the diversity of women: multiculturalism, culturally sensitive care, intersectionalities of identities, anti-racism, postcolonial feminism, anti-oppression, eco-systemic frameworks and social determinants of health. While not all fall under the umbrella of critical theoretical perspectives, most of these approaches to exploring women's health challenge ethnocentric, racist and androcentric theoretical, research and practice paradigms and, therefore, have some common elements. These perspectives have been used in various practice settings to improve care to women of diverse backgrounds. Our intention is to provide a basic understanding of each approach. We refer the reader to the original works for in-depth information about each, and to the relevant chapters in this book for insights into how some of these perspectives and frameworks can be used to analyze a range of issues that women face in the context of immigration and settlement. Throughout, we look at how power and oppression influence immigrant women's health, as well as the care women receive. The chapter concludes with strategies for mental health professionals to apply these perspectives to their work with clients.

Multiculturalism

Canada's Aboriginal communities claim many cultural and language traditions. With the arrival of English and French settlers, institutions based on European models replaced institutions of Aboriginal communities, and English and French were eventually enshrined as Canada's official languages, with English becoming the dominant language. The multiculturalism policy was introduced by the Liberal government in 1971, within a bilingual framework, with the intent to recognize pluralism in Canadian society (Esses & Gardner, 1996; Henry et al., 1995; James, 1996). The multicultural model is based on the notion of acceptance of difference and recognition that people from different cultures have a right to retain their cultural identity (unlike the melting pot model of the United States that promoted assimilation). In the early 1970s, this led to a period of celebration and preservation of religious and ethnic identities. This was followed by a shift in focus in the late 1970s, from one of celebration to exploring ways to understand diverse cultural groups and focus on group relations (Elliot, 1999).

With the increase in immigrants and refugees from Asia, Africa and the Caribbean in the 1980s—and changes in the accompanying ethnic mix of the country—came a need to address issues related to equity and racism. The Canadian Charter of Rights and Freedoms was passed in 1982, protecting equality and freedom from discrimination. The Canadian Multiculturalism Act, passed in July 1988, promoted an understanding of the cultural diversity of Canadian society and acknowledged the freedom of all members to preserve, enhance and share their cultural heritage (Goodrich, 2002). More recently, the objectives of the multiculturalism program at the Department of Canadian Heritage include fostering cross-cultural understanding, combating racism and discrimination, promoting shared citizenship, and making Canadian institutions more reflective of Canadian diversity (Canadian Heritage, 2004).

Bannerji (2000) cautions us to examine how Canadian multiculturalism is being used "to manage a colonial history, an imperialist present, and a convoluted liberal democracy" (p.10). She analyzes how multiculturalism as an official policy appeared during a period of intense English-French rivalry, when Canada's Aboriginal population had demonstrated a growing interest in struggle for land claims. Within such a context, multiculturalism could be seen as a "diffusing or muting device" that redirected these groups' concerns and demands into a "cultural" issue that helped to maintain the hegemonic Anglo-Canadian national state and culture (Bannerji, 2000). The main criticisms of the multiculturalism policy falls into four areas: a) its failure to address the inequalities of power and privilege in a stratified society; b) its failure to address racial discrimination and systemic inequalities that are often inherent in institutional policies; c) the obvious exclusion of racial minorities from participating in positions of power; and d) limited access to resources and supports to racialized groups. In addition, issues related to gender and race are not articulated in the larger discourse on multiculturalism, even though they are central to debates on pluralism in Canadian society (Henry et al., 1995). As Bannerji (2000) has noted, "The Canadian state, for example, has a lot of work to do. It not only has to mediate and express the usual inequalities of a class and patriarchal society but also the ones created through colonialism and racism through which inflect class and patriarchy" (p. 5). Regardless of its limitations, the Canadian multiculturalism policy has had a major impact not only on Canada but also on other countries that receive immigrants such as England, Australia and the United States.

Culturally Sensitive Care

Since the 1960s, health care professionals from various disciplinary backgrounds including social work, nursing and psychology have come to acknowledge the limitations of "traditional" health care models in meeting the needs of changing health care consumers (Minors, 1996; Tator, 1995; Tsang & George, 1998). Some health care professionals have embraced a culturally sensitive approach to their practice that is based on a multicultural perspective. With this approach, health care professionals provide care that acknowledges and respects the cultures and cultural practices of their clients, and tend to develop awareness of their own cultural values and beliefs that shape health care encounters.

Nursing, in particular, has embraced the work of Madeline Leininger, an American nurse anthropologist who encouraged nurses to develop in-depth knowledge of their patients' cultures in order to provide culturally sensitive care. She introduced the notion of transcultural nursing, which was based on culture care theory and depicted by the Sunrise model (see below). It focused on care, health and illness patterns of individuals and groups with respect to differences and similarities in their cultural values, beliefs and practices (Leininger, 1978).

FIGURE 2-1

Leininger's Sunrise Model to Depict the Theory of Culture Care Diversity and Universality

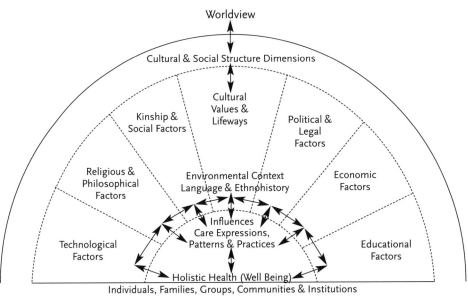

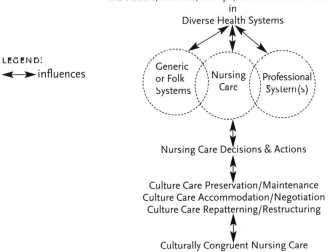

Source: Leininger, M.M. (Ed.) 1991. *Culture Care Diversity and Universality: A Theory of Nursing.* New York: National League for Nursing Press. Reprinted with permission of the National League for Nursing, New York, NY.

Leininger provides an extensive list of premises about culture care (1995a; 1995b), out of which we have extracted a few that are relevant to our discussion:

- Care is the essence of nursing and the distinct, dominant, central and unifying focus of nursing.
- Care (caring) is essential to well-being, health, healing, growth and survival and to confronting illness and/or death.
- Care takes place in cultural contexts.
- Culture care meanings, expressions, processes and structural forms reflect differences and similarities among all cultures of the world.
- Culture care values, beliefs and practices are influenced by and tend to be embedded in the worldview, language, religious (or spiritual), kinship, legal, educational, economic, historical and environmental contexts of a particular culture.

She noted that in order to provide culturally sensitive care to clients, it is critical for nurses to learn about similarities and differences among cultures, their own as well as their clients'.

Health care professionals, especially those in major cities across Canada, have gained insights on caring for clients from diverse cultures by using culturally sensitive care frameworks. Often problematic in a "culturally sensitive framework," however, are the underlying notions that: a) "cultures" or "cultural values and beliefs" can be learned or mastered (an approach hardly possible given the diversity of clients one might see on any given day); b) cultures are homogeneous; c) cultures are static (when cultures across the world are changing as a result of globalization); and d) "Canadian culture" is to be considered the norm against which all other cultures and their values and beliefs are compared. Further, culturally sensitive care frameworks often fail to acknowledge intersecting identities such as race and gender (Bannerji, 2000; Barbee, 1993), and until recently, did not incorporate the impact of systemic and structural inequalities that contribute to ongoing power and dominations. (See also Chapter 3 for further discussion on the culturally sensitive approach to care).

Intersecting Identities

A range of identities intersect and change in various social contexts to shape women's experiences. As such, it is critical that mental health professionals consider women's unique experiences, rather than focusing on commonalties based on gender alone. They also need to understand social locations in which identities are constructed, the fluidity and flexibility of identities, and the salience of different identities in different social situations (or when people move across borders, for example, from rural to urban communities and from developing to developed countries) (Agnew, 1996; Mohanty, 1997). There is a growing body of literature on intersectionality and intersectionalities of identities (Bannerji, 1995; Crenshaw, 1991; Guruge & Khanlou, 2004; Hill Collins, 2000; hooks, 1984; Rummens, 2004a; 2004b). Intersectional analyses in the context of health involve examining how intersections of gender, race, ethnicity, class and other axes of difference have an impact on women's health. According to Weber and Parra-Medina (2003 noted in Hankivsky, 2007, p. 80), the broad questions that drive an intersectional analysis are:

- What is the meaning of race, ethnicity, class, sexuality and other systems of inequality across the ideological, political and economic domains of society, in institutional structures and in individual lives?
- How are these co-constructed systems of inequity simultaneously produced, reinforced, resisted and transformed—over time, in different locations and in different institutional domains (e.g., health, education, religion, politics)?
- How can our understanding of the intersecting dynamics of these systems guide us in the pursuit of social justice?

Gender relations form the basis for organizing social relations in all societies throughout the world. Across almost all societies women tend to be assigned subordinate positions to men. However, gender is experienced differently by women in different social contexts, depending on historical, socio-economic and cultural experiences (Ng, 1988). Race becomes salient in stratifying people and assigning positions of economic, political and social privilege. For example, white men occupy the most powerful positions in society especially in the arenas of economy, business, law and politics, and white women are second only to white men in the social hierarchy of power and privilege. In her paper *White Privilege: Unpacking the Invisible Knapsack*, McIntosh (1990) discussed taken-for-granted privileges that are enjoyed by white people and denied to blacks and other minorities. She includes in her metaphoric knapsack the right to access equitable standards in education, housing, safety, health and employment. Various systemic practices are in place to ensure such positions are maintained within these hierarchies. Immigrant women, refugee women, women of colour and "illegal" women of colour with "psychiatric disorders" are often assigned lower social statuses (frequently in the order listed). Similarly, certain forms of knowledge production and various discourses are used to justify an inequitable distribution of resources.

Ng (1988) noted that immigrant women are treated as a homogeneous group that ignores their many differences based on education, class and social position. Racialized women who were highly competent in their own societies are rendered incompetent when they are given certain socially ascribed positions in the Canadian labour market. For example, when a pediatrician who is a well respected member of her community in India migrates to a country such as Canada, she might only be allowed to practise as an auxiliary health care worker. Downward professional and social mobility and the associated socio-economic losses that she might experience in Canada—combined with her accent, dress and skin colour—might be further used to reinforce stereotypic identities about immigrant women being "uneducated." While immigrant women develop strategies that enable them to adapt to new situations and to challenge various oppressive encounters (involving for instance, racism and sexism) (Giroux, 1991; Omi & Winant, 1993), these oppressive social relations can lead to the development of mental health problems.

Anti-Racism

Because of the failure of multiculturalism and culturally sensitive care frameworks to address inequalities in society based on other identities, academics and community activists in the 1980s introduced alternative frameworks, one of which was anti-racism. While proponents of anti-racism frameworks acknowledge the influence of intersecting social identities, they emphasize that race is central to assigning or denying power (Dei, 2000; Omi & Winant, 1993). Although there is no scientific justification for the concept of race, it continues to be used as a social marker that identifies and stratifies people into groups, with white people being considered as superior (Omi & Winant, 1993). *Racism* refers to actions of individuals and/or groups that exclude people from resources and privileges on the basis of race. *Systemic racism* refers to organizational practices that lead to people being excluded or discriminated against based on their race. While systemic racism may be embedded in day-to-day functioning, norms and practices of social institutions, these norms and practices may not be perceived as expressions of racism (Anthias & Yuval-Davis, 1992). Everyday racism "is the interweaving of racism in the fabric of the social system" (Essed, 1991, p. 37), and refers to institutional practices that are taken as normal and are used to justify privileges to some, while denying them to others (Essed, 1991; Henry et al., 1995; James, 1996). Dominant groups in Eurocentric societies have access to power and privilege based on a social construction of "whiteness" that forms the basis for economic, social and political dominance (Bedard, 1994; Roman, 1993). Power and dominance associated with whiteness that were produced in historical and social contexts continue to be reproduced in contemporary social relations.

Key premises of anti-racism include a need to interrogate whiteness as a source of dominance within society and the need for power-sharing and bringing about social justice and equity for all members of society (Dei, 2000). Anti-racism strategies are based on the premise that institutions, organizations and individuals are dynamic and are capable of changing to include aspirations of minority groups (James, 1996). People are expected to engage in collective action to challenge the status quo, and bring about social, political and economic changes (James, 1996).

This framework provides a more realistic approach than a culturally sensitive approach to addressing mental health and illness concerns of immigrant women who experience everyday racism and various social inequities based on systemic racism. At the individual level, some mental health professionals have used anti-racism frameworks in shaping their practice. Some health care disciplines such as social work have also adopted anti-racism frameworks in academic and practice settings (Tsang & George, 1998).

Health care workers and others have criticized anti-racism frameworks, arguing that there is no scientific basis for race, so the concept should be discarded. The principle of fairness and justice in health and social services and other organizations comes from the ideology that underlies social relations in Canada. Social systems are premised on the colour-blind approach, which claims to treat all people alike and disregard their differences. Even though there is considerable evidence of racism in Canadian society, people continue to deny that it exists (Henry et al., 1995). As a result, much work has yet to be accomplished in bringing about organizational change to reflect the needs and interests of racialized groups of women.

Postcolonial Feminist Perspectives

Early feminist movements brought about significant changes in redressing gender oppression, gaining entry into male-dominated occupations, and improving work and social conditions for white middle class heterosexual and able-bodied women in developed countries such as England, the United States and Canada. In spite of these changes, gender discrimination remains a reality for women in such countries, with gains being inequitably distributed across diverse groups of women. Early feminist movements were primarily concerned with dismantling patriarchal conventions, assumptions and domination that were seen as the root of all forms of oppression. Throughout the first wave of the feminist movement in the 1950s and most of the second wave of the movement in Europe and North America in the 1960s and 1970s, white middle class women were primarily concerned with issues around sexuality, reproduction and abortion; with challenging the notion that women's biology makes them mentally and physically inferior to men; with issues related to violence against women, birth control, public health and poverty; and with engaging in civil rights, labour and peace movements.

Although issues such as housing, employment and social services were of concern to new immigrant women from Asia, Africa and the Caribbean, most immigrant women were not motivated to join the feminist movement in North America as issues such as racism, discriminatory immigration policies, un/underemployment and lack of language training were not evident in feminist discourses at the time. Furthermore, white middle class feminists embraced racist views of the larger society that tacitly contributed to the oppression of women of colour (Agnew, 1996). However, immigrant women were actively working in their communities and organizing in a significant way to actively challenge racism, sexism and classism in Canada, as they did through the organization *Women Working with Immigrant Women* in Toronto (Das Gupta, 1999). Immigrant women were also a driving force behind academic work that critiqued earlier feminists' works for their naïve notion of shared sisterhood, and the belief that patriarchy was the main source of oppression among women (Anzaldua & Moraga, 1981; Bannerji, 1993; hooks, 1981, 1988). As a result, one of the new discourses put forward by the third wave feminists in the 1980s was postcolonial feminism, which critiqued the role of colonialism and its ongoing effects on people of racialized communities.

Postcolonial perspectives include a wide range of positions, many of which present complex, critical and sometimes contradictory perspectives. One of the most commonly noted contestations has been about the term "post" in postcolonialism.

While some have interpreted "post" to mean "after" colonialism, this is a narrow under-standing of the term. Most users of this terminology (and perspective) take a broader understanding to include the ongoing effects of both colonial and neo-colonial rela-tions on the lives of people living in previously colonized countries as well as in the experiences of people within "first world colonial powers" (Reimer-Kirkham & Anderson, 2002). In their introduction to the volume *Post-Colonial Studies,* Ashcroft et al. (1997) stated that:

> Post-colonial theory involves discussion about experiences of various kinds: migration, slavery, suppression, resistance, representation, difference, race, gender, place and responses to influential master discourses of imperial Europe such as history, philosophy, and linguistics and the fundamental expe-riences of speaking and writing by which all these come into being. (p. 2)

The following diagram represents a synthesis of concepts cited by postcolonial feminist writers to address these oppressions.

FIGURE 2-2

Relationships of Key Concepts in Postcolonial Feminism

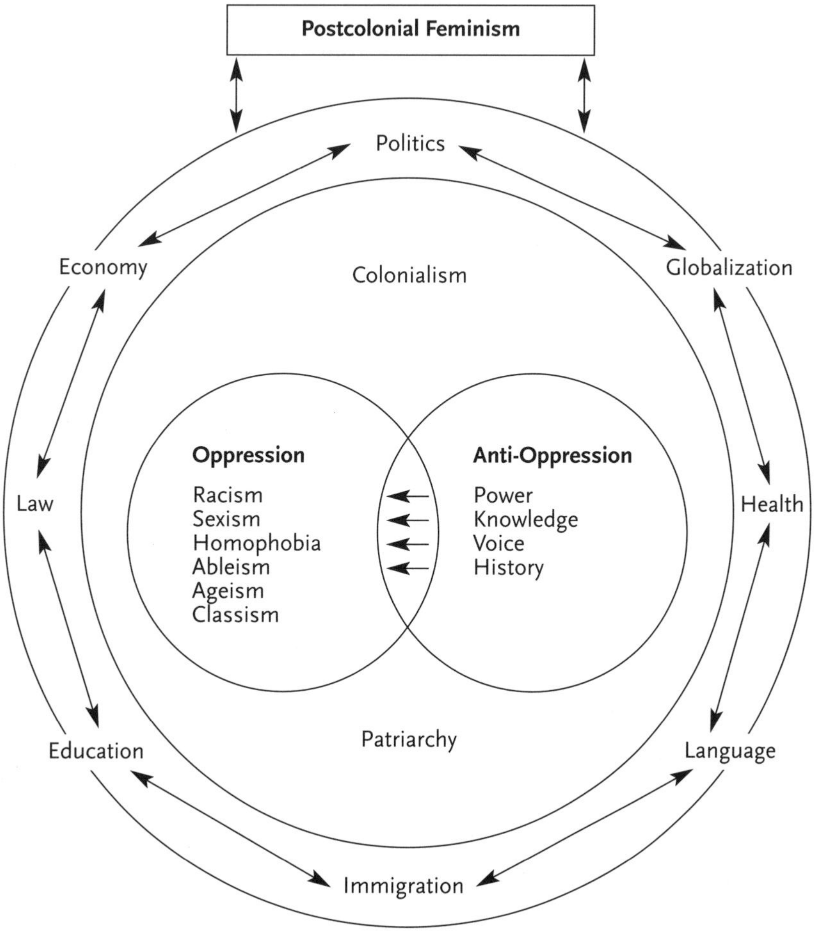

Postcolonial feminist scholars argue that oppression is not accidental, but occurs through systematic processes associated with multiple and intersecting identities. Structural systems in society create hierarchies, whereby some sectors enjoy power and privilege while others are marginalized (Hill Collins, 1991; Mohanty, 1991; Razack, 1998). As bell hooks (1988) stated: "We must understand that patriarchal domination shares an ideological foundation with other forms of group oppression, that there is no hope that it can be eradicated while these systems remain intact" (p. 22). She contends that there is a need for all groups in society to confront intersecting oppressions, such as gender, race, class and sexuality, and to work collectively to eradicate them. Both men and women should be cognizant of their position as both oppressors and the oppressed and how their positions may change from one situation to another. For example, women often experience violence in their homes and in intimate relationships by men who experience racism and other forms of oppression in the public sphere. Postcolonial feminists advocate multi-faceted strategies to dismantle all forms of oppression and to create a just and equitable society for all people.

The production and control of knowledge are central themes in postcolonial discourses. "Mainstream" knowledge generated by academic research, publication and media is controlled by elite groups who are invested in maintaining the status quo and their privilege (van Dijk, 1993). Postcolonial feminists ask questions such as: What counts as legitimate knowledge? Who has the right to produce knowledge? The idea of "subjugated knowledge"—a term borrowed from postmodernist/post-structuralist perspectives—is central to debates around production and control of knowledge. People who have experienced oppression demand to be heard, and to have subjugated knowledge (knowledge that was previously dismissed as backward or not worthy of attention) acknowledged as legitimate (Spivak, 1997). Dei and Rosenberg (2002) argue that "[t]he negation, devaluation and denial of indigenous knowledges, particularly those of women, is the result of deliberate practices of establishing hierarchies of knowledge" (p. 4). These hierarchies of knowledge support the interests of elite groups who benefit from unequal power relations created by race, class, gender, economics and other forms of oppressions (Hill Collins, 1998; van Dijk, 1993).

Women who have been silenced by experiences of colonization and patriarchy are creating new ways of thinking and viewing their world. Postcolonial feminists consider the impact of globalization on experiences of women in social contexts. Bell hooks (1988) stated that we live in a world that is governed by domination, where superior groups rule over inferior ones. In this environment, disastrous consequences—systematic dehumanization, worldwide famine, ecological devastation and industrial contamination—are possible and can negatively influence women's mental health. Immigrant women may come to Canada to escape such situations, only to experience added forms of oppression—such as racism, unemployment/underemployment and chronic poverty—during resettlement in Canada (Agnew, 1996, Mojab, 1999). Third wave feminists, such as Lorde (1984), hooks (1984) and Mohanty (1991), thus encourage scholarship that goes beyond gender oppression to include and focus on the realities of women's lives that are shaped by intersecting oppressions, such as race, class, gender, culture, history, religion and sexual orientation.

New bodies of knowledge are emerging and claiming space in academia. For example, Canadian feminist scholars such as Agnew (1996), Bannerji (1993) and Ng (2002, 1988) have demonstrated how immigrant women of colour in Canada are responding to their experiences of oppression. In "Talking back," bell hooks (1989) discusses the barriers and struggles that black women experience in writing and sharing their stories and eventually coming to "voice." For those who gain confidence to speak out about their experiences, the process is liberating. She states poignantly:

> Moving from silence into speech is for the oppressed, the colonized, the exploited, and those who stand and struggle side by side, a gesture of defiance that heals, that makes new life and new growth possible. It is that act of speech, of "talking back," that is no mere gesture of empty words, that is the expression of our movement from object to subject—the liberated voice. (bell hooks, 1989, p. 16)

In her book entitled *Black Feminist Thought* (1991) and her later work *Fighting Words, Black Women and the Search for Justice* (1998), Hill Collins analyzes women's experiences and demonstrates how interlocking oppressions are created and maintained within society through ideology, the economy and politics. She contends that the undervaluing of black people's labour was a strategy that served to maintain power and privilege among elite white groups. Hill Collins noted that while the concept of coming to voice became popular in the feminist movement of the 1970s, black women have historically spoken out against oppression. By informally sharing their experiences in "kitchen table conversations," and by challenging "mainstream" discourses, black women began to break their silence and find ways to reclaim their humanity. Collectively their stories created greater awareness of their oppression and bolstered their ability to confront these oppressions, and contribute significantly to feminist scholarship.

Postcolonial feminist perspectives recognize the need for knowledge to be constructed from the point of view of marginalized women whose voice has been silenced "in the knowledge production process" (Reimer-Kirkham & Anderson, 2002; Tuhiwai Smith, 2001). By learning from the perspective of marginalized immigrant women, we are able to see how "some of the systemic practices and structural barriers in the host country reduce the space for resistance and hope on the part of immigrant and refugee women, and that migration to a country of the North does not necessarily improve a woman's status both within and outside the home" (Guruge & Khanlou, 2004, p. 37). Thus, postcolonial feminist perspectives help us to see how the complex historical, political, cultural and socio-economic context affects immigrant and refugee women's health and illness, and their access to quality care (Guruge & Khanlou, 2004).

Anti-Oppression Perspectives

Anti-oppression advocates posit that oppression is socially constructed and operates in various contexts, creating consequences for both individuals and for society. Anti-oppression perspectives recognize how multiple forms of oppression operate through intersecting social identities based on age, gender, race, class, sexuality and ability (Hill Collins, 1991 & 1988; hooks, 1988). The focus of anti-oppression analysis, therefore, "is apparent in the stand that theorists take against all forms of oppression," rather than on "singular social identities, such as gender or race" (Moosa-Mitha, 2005, p.62). Today, anti-oppression approaches involve adopting a critical stance and contesting "mainstream" theories that characterize "difference" as problematic or inferior (Dominelli, 2002).

In line with anti-racist, disability, Aboriginal and other social identity-based movements, anti-oppression discourse analyzes processes by which certain groups in society maintain power and privilege while less powerful individuals and groups are dominated and marginalized (van Dijk, 1993). Groups of people who display certain socially defined characteristics are placed in categories that are less valued in society. Anti-oppression perspectives claim that people can be either oppressed or oppressors, depending on the social context in which they are situated (Razack, 1988). For example, based on the social context, both men and women can be oppressed while being oppressors; therefore, there is a need to work together to confront differences. Proponents of anti-oppression believe that to create a society where social justice and equity are achievable for all, multi-pronged strategies must be used to unravel all forms of oppression (Hill Collins, 1998; hooks, 1988). Therefore, actions to challenge intersecting oppressions such as sexism, racism, ageism and homophobia are all part of a multi-faceted approach in anti-oppression work. Within this approach, difference is complicated—multiple, fluid and changing—rather than being fixed and reduced to a single position (Yuval-Davis, 1999).

Ecosystemic Frameworks

The ecosystemic (or ecological) framework has often been used in various disciplines, such as psychology, social work and nursing. It was originally used to help organize research findings on the etiology of child abuse (Belsky, 1980), but more recently has been widely used to address the factors contributing to intimate partner violence (see for example, Dutton, 1988; Edleson & Tolman, 1992; Guruge, 2007). Seminal work by Garbarino (1977), Bronfenbrenner (1977; 1979) and Belsky (1980) proposed that in order to understand human behaviour, one needs to move beyond the individual to examine the context or environment within which the individual is located. The context or environment, in turn, is perceived to consist of a series of settings or systems, each nested within the broader setting or system to include the micro-environment of the immediate and extended family, the meso-environment of the immediate social network (that is, schools, workplaces and neighbourhoods) and the macro-environment of the society at large.

A modification of the widely used diagram (as presented in Guruge, 2007) is provided below. It captures the migration contexts.

FIGURE 2-3

Depiction of an Ecosystemic Framework in the Context of Immigration and Resettlement

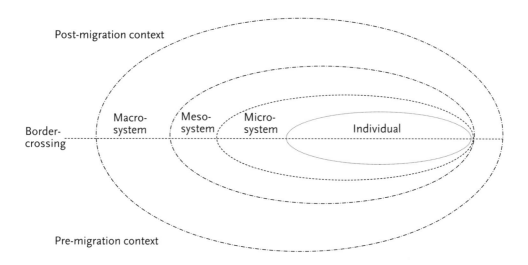

The transactions between these systems are seen as continuous and reciprocal. "Although there appears to be room for interpretation and debate as to exactly where a particular factor might fit within the framework, more important than the location of any single factor is the dynamic interplay between factors operating at multiple levels" (Guruge, 2007, p. 69). Ecosystemic frameworks provide a basis for analyzing the complex issues at the intersection of various social identities (both imposed and assumed) and the interaction of these with micro-, meso- and macro-level factors (Guruge & Khanlou, 2004). In analyzing the application of ecosystemic frameworks to social work practice, Tsang and George (1998) have pointed out that micro levels of practice do not operate independent of societal and institutional contexts. Mental health professionals who choose to view their practice from an ecosystemic framework can see how macro systems such as the politics and economics of the health care system influence encounters between the client and health professional.

The Social Determinants of Health Approach

According to Raphael (2004), an understanding of social determinants of health dates back to the 1800s when a German physician, Virchow, and Engels explored the mechanisms by which political and social lives and material conditions shaped people's health.

Social determinants of health are the social and economic conditions that positively or negatively affect the health of individuals, their families and communities. Health Canada's Population Health Approach (2002) has recognized income and social status, education, employment and working conditions, physical environments, social environments, social support networks, personal health practices and coping skills, healthy child development, biology and genetic endowment, health services, gender and culture as social determinants that affect health. Increasing evidence from the United States, the United Kingdom and Sweden, for example, supports the need to understand health holistically, and to recognize that social, cultural, economic and physical circumstances of individuals and groups can be even more important than personal health behaviours in influencing people's health (Donovan et al., 1992; Raphel, 2004; Stephen et al., 1994). There is strong and growing evidence that higher socioeconomic status is associated with better living conditions, such as safe housing and ability to afford sufficient and healthy food (Raphel, 2004). Similarly, un/underemployment, stressful and unsafe work conditions, and barriers to accessing affordable and quality care are associated with poorer health (Health Canada, 2002). These factors explain why some people are healthy and others are not. The impact of these conditions is magnified by such forms of oppression as racism, sexism and ageism.

Social determinants of health—including immigration status itself—affect immigrants through the process of immigration and resettlement. Several health researchers have explored the topic of social determinants of health in relation to immigration and settlement and, in particular, in relation to immigrant women's health (see for example, Hyman, 2002; Hyman & Guruge, 2006; Oxman-Martinez et al., 2000; Vissandjée et al., 2001). Many newly arrived immigrant women are disadvantaged by poverty, discrimination and immigration status. Certain determinants—such as "social isolation, language barriers, separation from family, change in family roles and norms, lack of information about available resources, and unemployment"—are critical to the health of immigrants and refugees (Fowler, 1998, p. 389). Furthermore, some women may have experiences of living through war, slavery and violence (Tsang & George, 1998). These experiences have profound effects on the mental health of women during post migration and settlement, especially considering the added effects of separation from familiar culture and community.

Strategies for Incorporating Theoretical Frameworks into Mental Health Practice

Here we present some strategies to help mental health professionals enhance the care they provide to immigrant women:

- Recognize that there are many ways of knowing and creating meaning (Arslanian-Engoren, 2002), and consider frameworks for care that are appropriate for each woman's individual situation.
- Gain a broader understanding of the causes of mental health problems to include social determinants of mental health throughout the migration process.
- Broaden awareness of the unique meaning of mental health and illness within the context of women's cultural, historical and social frames of reference.
- Recognize that women's lives are shaped by multiple identities, which overlap and/or change in different social situations. Some women may be disadvantaged additionally because of new social identities assigned to them in post-migration contexts.
- Acknowledge the limitations of providing care that is based on the primacy of gender oppression, and incorporate into care an understanding of how women's lives are affected by intersecting oppression based on race, culture, class, citizenship, age, ability and sexual orientation.
- Understand that women in different social and economic contexts experience gender oppressions differently.
- Pay attention to the mechanisms that reinforce oppressive practices in Western, medical model-based institutional care.
- Develop awareness of your own power and privilege and how they can influence interactions with women during mental health encounters.
- Create opportunities for both practitioners and patients/clients/women to be learners and teachers.
- Provide women with information about all treatment options and care modalities, learn from the women what works (or not) in their situation, and together make the best choice(s) for the women and their families.
- Recognize the ability of women to resist oppression and support women to take control of their health.

Some questions that might be useful to mental health practitioners who work with immigrant and refugee women in their practice include:

- What has been the journey that brought her to seek mental health care?
- What past experiences may have an immediate or latent impact on her mental health?
- What is the woman's experience of violence? What is the nature of the violence?
- How does the woman view her strengths as well as vulnerabilities?
- How does she define family and community?
- What are her resettlement experiences?

- What are her experiences of racism, sexism and heterosexism in the resettlement process?
- What kinds of support and resources are needed and can be offered to address the impact of such experiences both in the short- and long-term?

Conclusion

Mental health professionals can use the theoretical perspectives and conceptual frameworks discussed in this chapter to inform their practice. Some practitioners may choose to work from an anti-oppression perspective, while also considering the unique experiences of women. Others may use a social determinants of health approach that attends to the broader determinants of health, such as social inclusion or exclusion, unemployment, underemployment, poverty and their impact on health. We recognize that some of the frameworks may be controversial and may even be challenged in certain practice settings. Similarly, there is some discrepancy in the literature about how certain key authors conceptualize the interrelationship between race and gender, along with other social identities (for example, whether someone is grounded in anti-racist feminist thought or postcolonial feminist scholarship). However, it is our hope that an understanding of these perspectives and frameworks will create a foundation for advancing mental health practice that reflects the diverse needs of women. We encourage mental health professionals to interrogate institutional practices that contribute to oppression in women's lives, and consciously promote practice strategies that enable women to take control of their lives. By adopting such a stance, mental health professionals can become advocates for equal benefits for women of all backgrounds.

References

Agnew, V. (1996). *Resisting Discrimination: Women from Asia, Africa and the Caribbean and the Women's Movement in Canada.* Toronto: University of Toronto Press.

Anzaldua, G., & Moraga, C. (Eds). (1981). *This Bridge Called My Back: Writings by Radical Women of Colour.* New York: Kitchen Table Press.

Anthias, F. & Yuval-Davis, N. (1992). *Racialized Boundaries: Race, Nation, Gender, Color and Class in the Anti-racist Struggle.* London: Routledge.

Arslanian-Engoren, C. (2002). Feminist post-structuralism: A methodological paradigm for examining clinical decision-making. *Journal of Advanced Nursing,* 37 (60), 512–517.

Ashcroft, B., Griffiths, G. & Tiffin, H. (1997). Introduction. In B. Ashcroft, G. Griffiths & H. Tifflin (Eds.), *The Post-Colonial Studies Reader,* (pp. 1–4). London: Routledge.

Baines, D. (1998). Everyday Practice of Race, Class and Gender. Unpublished doctoral dissertation, Toronto: University of Toronto.

Bannerji, H. (1993). Returning the gaze: An introduction. In H. Bannerji (Ed.), *Returning the Gaze, Essay on Racism, Feminism and Politics* (pp. ix–xxiv). Toronto: Sister Vision Press.

Bannerji, H. (1995). *Thinking Through: Essays on Feminism, Marxism, and Anti-Racism.* Toronto: Women's Press.

Bannerji, H. (2000). *The Dark Side of the Nation: Essays on Multiculturalism, Nationalism, and Gender.* Toronto: Canadian Scholars' Press.

Barbee, E. (1993). Racism in U.S. nursing. *Medical Anthropology Quarterly, 7* (4), 346–362.

Bedard, G. (1994). Quebectitude: An ambiguous identity. In C. James & A. Shadd (Eds.), *Thinking about Difference: Encounters in Culture, Language and Identity.* (pp. 23–28). Toronto: Between the Lines Press.

Belsky, J. (1980). Child maltreatment: An ecological integration. *American Psychologist, 35,* 320–335.

Bronfenbrenner, U. (1977). Toward an experimental ecology of human development. *American Psychologist, 32,* 513–531.

Bronfenbrenner, U. (1979). *The Ecology of Human Development.* Cambridge, MA: Harvard University Press.

Canadian Heritage (2004). Annual report on the operation of the Canadian Multiculutral Act, 2002-2003. Available: www.pch.gc.ca/progs/multi/new/index_e.cfm. Accessed February 18, 2008.

Crenshaw, K.W. (1991). Mapping the margins: Intersectionality, identity politics, and violence against women of color. *Stanford Law Review, 43* (6), 1241–1299.

Das Gupta, T. (1999). The politics of multiculturalism: "Immigrant women" and the Canadian state. In E. Dua & A. Robertson (Eds.), *Scratching the Surface: Canadian Anti-Racist Feminist Thought.* Toronto: Women's Press.

Dei, G. (2000). Toward an anti-racism discursive framework. In G.J.S. Dei & A. Calliste (Eds.), *Power, Knowledge and Anti-Racism Education: A Critical Reader* (pp. 23–40). Halifax, NS: Fernwood.

Dei, G. & Rosenberg, D. (2002). Introduction. In G. Dei, D. Rosenberg & B. Hall, *Indigenous Knowledges in Global Contexts. Multiple Readings of Our World* (pp. 3–17). Toronto. University of Toronto Press.

Doane, G. & Varcoe, C. (2005). *Family Nursing as Relational Inquiry: Developing Health Promoting Practice.* Philadelphia: Lippincot, Williams & Wilkins.

Dominelli, L. (2002). *Anti-Oppressive Social Work Theory and Practice.* London: Palgrave.

Donovan, J., d'Espaignet, E., Metron, C. et al. (Eds.). (1992). *Immigrants in Australia: A Health Profile.* Canberra: Australian Government Publishing Service.

Dutton, D.G. (1988). Profiling of wife assaulters: Preliminary evidence for a trimodal analysis. *Violence and Victims, 3* (1), 5–29.

Edleson, J. & Tolman, R.M. (1992). *Intervention for Men Who Batter: An Ecological Approach.* Newbury Park, CA: Sage.

Elliot, G. (1999). Cross-cultural awareness in an aging society: Effective strategies for communication and caring. Hamilton, ON: McMaster University, Office of Gerontological Studies.

Essed, P. (1991). *Understanding Everyday Racism: An Interdisciplinary Theory.* Newbury Park, CA: Sage.

Esses, V. & Gardner, R. C. (1996). Multiculturalism in Canada: Context and current status. *Canadian Journal of Behavioural Science, 28* (3), 145–154.

Freire, P. (1989). *Pedagogy of the Oppressed.* New York: Continuum.

Fowler, N. (1998). Providing primary health care to immigrants and refugees: The North Hamilton experience. *Canadian Medical Association Journal, 159,* 388–91.

Garbarino, J. (1977). The human ecology of child maltreatment: A conceptual model for research. *Journal of Marriage and the Family,* 39 (4), 721–735.

Giroux, H. (1991). Postmodernism as border pedagogy: Refining the boundaries of race and ethnicity. In. H. Giroux (Ed.), *Postmodernism, Feminism and Cultural Politics: Redrawing educational Boundaries* (pp. 217–256). Albany: State University of New York Press.

Goodrich, J. (2002). Mulitculturalism in Canada, Canadian Studies at Mount Allision University. Available: www.mta.ca/faculty/arts/canadian_studies/english/about/multi/index.htm. Accessed February 18, 2008.

George, U. & Tsang, A. (1999). Toward an inclusive paradigm in social work: The diversity framework. *Indian Journal of Social Work,* 60 (1), 57–68.

Guruge, S. (2007). The influence of gender, racial, social, and economic inequalities on the production of and responses to intimate partner violence in the post-migration context. Unpublished doctoral dissertation, University of Toronto, Toronto.

Guruge, S. & Khanlou, N. (2004). Intersectionalities of influence: Researching the health of immigrant and refugee women. *Canadian Journal of Nursing Research,* 36 (3), 32 –47.

Gustafson, D. (2000). Introduction: Health care reform and its impact on Canadian women. In D. Gustafson (Ed.), *Care and Consequences: The Impact of Health Care Reform* (pp. 1–24). Halifax: Fernwood Publishing.

Hankivsky, O. (2007). More than age and biology: Overhauling lifespan approaches to women's health. In M. Morrow, O. Hankivsky & C. Varcoe (Eds.), *Women's Health in Canada: Critical Perspectives on Theory and Policy.* Toronto: University of Toronto Press.

Health Canada (2002). *Population Health.* Ottawa. Available: www.phac-aspc.gc.ca/ph-sp/phdd/determinants/index.html#determinants. Accessed February 18, 2008.

Henry, F., Tator, C., Mattis, W. & Rees, T. (1995). *The Color of Democracy: Racism in Canadian Society.* Toronto: Harcourt Brace.

Hill Collins, P. (1998). *Fighting Words: Black Women and the Search for Justice.* Minneapolis: University of Minnesota Press.

Hill Collins, P. (1991). *Black Feminist Thought: Knowledge, Consciousness and the Politics of Empowerment.* New York: Routledge.

Hill Collins, P. (2000). *Black Feminist Thought: Knowledge Consciousness, and the Politics of Empowerment,* 2nd ed. New York: Routledge.

hooks, b. (1981). *Ain't I a Woman: Black Women and Feminism.* Boston: South End Press.

hooks, b. (1984). *Feminist theory: From Margin to Center.* Boston: South End Press.

hooks, b. (1988). *Talking Back: Thinking Feminist, Thinking Black.* Boston: South End Press.

hooks, b. (1989). Talking back. In A. Kesselman, L. McNair, N. Schniedewind (Eds.), *Women: Images and Realities: A Multicultural Anthology* (pp. 13-16). Mountainview, CA: Mayfield.

Hyman, I. & Guruge, S. (2006). Immigrant women's health. In R. Srivastava (Ed.), *The Health Care Professional's Guide to Clinical Cultural Competence* (pp. 264-280). Toronto: Elsevier Canada.

Hyman, I. (2002). Immigrant and Visible Minority Women. In D.E. Stewart, A. Cheung, L.E. Ferris, I. Hyman, M.M. Cohen & L.J. Williams (Eds.), *Ontario Women's Health Status Report.* Toronto: Ontario Women's Health Council.

James, C. (1996). Race culture and identity. In C. James (Ed.), *Perspectives on Racism and the Human Services Sector: A Case for Change* (pp. 15–35). Toronto: University of Toronto Press.

Leininger, M. (1978). *Transcultural Nursing: Concepts, Theories, Research & Practices.* New York, John Wiley & Sons

Leininger, M. (1995a). Culture care theory, research and practice. In *Nursing Science Quarterly,* 9 (2), 71–78.

Leininger, M. (1995b). Transcultural nursing perspectives: Basic concepts, principles, and culture care incidents. In M. Leiniger & M.R. McFarland (Eds.), *Transcultural Nursing: Concepts, Theories, and Practice,* 2nd ed. (pp. 57–92). New York: McGraw Hill.

Lorde, A. (1984). *Sister Outsider Freedom.* CA: Crossing Press.

McIntosh, P. (1990, Winter). White privilege: Unpacking the invisible knapsack. *Independent School,* 31–36.

Minors, A. (1996). From uni-versity to poly-versity: Organizations in transition to anti-racism. In C. James (Ed.), *Perspectives on Racism and the Human Services Sector: A Case for Change* (pp. 196–208). Toronto. University of Toronto Press.

Mohanty, C.T. (1991). Under Western eyes: Feminist scholarship and colonial discourses. In C.T. Mohanty et al. (Eds.), *Third World Women and the Politics of Feminism.* Bloomington: Indiana University Press.

Mohanty, C.T. (1997). Under Western eyes: Feminist scholarship and colonial discourses. In B. Ashcroft, G. Griffiths, & H. Tifflin (Eds.), *The Post-Colonial Studies Reader* (pp. 259–272). London: Routledge.

Mojab, S. (1999). De-skilling immigrant women. *Canadian Woman Studies/Les Cahiers De La Femme, 19* (3), 123-127.

Moosa-Mitha, M. (2005). Situating anti-oppressive theories within critical and difference-centred perspectives. In L. Brown and S. Strega (Eds.), *Research as Resistance. Critical, Indigenous and Anti-Oppressive Approaches* (pp. 37–72). Toronto: Canadian Scholars' Press.

Nelson, E. & Robinson, B. (1999). *Gender in Canada.* Scarborough, ON: Prentice Hall.

Ng, R. (1988). *The Politics of Community Services: Immigrant Women, Class and State.* Toronto: Garamond.

Ng, R. (2002). Toward an embodied pedagogy: Exploring health and the body. In G. Dei, B. Hall & D. Rosenberg (Eds.), *Indigenous Knowledges in Global Contexts: Multiple Readings of Our World* (pp. 167–183). Toronto: University of Toronto Press.

Omi, M. & Winant, H. (1993). On the theoretical concept of race. In C. McCarthy & W. Crichlow (Eds.), *Race, Identity and Representation* (pp. 3–10). New York: Routledge.

Oxman-Martinez, J., Abdool, S.N. & Loiselle-Leonard, M. (2000). Immigration, women and health in Canada. *Canadian Journal of Public Health, 91* (5), 394–395.

Raphel, D. (2004). *Social Determinants of Health: Canadian Perspectives.* Toronto: Canadian Scholars' Press.

Razack, S. (1998). *Looking White People in the Eye: Gender, Race and Culture in Courtrooms and Classrooms.* Toronto: University of Toronto Press.

Reimer-Kirkham, S. (2002). The politics of belonging and intercultural health care. *Western Journal of Nursing Research, 25,* 762–780.

Reimer Kirkham, S. & Anderson, J. (2002). Postcolonial nursing scholarship: From epistemology to method. *Advances in Nursing Sciences, 25* (1), 1–17.

Roman, L. (1993). White is a color; white defensiveness, post modernism and anti-racist pedagogy. In C. McCarthy & W. Crichlow, *Race, Identity and Representation in Education* (pp. 71–87). New York: Routledge.

Rummens, J. A (2004a). Intersectionality. *Canadian Diversity, 3* (1), 3–4.

Rummens, J. A (2004b). Overlapping and intersecting identities. *Canadian Diversity*, 3. (1), 5–8.

Said, E. (1997). Orientalism. In B. Ashcroft, G. Griffiths, & H. Tiffin (Eds.), *The Post-Colonial Studies Reader* (pp. 87–91). London: Routledge.

Spivak, G. (1997). Can the subaltern speak? In B. Ashcroft, G. Griffiths & H. Tiffin (Eds.), *The Post-Colonial Studies Reader* (pp. 24–28). London: Routledge.

Stephen, E.H., Foote, K., Hendershot, G.E. et al. (1994). Health of the foreign-born population. *Advance Data from Vital and Health Statistics, 241,* 1–10.

Tator, C. (1995). Anti-racism and the human services delivery system. In C. James *Perspectives on Racism and the Human Services Sector: A Case for Change* (pp. 152–170). Toronto. University of Toronto Press.

Tsang, A.K.T. & George, U. (1998). Towards an integrated framework for cross cultural social work practice. *Canadian Social Work Review, 15* (1), 73–93.

Tuhiwai Smith, L. (2001). *Decolonizing Methodologies: Research and Indigenous Peoples.* Dunedin, NZ: University of Otago Press.

Van Dijk, T.A. (1993). Elite discourse on racism. *Series on Race and Ethnic Relations*, Vol. 6. Newbury Park, CA: Sage.

Vissandjée, B., Weinfeld, M., Dupere, S. & Abdool, S. (2001). Sex, gender, ethnicity, and access to health care services: Research and policy challenges for immigrant women in Canada. *Journal of International Migration and Integration, 21* (1), 55–75.

Yuval-Davis, N. (1999). Ethnicity, gender relations and multiculturalism. In R.D. Torres, J.X. Inda & L.F. Miron, *Race, Identity and Citizenship: A Reader* (pp.112–125). Oxford: Blackwell.

Chapter 3

Are Sensitivity and Tolerance Enough?

Comparing Two Theoretical Approaches to Caring for Newcomer Women with Mental Health Problems

DIANA L. GUSTAFSON

As nurses, social workers, psychologists, physicians and other mental health practitioners concerned about professional competence and quality care, we must regularly update our knowledge and skills to meet the changing composition and needs of the communities we serve. One factor contributing to community transformation is the entry into Canada of diverse groups of newcomer[1] women and their families. This chapter presents two theoretical approaches to working with newcomer women with mental health problems: the cultural competence approach and the critical cultural approach.

The *cultural competence approach* is arguably the better known of the two approaches in the health care sector. Proponents of this approach encourage the practitioner to become culturally competent by acquiring a quantifiable set of attitudes, and communication and practice skills (Campinha-Bacote, 2002). The culturally competent practitioner is said to be better equipped to negotiate the similarities and differences

---

1. "Newcomer" is a general term referring to both immigrants and refugees. The terms "newcomer," "immigrant" and "refugee" are used throughout this chapter to describe populations that share a single characteristic, that is, an international move. The problem with using such terms is that they falsely homogenize these diverse groups into a single category obscuring the significant differences within these populations.

expressed in the client-provider relationship and help the client with her or his daily health and living needs. Critics of this approach argue that the humanistic focus on individual cultural characteristics and behaviours depoliticizes social and human difference. That is to say, the cultural competence approach tends to divert our attention away from the political power inherent in the social practices and relations that produce social and human differences and the health inequalities evident across diverse populations (Fernando, 2003; Gustafson, 2005).

The *critical cultural approach*, as the name suggests, has its roots in critical cultural studies (Fernando, 2003; McGibbon, 2000; Razack, 2002). Proponents of this approach challenge the assumption that cultural identity is an easily identifiable, fixed set of beliefs and practices that exist in a social and historical vacuum. Rather, cultural identities emerge from a dynamic interplay between *micro-level relations* (e.g., day-to-day interpersonal engagement between client and practitioner) and *macro-level relations* reflected in organizational policies and practices (e.g., professional standards of practice, diagnostic procedures and immigration laws). In other words, cultural identity (as theoretical concept and everyday practice) is continually being redefined and experienced, contested and modified in both personal practice and through collective action (Omi & Winant, 1994). Practitioners of this approach are politically and critically engaged with exposing the complex macro-level relations as an essential means to addressing the inequities that play out in the micro-level relations between practitioners and newcomer women.

Both the critical cultural approach and the cultural competence approach challenge our thinking by placing cultural diversity on our professional agenda and making these complex issues more eligible for discussion. Both approaches to diversity are presented in this chapter with examples that illustrate how a mental health practitioner might incorporate each approach into her or his practice. Care has been taken to expose the explicit and hidden assumptions in both approaches and in so doing, fairly represent the strengths and limitations of both approaches.

However, as I and others argue (Doane & Varcoe, 2005; Gustafson, 2005), there are consequences to our theoretical positions that play out in our everyday practice and make us (knowing) participants in the production and dissemination of knowledge. The following discussion intends to raise questions about using the cultural competence approach as a way of thinking, acting and understanding human and social differences. Thus, this chapter makes a case for moving beyond sensitivity and tolerance in our day-to-day engagement with individuals—a hallmark of the cultural competence approach—toward a critical cultural approach to diversity. This theoretical shift requires that we appreciate how dominant discourses of cultural diversity that are grounded in and emerge from institutional practices and processes create and sustain power dynamics that impact on the everyday work of engaging with newcomer women and their families. This shift allows us to recognize the limits of individual action and the need for implementing institutional practices that promote greater equity, fairness and social justice for newcomer women and their families.

This chapter:

- reviews health issues in newcomer populations
- provides an overview of the cultural competence approach and the critical cultural approach
- compares these two theoretical approaches to diversity, including their assumptions, their definitions of culture and how knowledge is acquired in each approach
- examines how each approach can be applied
- concludes with some recommendations for action.

Newcomers and Mental Health

To provide context for this discussion, the chapter begins with a broad overview of issues and terms relating to newcomer populations and health.

Recent statistics indicate that an average of 220,000 immigrants and refugees per year have made Canada their new home (Citizenship and Immigration Canada [CIC], 2005). Contrary to popular belief, community transformation by migration is not new. Newcomers have been a significant feature of Canadian population growth since the 1890s. For much of the 20th century, the majority of Canadian immigrants and refugees were white, and emigrated from Europe or the United States (CIC, 2003). Over the past two decades, newcomers from Europe and the United States account for only 17 per cent and 2 per cent, respectively, of migrants, with 52 per cent coming from South Asian and Pacific Asian countries and 20 per cent from African and Middle Eastern countries (CIC, 2005).

These demographic shifts have been used as evidence of increasing cultural diversity in Canada and the United States and constituted by some health researchers and policy-makers as a problem that needs to be addressed (Gustafson, 2005). However, a careful historical analysis illustrates that newcomer groups—Irish, Indian, Polish, Italian, Vietnamese, Jewish, to name a few—at various historical moments, have been categorized as visible minorities and populations that threaten the imagined homogeneous nation (Omi & Winant, 1994). Over time, these categories have been formed and transformed with some subsumed under or reduced to broader categories of difference. This observation suggests that racial or ethnic identity, religious affiliation and country of origin are not, in and of themselves, reasons why some newcomers are regarded as different from persons born in Canada. Rather it is how these categories of difference are taken up at particular historical moments that characterizes some newcomers as "like us" or "not like us," superior or inferior, and desirable or threatening.

Does this mean that some newcomer women are more likely than others to be regarded as different? The research says yes. In the minds of some Canadians, immigrants are persons of colour "who don't speak English or who speak English with an accent (other than British and American) . . . [and] who have certain jobs (e.g., a cleaning lady or a sewing machine operator)" (Ng, 1996, p. 22). Note also that being culturally different is often equated with being racially different. In this process of *racialization* (where race is the category of human difference used to define and enforce an unequal relationship between the *dominant* and the *subordinated* group[2]), some newcomer populations feel less welcomed as prospective citizens because they do not reflect the collective imagining of the so-called average Canadian. As Palmer (1998) points out in the book *"But Where Are You Really From?,"* the label of immigrant tends to adhere firmly to some newcomer groups even after their families have lived in Canada for generations. By contrast, the label of immigrant tends to fall away from those groups who are white and emigrated from the United Kingdom, Europe or the United States—and are therefore viewed as more desirable (Ng, 1996)—in favour of more positive labels such as "expatriate."

Newcomer experiences vary widely for other reasons also. How well newcomers make the transition to their adopted home depends on the circumstances that precipitated their move and the conditions under which they gained entry to Canada.[3] The functional and cultural adjustments to living in a new country can be complicated by separation from friends and family, fear and concern for those left behind, limited economic resources, past trauma, language barriers and social isolation. These factors can be made worse if newcomers also experience discrimination based on race, ethnicity, religion, gender identity, sexual orientation and country of origin (Guruge et al., 2000; Reitmanova & Gustafson, in press).

The same factors that affect newcomers' vulnerability to and capacity for dealing effectively with the transition to a new home are also linked to health outcomes (Public Health Agency of Canada, 2006). The complex intersection of the social determinants of health (such as income and social status, employment and working conditions, social support networks) can impact negatively on the mental well-being of newcomer families in general and newcomer women in particular. Newcomer women have varying abilities to access mental health services and lobby effectively to receive quality care for themselves and their families. Consider also that some women face difficulties in making themselves and their needs understood when they are seen by some health care providers as being different from Canadian-born clients (Guruge et al., 2000; Johnson et al., 2004; Reitmanova & Gustafson, in press).

Two Theoretical Approaches to Diversity

Even a cursory overview of the health care literature published in the last five years illustrates that more space is being devoted to the intersection of health and culture. Two approaches to cultural diversity stand out: the cultural competence approach to

2. At one time, the white middle class was referred to as the majority while labelling non-white groups as minorities. The white middle class is no longer the numerical majority, yet this group tends to have greater access to political power and social privilege than other social groups. For this reason, critical cultural theorists more commonly refer to these groups as the dominant group and subordinated or marginalized groups.

3. For a more in-depth discussion of how Canada's immigration policies affect health, quality of life and settlement experiences, go to the National Anti-Racism Council of Canada website at www.narcc.ca and click the "Immigration" link.

care and the critical cultural approach to social and human difference. This section provides a brief overview of both.

CULTURAL COMPETENCE APPROACH

The cultural competence approach is a theoretical and practical framework that uses a broadly defined concept of culture as a way to understand individuals and their responses to health and disease, and the client-practitioner relationship. *Culture* is understood to be a set of shared beliefs, values and behaviours held by a group that shares, for example, a common race, language, country of origin or religious affiliation. *Cultural competence* is defined as "the process in which the health care provider continuously strives to achieve the ability to effectively work within the cultural context of a client, individual or community" (Campinha-Bacote, 2002, p. 183).

This approach focuses on the individual, on interpersonal relations and on how the individual understands her or his cultural self and enacts cultural practices in practical, everyday interactions. The onus is on the practitioner to become aware of her or his culture, the client's culture and any similarities or differences between cultures that may negatively impact on the client's health and health practices, and the therapeutic relationship between client and practitioner.

The cultural competence approach has its theoretical roots in mid-20th-century anthropology and is linked with the sub-discipline of transcultural nursing that was conceived by Madeleine Leininger in the 1960s. Depending on the practice setting, this approach is variously referred to as culture care, transcultural care, culturally appropriate care, culturally responsive care, cultural sensitivity, cultural effectiveness, and so on (Cerny, 1997, as cited in Canadian Nurses Association [CNA], 2000). Although there are subtle differences in how these terms are used by nurses, physicians and other practitioners, all tend to share a similar focus on improving the individual care provider's respectful understanding and effective communication with a client who is viewed as culturally different from mainstream Canadian culture.[4]

Over the last decade, this approach gained considerable visibility and acceptance across Canada especially among nurses. For instance, in 1999 the College of Nurses of Ontario (CNO) issued a culture care standard of practice making cultural sensitivity a requirement of quality care. Subsequently, the Registered Nurses Association of Ontario (RNAO) linked this standard to their *Client Centred Care: Nursing Best Practice Guidelines* (RNAO, 2002). Recently, the Canadian Nurses Association (CNA, 2000) recommended that questions about cultural competencies be included in provincial licensure examinations.

Similarly, other professional associations such as the Canadian Psychological

---

4. "Mainstream" is an amorphous term that suggests the ordinary or typical Canadian identity and usually reflects white, middle-class beliefs, values and practices. Terms such as mainstream hide the power a dominant group exercises when defining itself and its culture as the norm (Henry & Tator, 2005).

Association (2000) and the Society for Obstetricians and Gynaecologists of Canada (Smylie, 2001) provide guidance about cultural sensitivity in their code of ethics and policy statement, respectively. Researchers are also using cultural competence as a conceptual framework when studying health among newcomer, settler[5] and Aboriginal populations (see D'Avanzo & Geissler, 2002; Majumdar et al., 1999; Tucker et al., 2003). Such institutional support lends credibility to this approach to diversity.

CRITICAL CULTURAL APPROACH

The critical cultural approach assumes an explicitly political standpoint that encourages practitioners to engage with ideas about human and social difference and the context in which they operate. To be *critical* means to be concerned with exposing and transforming dominant ways of thinking, knowing and doing (Dei, 1996, p. 10). In contrast to the cultural competence approach, cultural knowledge and practice are not regarded as politically neutral but as reflecting the beliefs and values of those who have the power to promote a particular theoretical perspective, produce knowledge, and enforce and evaluate social practices.

This approach will be more familiar to social workers and other health care practitioners whose knowledge draws on cultural studies, post-colonialist and radical feminist literature.[6] According to Fernando (2003), the critical cultural approach may be less familiar to some psychologists, psychiatrists and nurses. Barbee's (2002) search of the Cumulative Index to Nursing and Allied Health Literature, for example, revealed few references in the health literature dealing explicitly with racism or more specifically with racism in psychiatric nursing. The muted discussion of racism, sexism and other *systemic oppressions*[7] may be attributed to the pervasiveness of the cultural competence approach. As I argue elsewhere, a broadly defined but narrowly applied definition of culture is visible in such texts where culture "stand[s] in for and operate[s] as a code word for race and ethnic differences" (Gustafson, 2005, p. 8).

Unlike the cultural competence approach, cultural identity is not simply a way that an individual makes sense of her or his membership in a social group. Nor is culture an easily identifiable, fixed set of beliefs and practices that exists in a social and historical vacuum (Fernando, 2003; McGibbon, 2000; Razack, 2002). Rather, cultural identity is

---

5. "Settler" is a term that reminds us that the land originally inhabited by indigenous peoples was colonized (invaded) by white immigrants. Using this post-colonialist language challenges the romantic notion that Canada is a nation of immigrants and points to the contradictory attitudes we hold about newcomers and immigration.

6. Frantz Fanon, Edward Said, Homi Bhabha, bell hooks and others wrote foundational works in these fields that challenged the legacy of colonialism while reclaiming or talking back to the cultural identities that had been constructed and used by colonizers to subordinate and marginalize indigenous peoples.

7. A systemic oppression is a set of deeply-held beliefs and values that are assumed to be universal, that are embedded in institutional policies and practices, and that tend to marginalize, silence or exclude another group with often radically different beliefs and values. The social inequities associated with racism, sexism and homophobia, for example, are visible and deeply felt by those who are subordinated by these systemic oppressions but tend to be less visible to members of the dominant group.

understood as a complex, flexible system of world views that is continuously being negotiated from both within and beyond the group.

Cultural identities result from a dynamic interplay between *micro-level relations* (e.g., day-to-day interpersonal engagement between client and practitioner) and *macro-level relations* (e.g., professional standards of practice, diagnostic procedures and immigration laws). This interplay modifies both the idea of cultural identity and how that identity is experienced and expressed. Consider the following two examples:

> *Example:* Some groups, for instance, English-speaking, white, male psychiatrists, have greater power to assert their own identity and represent themselves and their world view as the norm. In contrast, other groups, such as Arabic-speaking newcomer women from Sudan, may have less power to assert themselves in a social situation and represent their world view as valid. Although the power imbalance between practitioners and these newcomer women plays out in micro-level relations, the power available to each individual comes from their *social location*—a composite of social identities (race, gender, country of origin, language)—and social roles and relationships. Taken one interaction at a time, the power inequity between practitioner and client may be managed in an act of sensitivity and tolerance or mismanaged and disregarded in an act of racial or sexual marginalization or discrimination. When multiple micro-aggressions are considered collectively in the context of macro-relations, the limitations of individual action become apparent. Practitioners recognize the need to attend to the macro-level mechanisms that structure their day-to-day interactions.

> *Example:* Exploring power dynamics is considered foundational to understanding the interplay between micro-level and macro-level relations and the expression and interpretation of human and social difference. Power dynamics that are part of systemic oppressions such as sexism and racism function within and beyond any given group to generate and enforce *cultural meanings*—those widely held beliefs about a group or a social practice. Consider how the bombing of the Twin Towers in New York on September 11, 2001, impacted on cultural identities. This event brought about many changes in airport procedures, policing and security activities intended to identify terrorist threats and promote national safety. Over time, the acts of some Muslim extremist organizations began leaking into media representations of Muslims and South Asians more broadly, whose appearance, dress and practices became the object of closer examination. There were reports of racial profiling at airports, as officials searched for potential

terrorists. Many South Asians (both newcomers and long-time residents) experienced harassment and increased scrutiny at work and in their neighbourhoods. To appear less visibly different, some South Asian women stopped wearing bindis (the small, usually red, forehead mark worn by some Hindu women) and put away their saris in favour of Western-style clothing. Some newcomers felt pressure to express their patriotism more overtly to distinguish themselves from extremists (Kalita, 2005).

The preceding examples illustrate three related points:
- Cultural identity (as theoretical concept and everyday practice) is continually being redefined from within and from outside the group.
- Ways of thinking, talking and behaving in interpersonal engagements are influenced and justified by broader social discourses and institutional laws, rules and procedures. Changes in individual practices and expressed beliefs do not occur in a social vacuum. They are understandable responses to broader social discourses and the exercise of power at the macro-level.
- Culture is experienced and expressed through individual and collective action. A dominant group has greater power to represent and enforce its world view and identity as the norm while simultaneously representing other groups as different, inferior, suspicious, even dangerous. Such collective cultural beliefs are transmitted in individual acts that reinforce power imbalances among groups. Thus, culture is a matter of individuality and of collectivity.

Making these connections is important for provoking questions about who benefits from the construction and transmission of cultural knowledge about dominant and non-dominant groups.

Comparing Approaches

The theoretical starting point of each approach focuses attention differently on the issue of human and social difference. Each approach starts from an underlying set of assumptions about culture and human interaction. The strategies for achieving the identified goals of each approach emerge from those assumptions. This section poses three important questions that guide the comparison of these approaches to culture:
- What assumptions orient each approach to cultural diversity?
- How does each approach define culture as a category of difference?
- How does a mental health practitioner become more knowledgeable and skilled in each approach?

COMPARING UNDERLYING ASSUMPTIONS

The cultural competence approach to care is oriented toward the individual and improving cultural interactions between practitioner and client. The culturally competent practitioner is said to be better equipped to negotiate the similarities and differences expressed in the client-practitioner relationship and help the client with her or his daily health and living needs. This liberal orientation holds considerable appeal to caring professionals who value and promote individual rights and responsibility for health and well-being, self-awareness, tolerance, freedom of choice and the ethic of care (Browne, 2001; CNO, 1999).

Every person, whether a care provider or a care recipient, is said to have a unique culture (RNAO, 2002). Every situation is also regarded as unique and therefore, it is argued, there is no single right way to approach all individuals with the same cultural background. The culturally competent practitioner is aware of his or her own culture, the client's culture and the impact of both on the client-practitioner relationship (Campinha-Bacote, 2002). There is no overt attention to the macro-relational dynamics of unequal power distribution or to systemic oppressions.

Unlike the cultural competence approach, which attends to the individual and to individual identity formation, the critical cultural approach examines the social processes and practices through which group identities are reproduced over time and in different places, both from within the group and in response to representations created by those outside that group. Practitioners focus on understanding how power structures both social relations and the expression of social and human differences. Particular attention is directed at systemic oppressions such as sexism and racism and at the macro-level knowledge and practices that support these mechanisms. There is overt attention to the inequitable distribution of power and decision-making capacity, and to the unequal access to material and human resources. This is of particular interest to mental health practitioners who question psychopathological explanations for mental illness and attend to the social determinants of mental illness (Bryant-Davis & Ocampo, 2005; Fernando, 2003; Porter & Barbee, 2004).

The cultural competence approach regards cultural diversity as a problem that can be better managed in the context of the client-practitioner relationship. By comparison, the critical cultural approach focuses on how systemic oppressions and institutional policies and processes such as immigration laws, professional standards of practice and hospital admission procedures reinforce dominant ways of understanding social and other human differences and impact on newcomer women's mental health and the client-practitioner relationship.

COMPARING DEFINITIONS OF CULTURE

Both approaches are oriented toward culture but define culture differently. The cultural competence approach to care defines culture as a discrete set of learned attitudes, beliefs, biases, values and practices held by an individual or group and passed along from one generation to the next. Reminiscent of the writings of noted American anthropologist Margaret Mead, culture is said to be made up of and influenced by gender, sexual orientation, race, ethnicity, religion, language, socio-economic status and life experience (CNA, 2000). This power-neutral composite of attributes is believed to produce unique individual cultural identities and affect "the way people view and respond to their world and other people in it" (CNO, 1999, p. 4). According to this approach, the unequal valuing of and respect for different cultural identities leads to negative health outcomes and problems in delivering safe and effective health care.

According to critical cultural theorists, culture is a "flexible system of values and world views that people live by and recreate continuously" (Fernando, 2003, p. 11). The approach assumes that culture is a composite of race, religion, gender and sexual differences (to name a few) that are deeply interconnected social and political categories. Positive, negative and neutral meanings are attached to these categories. These meanings change over time and from place to place and have significant consequences for cultural groups. For some newcomer women, this means different and inequitable levels of access to employment, suitable housing, social networks and health care services (Ng, 1996; Reitmanova & Gustafson, in press).

Although the definitions of culture appear on the surface to be similar, the subtle but important differences have significant implications for knowledge production and practice.

The first definition assumes that culture is a discrete, fixed entity that is a matter of individuality. A practitioner who learns the objective cultural facts is supposed to be more knowledgeable about an individual member of that group. A knowledgeable practitioner is more likely to respect and value individual difference. For that reason, the medical and health literature offers practitioners recipe-like descriptions of various newcomer groups classified by country of origin, race and ethnicity (see D'Avanzo & Geissler, 2002; Leininger & McFarland, 2002). However, the continuing reiteration of cultural differences as if they were static, immutable facts has material consequences for practitioners and clients as individuals and groups (Bryant-Davis & Ocampo, 2005). The unreflective and continuing use of such tools penetrates everyday interaction, reproducing and sustaining the powerful political and social meanings attributed to cultural differences.

As mentioned earlier, a discussion of race and racism rarely appears in the cultural competence literature despite the central role these mechanisms play in structuring categories of difference. This is not to suggest that race and culture are synonymous. Race along with gender and other categories of difference are social not biological facts. Yet with few exceptions, the construction of social categories, the different social meanings attached to each category and the powerful ways these meanings work in concert to buttress values and beliefs about this group or that are seldom examined. Instead the focus is on more comfortable, celebratory aspects of human and social difference such as food preferences and folksy practices. Moreover, attention to the liberal values of tolerance and sensitivity simultaneously diverts attention away from the covert racist (and sexist) institutional practices that some newcomers must deal with every day (Bryant-Davis & Ocampo, 2005; James, 2000).

The critical cultural definition of culture highlights the fluidity of cultural identity across time and space. Belief systems and interpersonal relations are informed by and reproduce institutional knowledge and practices. Practitioners of the critical cultural approach challenge the fixed and bounded categories that purport to distinguish one group from another. Instead, categories of difference are regarded as "coercive and resilient" social and political facts (Dei, 1996, p. 59). The fluidity of cultural identity also enables the practitioner to attend to the differences within groups of newcomer women. We cannot assume that all women are the same because of their gender experience or their affiliation with a particular cultural group. Imposed categories of difference may not reflect variations in how individual women or groups of newcomer women think about themselves or would choose to represent themselves to the world. Thus, when discussing the mental health of newcomer women, the category of woman cannot be treated in isolation from other categories of human and social difference (Guruge & Khanlou, 2004). Social, economic and political factors are associated with health differences between:

- newcomer and settler women
- immigrant and refugee women
- recent newcomer women and those who immigrated more than a decade ago.

COMPARING HOW KNOWLEDGE IS ACQUIRED

The assumptions underlying our theoretical orientation and how we define culture have implications for how we acquire knowledge about cultural groups, and for what end.

The cultural competence approach emphasizes individual identity and interpersonal relations at the micro-level. Acquiring cultural knowledge is expected to provide the practitioner with a set of rules or guidelines for relating to an individual who is regarded as culturally different. This is the goal of becoming culturally competent. *Cultural competence* is a "process of becoming" rather than a state of being (Campinha-Bacote, 2002). The practitioner who continuously works on building a quantifiable set of knowledge, attitudes and skills is expected to be more effective in working across cultures (CNO, 1999). Information produced through research and appearing in professional journals and textbooks tends to be regarded as authoritative and legitimate because it is seen as rational, objective and emerging from a politically neutral space.

By contrast, the critical cultural approach assumes that knowledge is situated in a particular historical, institutional and social moment. All knowledge, most especially institutionalized or taken-for-granted knowledge, is eligible for critical examination. From there, we can begin to examine more critically how we name a mental health problem, the practice standards we use to structure our engagement with a client, the power we exercise and the resources we leverage in those moments.

The discussion that follows examines the limitations of two strategies for becoming culturally competent: acquiring cultural self-awareness and acquiring knowledge of cultural groups. The comparison reveals the limitations of the cultural competence approach to cultural diversity and offers alternative strategies.

Limitations of Acquiring Cultural Self-Awareness

According to the cultural competence approach, *cultural self-awareness* is a "process of cultural humility" in which a practitioner engages in continuous self-reflection about personal beliefs, values and practices (Campinha-Bacote, 2002, p. 183). We are considered ethnocentric if we are unaware of our cultural beliefs or how central our beliefs are to our worldview or if we believe that our beliefs are superior. A mental health practitioner who is *ethnocentric* tends to impose her or his cultural beliefs on the client with a different culture. As we become more aware of our *ethnocentrism*—that is, the valuing of our own cultural beliefs as superior—we move along the cultural competency continuum toward *ethnorelativism*, which is characterized by recognition, acceptance and respect for cultural differences.

The cultural competence approach suggests that by imagining ourselves in the shoes of someone who is different, we can become more aware of how our biases influence our interactions. For example, if we are caring for a Hindu woman living in an arranged marriage, we might ask ourselves: How do I feel about arranged marriages? How might these beliefs influence my communications with this client? What are my assumptions about her family relationships and intimacy? Then we might reflect on the meaning we attribute to the marriage ritual. How do my beliefs about marriage influence my attitudes toward the meaning of family relationships, communication, space, privacy and so on.

Although cultural self-awareness can produce some valuable outcomes (Browne et al., 2002), I raise three points of caution:

- The cultural competence approach tends to encourage an inward-facing exploration of our attitudes toward practices, in this case, arranged marriages, which we regard as different from our own. Doing so may be easier than investing energy in the outward-facing reflection that questions the social context for individually held beliefs.

  Critical self-awareness as promoted by the critical cultural approach encourages practitioners to engage in both critical inward and outward facing reflection. Outward-facing reflection involves questioning the assumptions underlying value systems that rank some practices as legitimate or superior to others. Challenging and discomforting, outward-facing reflection may expose, for example, the contradiction that the dominant Canadian discourse, on the one hand, advances love as the superior reason to marry while on the other hand, advances and supports a host of other reasons to marry. Consider that some non-Hindu Canadian-born women and their families "arrange" marriages as a response to unintended pregnancy or the prospect of a life alone, or to move up the social ladder or secure financial stability.

- Making explicit our personal beliefs about the marriage ritual, for instance, may not change our attitudes about the rightness or superiority of those beliefs and practices. We may continue to believe that those who practice arranged marriages are less "this" or more "that" than those who marry for love. Thus, being more aware of one's own cultural value system may have little impact on how we regard the value system of those newcomers we regard as different.
- A cultural competence approach to self-awareness starts from the assumption that every individual has a unique culture. This assumption is explicitly stated in some health professional literature (see CNO, 1999). Such an understanding ascribes difference to everyone and to everyone equally, creating an essential commonality of identity across human experience. If every person is differently different, it follows that the goal is to learn to recognize and respect those differences. Some educators have created cultural self-awareness labs where students reflect on how they would behave if they were members of a minority group in a clinical or everyday situation (see Pruitt et al., 1999).

  This exercise assumed that it is possible and even desirable to step in and out of a marginalized position. Critics of this exercise recognize that those of us who are Canadian-born with white skin, for example, cannot deny the privilege and power that our social location accords us regardless of whether we asked for that power and privilege or not. Nor can we shed that privilege for the purposes of a learning exercise or as matter of political choice.

The critical cultural approach understands cultural diversity this way: all of us operate in a society structured by gender, race, class and other social differences; those differences locate each of us differently in relation to those social hierarchies. For example, a Black Canadian-born social worker may have more power than her elderly Chinese-born client seeking treatment for depression but less power than the white woman who leads the care team. Thus, our social location (the politically laden composite of social identities and social roles) accords some of us more power and privilege in some situations than in others.

As mental health practitioners, it is important to understand how we are located in relation to our clients and to each other. Those of us who are Canadian-born with white skin are positioned in a world that gives us greater access to power and privilege than those of us who are not white, whether Canadian-born or not. Therefore, if we examine how our social location is linked to the cultural meanings that are embedded in everyday talk and organizational policies and practices and in turn the working of systemic oppressions (racism, sexism and so on), we can reflect on the power and privilege that some of us have over others and on how these play out in micro-level relations between client and practitioner. This critical awareness can be used to bring about change at both the interpersonal and the institutional levels (Gustafson, 2007).

To summarize, it is not cultural self-awareness per se that is the problem with the cultural competence approach to becoming more knowledgeable. Rather the problem is the emphasis on inward-facing self-reflection that ignores the social, historical and political context from which cultural beliefs and practices emerge. Critical cultural self-awareness goes beyond individualized psychological self-reflection to include an exploration of power relations, how we are socially located in the world, and how we occupy and wield power accorded by those social locations.

Limitations of Acquiring Cultural Knowledge

Acquiring cultural knowledge is another strategy for becoming culturally competent (Campinha-Bacote, 2002). This strategy assumes that it is both possible and necessary to have a knowledge base about how various cultural groups view the world. Although a practitioner is not expected to have an in-depth knowledge of all cultures, she or he is expected to acquire *cultural knowledge* about the beliefs, values and practices held by a particular group that affects how clients perceive their health, illness, suffering, hospitals, health care providers and so on. Two strategies for acquiring cultural knowledge are encouraged: drawing on text-based knowledge and engaging in cultural encounters.

TEXT-BASED KNOWLEDGE

A considerable body of reference books and journal articles on cultural competence has developed over the last four decades. These resources are intended to provide information about health and illness patterns of various cultural groups. Many published in the 1980s and 1990s are reminiscent of cookbooks with recipes for culture care (Gustafson, 2005). An indicator of the sturdiness of this perspective, some of these texts are now in their third and fourth editions for today's practitioners (see D'Avanzo & Geissler, 2002; Leininger & McFarland, 2002). These texts classify cultural groups into fixed categories based on a shared language or heritage of a language, shared historical experiences, pseudo-biological characteristics and so-called "culturally based health-illness patterns" (Leininger & McFarland, 2002, p. 325). More recent editions of these books have eliminated stark charts in favour of more detailed prose about biological variations, and differences relating to time, space and social organization in specific racialized groups (see Leininger & McFarland, 2002; Stanhope & Lancaster, 2002).

Critics note a couple of ways that this approach to cultural diversity reinforces rather than challenges cultural stereotypes and unequal power relations across groups (Fernando, 2003; Gustafson, 2005). Cultural knowledge is generated through research often done by dominant groups about those who are considered different from the imagined norm (Henry & Tator, 2005; Stanfield & Dennis, 1993). To be credible and legitimate, truth claims are advanced as objective, politically neutral and generalizable across time and space. Known as *positivism*, this way of generating knowledge is highly valued in the health sciences (Browne, 2001). Research data are used in the writing of diagnostic manuals, textbooks, educational curricula, institutional policy and procedures, and the professional standards of practice that practitioners turn to for guidance on how to be culturally competent. Knowledge reproduced in textbooks and journal articles has a higher degree of legitimacy and authority. What we learn from published materials based on this research reinforces a particular understanding about this group or that (Porter & Barbee, 2004).

Some positivist, medical and health care research, however, furthers cultural stereotypes and racist and sexist thinking by labelling people according to physical, genetic and other pseudo-biological characteristics despite the lack of evidence to support these categorizations (Barbee, 2002; Fernando, 2003; Omi & Winant, 1994; Porter & Barbee, 2004). Broad categorizations convey the message that culture is easily reduced to a set of definitions, is stable over time and is applicable to all individuals. Information that homogenizes, for example, the beliefs of all white Europeans, all Africans or all Pacific Asians into rigid categories perpetuates stereotypes that negatively impact on what we learn and how we engage with newcomer populations. Typically, authors of such materials caution the reader against stereotyping, faulty overgeneralizations or using these texts in a formulaic or prescribed way. However, the implicit message conveyed by these classifications is as important as the explicit one. The following examples illustrate how labels and stereotypes gain their power.

> *Example:* Some texts describe "cultural-bound illnesses," giving the example of Mexican-Americans with alcoholism and other drug abuse problems, and Chinese-Americans with tuberculosis (Campinha-Bacote, 2002, p. 185). Research is cited to support the credibility of these assertions. The implicit message is that the cause and treatment of such illnesses is located in the biology of individuals and groups. Social determinants such poverty, crowded living conditions and social alienation that give rise to these health outcomes are not mentioned.

> *Example:* Current mental health research is investigating a biological basis for aggression among Blacks or a cultural explanation for the disproportionate incidence of schizophrenia among Blacks. This literature is reminiscent of past research that linked personality disorders with inferior brains and mental capacity (Barbee, 2002; Fernando, 2003). While current research is more subtle than the overtly racist research of the past, linking psychopathologies with race, ethnicity or other cultural differences grants continuing credence to these categories as biological facts rather than socially constructed and socially significant categories. Barbee calls this "nothing more than a sophisticated form of 'victim blaming'" (2002, p. 195). Thus research and textbooks must be critically examined to evaluate whose interests are served by the advancement of some pieces of cultural knowledge.

CULTURAL ENCOUNTERS

The cultural competence approach also advocates acquiring cultural knowledge by engaging in *cultural encounters*. Cultural encounters permit the learner to communicate with someone from another culture in a field or practice setting to "practice cultural assessment techniques and gather information about individual and group attitudes toward health care" (Marcinkiw, 2003, p. 8). Consider critically the implications of this learning activity:

> Let's assume that a mental health practitioner wants to learn more about how Islamic religious beliefs influence a woman's beliefs and practices about modesty and the body. The learner may set up an encounter in the practice setting with a Muslim newcomer to learn more about why she wears a hijab or headscarf. In this case, the encounter focuses on a single marker of difference, in this case, a piece of clothing. A *marker* is a symbol, social practice or physical trait such as skin colour that conveys or signifies positive or negative meanings associated with difference.

Such an encounter may enable the learner to understand the meaning that a religious practice holds for one individual and certainly, an individual woman's perspective needs to be heard and valued. However, acquiring cultural knowledge by talking with individual members of newcomer groups will not necessarily help the learner understand how inequitable access to sustained employment and a reliable income disadvantages some Muslim newcomers and shapes their mental health experiences (Reitmanova & Gustafson, in press). I raise the following concerns:

- This attention to individual performance of social practices may not help the learner view the larger dynamics that accord meaning to markers of social and human difference. In this example, asking a Muslim why she wears a hijab pays little attention to the negative meanings attached to this practice by some non-Muslims or to the impact of that negative meaning on the everyday safety and mental well-being of Muslim women. Thus, a cultural encounter may not reveal the multiple ways that social meanings are attached to any given practice.

- In a related point, the cultural encounter assumes that cultural meaning-making is an individual activity without social, historical or political context. Engaging in a cultural encounter is unlikely to reveal the mechanisms by which some world views and health practices are deemed appropriate, scientifically based and legitimate, while others are labelled as folksy, sexist, inappropriate or even barbaric. Moreover, a newcomer may be unable to distinguish the broader cultural meanings from her individual preferences and beliefs *and* may not be prepared to explain at length these differences to someone who regards her as culturally different.

- Culture encounters may also contribute to a process referred to by critical cultural theorists as othering. *Othering* reinforces positions of dominance and subordination by identifying and marginalizing those who are thought to be different from the norm, in this case, a newcomer woman wearing a hijab (Johnson, Bottorff et al., 2004). A learning objective that requires the cultural other to perform her difference under the gaze of a member of the dominant group is a powerful one. Practices such as cultural encounters increase scrutiny of newcomer groups making them responsible for educating those of us in a position to make such demands. By contrast, consider that those of us who are Canadian-born Christian women, for instance, are seldom tokenized in this way and asked to explain our religious beliefs and practices on behalf of all Canadian-born Christian women.

- Taking this one step further, engaging in a cultural encounter also assumes that a newcomer could or would feel safe identifying those distinguishing cultural elements to a practitioner in a practice setting characterized by multiple social inequities. A newcomer woman may believe she has little to gain from a cultural encounter that is intended to benefit the practitioner's learning objectives. Thus, cultural encounters may be counterproductive. The potential benefit to the learner may be outweighed by the potential harm to the newcomer that results from the inappropriate exercise of power, being the object of the dominant gaze, and the persistent reminder that one is different.

- Engaging in cultural encounters also does little to reveal the everyday institutional processes of assessing, planning and implementing a mental health care intervention that influence the relationship between client and practitioner. Such processes are based on a best practices model or evidence-based research that can be deeply flawed by omission and commission. As Campinha-Bacote (2002) points out, these practice and research models tend to draw on dominant cultural beliefs without reflecting on cultural considerations and their meanings.

To summarize, the cultural competence approach is a micro-level framework that advocates cultural self-awareness, enhanced knowledge about diverse cultures and greater respect, sensitivity and tolerance for diverse cultures. This approach is limited because it fails to locate interpersonal relations in the broader social context that gives meaning to those relations. In particular, developing cultural self-awareness may not enable the practitioner to understand how social meanings are rooted in power relations and covert racist and sexist practices that shape the day-to-day engagement with newcomer women. Acquiring cultural knowledge and engaging in cultural encounters may not help practitioners see beyond the individual to the systemic or social causes of mental health problems among newcomer women.

Situated Knowledge

The critical cultural approach advances an alternative way of understanding and acquiring knowledge. *Situated knowledge* is a concept that is grounded in sociology, anthropology or anti-racism frameworks. Rather than thinking about knowledge as objective and politically neutral, knowledge is understood as socially constructed. In other words, things are knowable only from the socio-cultural contexts in which they are identified and operate. Reality exists but the meaning of that reality is constantly being mediated, negotiated, responded to and resisted through social processes and interactions. Taking that one step further, culture (and race and gender) exist, not as biological facts, but as social and political realities that are powerful determinants of life experience and mental health (Bryant-Davis & Ocampo, 2005).

There is also a concern for how knowledge is produced, by whom and for what outcome. What would it look like if mental health practitioners created space for more substantial and critical conversations about the power of white, Canadian-born subjects to advance a particular view of the world? Currently, knowledge about immigrants and refugees in general, and newcomer women in particular, tends to be produced from the dominant perspective in academic and non-academic forums. Because there is a disproportionate representation of dominant (white, middle-class, straight, Christian) women and men working as mental health care providers, managers, researchers and educators, existing mental health knowledge tends to advance the beliefs and values of this group (Turrittin et al., 2002). Critical cultural theorists argue that knowledge that is truly inclusive of marginalized groups must be developed by, about and in the self-defined political interests of marginalized groups (Guruge & Khanlou, 2004; Porter & Barbee, 2004).

The critical cultural approach challenges mental health practitioners to explore the cultural specificity and political situatedness of institutionalized knowledge. This means questioning the taken-for-grantedness of mental health knowledge, diagnostic categories and standards of professional practice. Instead of encouraging mental health practitioners to acquire knowledge of the other, it may be more useful to explore who, why, how and for what purpose, race, sex and other markers of human difference are used. As James (2000) notes, difference takes on significant meaning in the lives of those who are constructed as culturally other. Our responsibility as practitioners is to reflect critically on how we (individually and as participants in a hierarchically ranked society) mark cultural groups as different and attribute meanings to those differences. Taking up this challenge requires greater emotional and intellectual honesty than slotting an individual woman or a group of women into a rigid cultural category.

The critical cultural approach supports the goal of making culture more than a marginal sub-theme in the development of mental health care knowledge. This recommendation is different from integrating more cultural data into health educational programs, in-services and everyday care plans or what is sometimes referred to as the "add and stir" method. Research by Browne et al. (2002) illustrates an alternative approach that critically reflected on the operation of racism and sexism in the everyday engagement between South Asian women and their health care providers. Explicit discussions of power relations, systemic oppressions and the history of exploitation, violence and colonialism facilitate practitioners' learning about human and social difference at the macro-level. These insights move us to the next section on translating cultural knowledge into practice.

From Knowledge to Practice

These preceding observations about the strengths and limitations of two approaches to cultural diversity raise important issues about how knowledge translates into everyday practice with newcomer women.

APPLYING THE CULTURAL COMPETENCE APPROACH

In practice, providing culturally competent care might look something like this: A psychiatric nurse meets a client in the clinic and begins a systematic assessment. In that and subsequent meetings, the nurse uses her knowledge and skills to collect culturally relevant information about the client's health history and presenting symptoms. She listens with interest and remains non-judgmental as the client describes her condition. Together the nurse and the client establish mutually acceptable goals for care and treatment. If the nurse recognizes a conflict between her cultural beliefs and those of the client, she works to integrate the client's beliefs and practices into the plan of care. If she determines that the client's beliefs and practices put the client (or anyone else) at risk of harm, the nurse helps the client to adopt new patterns of behaviour. If the nurse finds that her personal biases prevent her from providing culturally sensitive care to the client, she addresses these deficits through the continuous process of becoming culturally competent.

Some studies that describe formal cultural sensitivity training for care providers report positive learning outcomes in the short term (Majumdar et al., 1999; St. Clair & McKenry, 1999). However, a review of health literature found little evidence to indicate that acquiring and applying cultural knowledge to the practice setting translates into real and meaningful changes in the health of marginalized groups. Brach and Frasier claim that while there is "substantial research evidence to suggest that cultural competency should in fact work, health systems have little evidence about which cultural competency techniques are effective [in reducing health disparities] and less evidence on when and how to implement them properly" (2000, p. 181). They go on to say that the literature on cultural competency has "by and large, not linked cultural competency activities with the outcomes that could be expected to follow from them" (p. 181). Thus, despite the long-standing (four decades) visibility and popularity of the cultural competence approach to care, there is little evaluation or evidence of the long-term effectiveness of this approach for improving client-practitioner relationships, reducing health disparities or improving mental health outcomes.

APPLYING THE CRITICAL CULTURAL APPROACH

Mental health practitioners operating from a critical cultural approach consider how everyday work is situated within dominant health care structures and practices. The practice knowledge we bring to work and how we make sense of our daily interactions is fluid and ever changing, in part, because the broader context of our lives is fluid and ever changing. The mental health practitioner considers how her or his knowledge, beliefs and ideas are situated in a social context that is dynamically connected to the macro-relations at the institutional and societal levels (Bryant-Davis & Ocampo, 2005; Guruge & Khanlou, 2004; McGibbon, 2000). Similarly, the health and illness experiences of newcomer women making the functional and cultural adjustments to a new home are located in a particular time and place (Guruge & Khanlou, 2004). How women make meaning of and negotiate these experiences is constantly being responded to, and resisted through their interactions in and beyond mental health settings.

If we accept these assertions, the next step is to begin examining how we, as mental health practitioners, are implicated in the institutionalization of oppressive practices. For instance, the fourth edition of the *Diagnostic and Statistical Manual of Mental Disorders* (DSM-IV) is a widely used set of criteria for diagnosing mental disorders. Over the years, however, this tool has been challenged for pathologizing gender and sexual roles and behaviours, reproducing cultural stereotypes and reinforcing sexist, homophobic and racist thinking (Bryant-Davis & Ocampo, 2005; Fernando, 2003; Kupers, 1995). The continuing and unreflective use of this tool has implications for those who are diagnosed as mentally ill.

Thus, applying a critical cultural perspective to education programs, in-services, and intake and evaluation procedures (to name a few specifics) means challenging underlying assumptions and ways of thinking about, interpreting and performing human and social differences.[8] Let's consider these questions[9] for redirecting our attention toward situated practice:

- How does my power and privilege as a white woman situate me in relation to a newcomer from Ghana?
- How does a refugee woman attribute meaning to her experiences of being marginalized at home, at work and in the community?
- How does my position as a third-generation Chinese-Canadian result in my being seen as an "expert" on all things deemed cultural? Why am I asked to act as an interpreter when I speak only English?
- How does my status as a white, male psychiatrist in a mental health clinic give me greater power and privilege in relation to clients and other staff? How does that affect my clients' interactions with me?
- How does my position as a hockey-dad with a savings account for my children's education influence my understanding of a refugee woman who had been raped in front of her children in Rwanda?

8. Differences are performed in everyday interactions such as when a physician puts on a white lab coat that signifies her professional status, when a nun wears a habit to signify her religious affiliation or when a woman checks off "female" on an immigration form. Differences are also performed as collective action, such as the Toronto Caribbean Carnival (Caribana), a gay pride parade or the Olympics. At the individual and collective levels, performance highlights human and social differences that distinguish individuals and groups from each other while simultaneously reinforcing the boundaries.

9. I gratefully acknowledge the contributions Sylvia Reitmanova made to this section.

- How do media descriptions of terrorism and Islamic extremists influence the health and social experiences of Muslim women working or shopping in public spaces? How do such stories influence my ability as a health care practitioner to interact with a Muslim woman?
- How do news reports of crime and assault affect the mental health of immigrant women living in high-density, high-rise housing in urban spaces?
- How does my experience as a Canadian-born woman shape my ability to understand the beliefs and experiences of a refugee woman who fears deportation?
- How does my privilege of having a steady job situate me in relation to an educated woman who is not entitled to work in Canada?
- How does the DSM-IV organize how I assess an immigrant woman's mental health? How do dominant (white, male) understandings of women and mental health influence the DSM-IV classifications?
- How does my experience growing up in a safe, rural community impact on my ability to understand what constitutes normal in a war-torn country?
- How does my position of being a middle-aged mother embracing her family over a Thanksgiving dinner impact my view of a newcomer woman who has not seen her family for years?

The willingness to assume an explicitly political stance and the foundational focus on power relations and systemic oppressions distinguish the critical cultural approach from the cultural competence approach. One of the distinct challenges is communicating this approach in a way that enables practitioners to put it into practice. This involves translating complex radical feminist and post-colonialist ideas into language and practices that make sense. Moreover, taking up an overtly political stance is not only dangerous (more so for marginalized groups than for dominant groups) but it is also regarded as contrary to the supposed neutrality of professional practice.

Summary

Moving family, house and home is challenging for most of us. An international move can be especially difficult. The critical cultural approach and literature on cultural competence offer two distinct models for addressing human and social differences. Both approaches affect and reflect the changing social times and the social locations of theorists and practitioners who produce and use them. Both approaches offer mental health practitioners ways to interpret and address cultural diversity in the workplace.

The cultural competence approach is a theoretical and practical framework that helps the individual practitioner to identify the problems and possible solutions for managing the care of people who are regarded as different. The strength of culturally sensitive care is its emphasis on the individual and the space this approach creates for agency and personal change. This approach also enables practitioners to start from where they are in bringing about changes in the everyday health experiences of clients. This strength is also its main weakness.

This approach to diversity is weakened by the persistent and depoliticizing emphasis on the individual and the liberal values of tolerance and sensitivity that obscure the institutionalization of oppressive practices. This approach keeps the practitioner narrowly focused on a static and decontextualized concept of culture. Action rests with individual practitioners who are accountable for their practice, for being tolerant of difference and for providing culturally sensitive care to newcomer women. The cultural competence approach to care does not question the political significance of difference, the way that dominant ideas deeply penetrate our professional knowledge and practice standards, and how this larger social context positions us and impacts how we individually and collectively engage in everyday practice (Gustafson, 2005; 2007).

The critical cultural approach re-imagines the cultural self in a broader social, political and historical context rather than in an identity grounded solely in individual subjectivity. The foundational focus on power relations and the operation of systemic oppressions shifts how we understand the connections between institutionalized cultural knowledge and everyday caregiving activities. Making this connection is important for provoking questions about who benefits from the construction and transmission of cultural knowledge.

Everyday caregiving activities are embedded in and transmitted through professional knowledge, educational materials and institutional policies. These sources of knowledge about cultural differences maintain the beliefs, values and political interests of those who produce and use this knowledge. In our role as users and reproducers of knowledge, mental health practitioners participate in political acts that are linked to broader power relationships. The critical cultural approach is a formal theoretical and practical process for taking action that questions the use of power: power to define human and social difference; power to produce cultural knowledge; and power to implement and evaluate professional standards and practices.

Conclusion

This comparison of these two theoretical approaches recognizes the limits of individual action and the necessity of advocating for institutional change in support of newcomer women and their families as well as health care providers who are members of marginalized groups. Mental health practitioners are invited to take action that acknowledges the importance of caring interpersonal relations that respect individual cultural differences while simultaneously paying overt attention to how power works in institutionalized knowledge and practices.

Action may include:

- speaking openly about sexism, racism and other systemic oppressions that impact on the mental health of newcomer women
- challenging dominant knowledge claims about those who are regarded as different
- detecting absences and erasures in dominant mental health knowledge
- challenging the applicability of tools and practices for assessing, planning and

implementing mental health interventions for newcomer women
- lobbying for fairer representation of newcomers in the professional caregiver groups
- pressing for more equitable distribution of power and community resources that support the mental health of newcomer groups adjusting to life in Canada.

References

Barbee, E. (2002). Racism and mental health. *Journal of the American Psychiatric Nurses Association, 8* (6), 194–199.

Brach, C. & Frasier, I. (2000). Can cultural competency reduce racial and ethnic health disparities? A review and conceptual model. *Medical Care Research and Review, 57* (Suppl. 1), 181–217.

Browne, A.J. (2001). The influence of liberal political ideology on nursing science. *Nursing Inquiry, 8* (2), 118–129.

Browne, A.J., Johnson, J.L., Bottorff, J.L., Grewal, S. & Hilton, B.A. (2002). Recognizing discrimination in nursing practice. *Canadian Nurse, 98* (5), 24–27.

Bryant-Davis, T. & Ocampo, C. (2005). The trauma of racism: Implications for counseling, research, and education. *The Counseling Psychologist, 33* (4), 574–578.

Campinha-Bacote, J. (2002). Cultural competence in psychiatric nursing: Have you "ASKED" the right questions? *Journal of the American Psychiatric Nurses Association, 8* (6), 183–187.

Canadian Nurses Association. (2000). Cultural diversity: Changes and challenges. *Nursing Now: Issues and Trends in Canadian Nursing*, No. 7. Available: www.cna-aiic.ca/CNA/documents/pdf/publications/CulturalDiversity_February2000_e.pdf. Accessed January 3, 2008.

Canadian Psychological Association. (2000). *Canadian Code of Ethics for Psychologists* (3rd ed.). Ottawa: Author.

Citizenship and Immigration Canada. (2003). *Serving Canada and the World*. Ottawa: Minister of Public Works and Government Services Canada.

Citizenship and Immigration Canada. (2005). *Facts and Figures 2004: Immigration Overview— Permanent and Temporary Residents*. Ottawa: Minister of Public Works and Government Services Canada. Available: http://dsp-psd.pwgsc.ca/collection/ci1-8-2004E.pdf. Accessed January 4, 2008.

College of Nurses of Ontario. (1999). *A Guide to Nurses for Providing Culturally Sensitive Care*. Toronto: Author.

D'Avanzo, C. & Geissler, E.M. (2002). *Guide to Cultural Assessment* (3rd ed.). St. Louis: Mosby.

Dei, G. (1996). *Anti-racism Education: Theory and Practice*. Halifax, NS: Fernwood Publishing.

Doane, G.H. & Varcoe, C. (2005). Toward compassionate action: Pragmatism and the inseparability of theory/practice. *Advances in Nursing Science, 28* (1), 81–90.

Dominelli, L. (1989). An uncaring profession: An examination of racism in social work. *New Community, 15* (3), 391–403.

Dominelli, L. (2002). *Anti-oppressive Social Work Theory and Practice*. Hampshire: Palgrave, Macmillan.

Fernando, S. (2003). *Cultural Diversity, Mental Health and Psychiatry: The Struggle against Racism*. New York: Brunner-Routledge.

Guruge, S., Donner, G.J. & Morrison, L. (2000). The impact of Canadian health care reform on recent women immigrants and refugees. In D.L. Gustafson (Ed.), *Care and Consequences: The Impact of Health Care Reform* (pp. 222–242). Halifax, NS: Fernwood Publishing.

Guruge, S. & Khanlou, N. (2004). Intersectionalities of influence: Researching the health of immigrant and refugee women. *Canadian Journal of Nursing Research, 36* (3), 33–47.

Gustafson, D.L. (2005). Transcultural nursing theory from a critical cultural perspective. *Advances in Nursing Science, 28* (1), 2–16.

Gustafson, D.L. (2007). White on whiteness: Becoming radicalized about race. *Nursing Inquiry, 14* (2), 153–161.

Henry, F. & Tator, C. (2005). *The Colour of Democracy: Racism in Canadian Society* (3rd ed.). Toronto: Nelson Thomson.

James, C.E. (2000). Grappling with difference. In C.E. James (Ed.), *Experiencing Difference* (pp. 14–24). Halifax, NS: Fernwood Publishing.

Johnson, J.L., Bottorff, J.L., Browne, A.J., Grewal, S., Hilton, B.A. & Clarke, H. (2004). Othering and being Othered in the context of health care services. *Health Communication, 16* (2), 253–271.

Johnson, R.L., Saha, S., Arbelaez, J.J., Beach, M.C. & Cooper, L.A. (2004). Racial and ethnic differences in patient perceptions of bias and cultural competence in health care. *Journal of General Internal Medicine, 19* (2), 101–110.

Kalita, S.M. (2003). *Suburban Sahibs: Three Immigrant Families and Their Passage from India to America.* New Brunswick, NJ: Rutgers University Press.

Kupers, T.A. 1995. The politics of psychiatry: Gender and sexual preference in DSM-IV. *Masculinities, 3* (2), 67–78.

Leininger, M.M. & McFarland, M.R. (2002). *Transcultural Nursing: Concepts, Theories, Research and Practice* (3rd ed.). New York: McGraw-Hill.

Majumdar, B., Keystone, J.S. & Cuttress, L.A. (1999). Cultural sensitivity training among foreign medical graduates. *Medical Education, 33* (3), 177–184.

Marcinkiw, K.W. (2003). The goal of nursing education. *Nursing Education Today, 23* (3), 174–182.

McGibbon, E. (2000). The "situated knowledge" of helpers. In C.E. James (Ed.), *Experiencing Difference* (pp. 185–199). Halifax, NS: Fernwood Publishing.

Ng, R. (1996). *The Politics of Community Services: Immigrant Women, Class and State.* Halifax, NS: Fernwood Publishing.

Omi, M. & Winant, H. (1994). *Racial Formation in the United States: From the 1960s to the 1980s* (2nd ed.). New York: Routledge and Kegan Paul.

Palmer, H., (Ed.). (1998). *"But Where Are You Really From?" Stories of Identity and Assimilation in Canada.* Toronto: Sister Vision Press.

Porter, C.P. & Barbee, E. (2004). Race and racism in nursing research: Past, present, and future. *Annual Review of Nursing Research, 22,* 9–37.

Pruitt, R.H., Gillespie, J. & Brown, K.M. (1999). Cultural awareness lab: First step toward competence. *Nurse Educator, 24* (2), 5, 10.

Public Health Agency of Canada. (2006). *What Determines Health?* Available: www.phac-aspc.gc.ca/ph-sp/phdd/determinants. Accessed January 5, 2008.

Razack, N. (2002). *Transforming the Field: Critical Antiracist and Anti-oppressive Perspectives for the Human Services Practicum.* Halifax, NS: Fernwood Publishing.

Registered Nurses Association of Ontario. (2002). *Client Centred Care: Nursing Best Practice Guidelines—Shaping the Future of Nursing.* Available: www.rnao.org/bestpractices/PDF/BPG_CCCare.pdf. Accessed January 5, 2008.

Reitmanova, S. & Gustafson, D.L. (in press). Mental health needs of visible minority immigrants in a small urban center: Recommendations for policy makers and service providers. *Journal of Immigrant and Minority Health.*

Smylie, J. (2000). SOGC policy statement: A guide for health professionals working with Aboriginal peoples—Cross cultural understanding (No. 100, February 2001). *Journal of the Society of Obstetricians and Gynaecologists of Canada, 23* (2), 157–167. Available: www.sogc.org/guidelines/public/100E-PS4-February2001.pdf. Accessed January 12, 2008.

St. Clair, A. & McKenry, L. (1999). Preparing culturally competent practitioners. *Journal of Nursing Education, 38* (5), 228–234.

Stanfield, J.H.I. & Dennis, R.M. (Eds.). (1993). *Race and Ethnicity in Research Methods.* Newbury Park, CA: Sage.

Stanhope, M. & Lancaster, J. (2002). *Foundations of Community Health Nursing: Community-Oriented Practice.* St. Louis, MO: Mosby.

Tucker, C.M., Herman, K.C., Pedersen, T.R., Higley, B., Montrichard, M. & Ivery, P. (2003). Cultural sensitivity in physician-patient relationships: Perspectives of an ethnically diverse sample of low-income primary care patients. *Medical Care Research and Review, 41* (7), 859–870.

Turrittin, J., Hagey, R., Guruge, S., Collins, E. & Mitchell, M. (2002). The experiences of professional nurses who have migrated to Canada: Cosmopolitan citizenship or democratic racism? *International Journal of Nursing Studies, 39* (6), 655–667.

Part 3

Current Realities for Immigrant Women and New Paradigms for Mental Health Practice

Chapter 4

Social Determinants of Depression among Immigrant and Refugee Women

FARAH N. MAWANI

Depression is a universal phenomenon (Kleinman, 1988; Beiser, 2003), but a great deal of evidence shows wide variations in prevalence, symptomatology and clinical presentation of depression both between countries around the world (Kirmayer & Groleau, 2001; Kirmayer, 2001) and between ethnic communities within those countries (Beiser et al., 1993; Fenta et al., 2004; Noh et al., 1999; Noh et al., 1992; Wu et al., 2003). Additional evidence shows wide variations in prevalence and symptomatology of depression between men and women across cultures (Salokangas et al., 2002). Despite the consistent finding that women are about twice as likely to experience depression as men, the reasons behind the striking difference remain poorly understood (Rodgers, 2002).

There are particular points along the life course in which women seem to be at increased risk for depression (e.g., premenstrual, postpartum, perimenopausal periods), which could partially explain the difference in prevalence of depression between men and women (Maughan, 2002; Salokangas et al., 2002). *Social determinants*, or the "social conditions in which people live and work" (Commission on Social Determinants of Health [CSDH], 2005, p. 4), may be partially responsible for the variations in the etiology (causation) of depression between men and women. Particular social factors affect the lives of immigrants and refugees in Canada and may shed light on the etiology of depression among immigrant and refugee women.

This chapter is an attempt to bring together disparate bodies of literature—one focused on inequities in depression between men and women and the other focused on

67

inequities in depression between immigrants and Canadian-born individuals—to explain social determinants and the pathways by which they may affect depression in immigrant and refugee women. This understanding will inform the subsequent recommendations for preventing depression in this population.

The chapter:

- clarifies the intended meaning of the category "immigrant and refugee" and the term "depression," which are used throughout this chapter
- describes the theoretical framework and conceptual model that form the basis of this chapter
- describes the epidemiology (population distribution and disease burden) of depression, with a focus on inequities based on gender, migration status, race and ethnicity
- reviews the literature on gender differences in the etiology of depression, including research focusing specifically on immigrants and refugees where relevant and possible[1]
- suggests strategies for mental health practitioners to address these determinants of depression, and thereby prevent the onset of depression, shorten episode duration, and prevent recurrence of depression in immigrant and refugee women.

Heterogeneity of Migrants

Immigrants and refugees are often distinguished from each other based on a combination of their choice in their migration process and their exposure to premigration trauma due to political violence, natural disaster, etc. Refugees are usually considered to be a particular group with no choice in their migration process due to exposure to premigration trauma. While this is often the case, it is important to be careful in making such distinctions as the context and reasons for migration are complex for both immigrants and refugees, and in particular for immigrant and refugee women.

In a study of recent immigrants to Quebec, more than 50 per cent of independent and sponsored immigrants cited the political situation in their country of origin as their primary reason for migration (Rousseau & Drapeau, 2004). Women, in particular, may not have a choice about their migration due to the dominance of their spouse or male family member(s) in decision-making. It is therefore important to consider migration choice and exposure to premigration trauma as important factors regardless of official migration status. Official migration status does, however, determine the particular policies that govern the settlement process of immigrants and refugees in Canada. Refugees face particular restrictions in accessing health care, education and employment; refugee claimants have even more limited access to services and resources; and

---

1. Research on gender differences in the etiology of depression in immigrants and refugees is limited. This review aims to highlight research gaps that are important to fill in order to clarify the levels and types of interventions needed to prevent depression in immigrant and refugee women.

non-status immigrants[2] face the most serious barriers to accessing the services, rights and protections enjoyed by most people living in Canada (Khandor et al., 2004).

It is important to recognize that in addition to reasons for migration, other factors—including country of origin, age at migration, fluency in an official language and length of time in Canada—influence the impact of migration on mental health.

Definition of Depression

The first challenge in studying as well as identifying, preventing and treating depression among immigrant and refugee women is the ongoing difficulty of defining depression.

The clinical definition of major depressive disorder (MDD) is:

> [A] common, disabling disorder characterized by a period of at least two weeks in which a person loses pleasure in nearly all activities and/or exhibits a depressed mood. Symptoms of major depression include feelings of sadness and hopelessness, diminished interest and pleasure, changes in weight and in sleep patterns, chronic fatigue, feelings of worthlessness or guilt and difficulty concentrating or thinking. These symptoms cause clinically significant distress or impairment in physical, social, occupational and other key areas of functioning. (Stewart et al., 2003, p. 1)

Individuals, however, can also suffer from dysthymia, a less severe but more chronic lowering of mood, as well as from depressive disorder, depressive phenomena or depressive symptoms (Maughan, 2002). For the purposes of this chapter, the term "depression" will be used to refer to the range of illness, from dysthymia to major depression.

Theoretical Framework

POPULATION HEALTH

This chapter applies a *population health approach*, defined as "an approach to health that aims to improve the health of the entire population and to reduce health inequities among population groups (PHAC, 2006)," to the study of depression among immigrant and refugee women. The following key elements of this approach inform the focus and recommendations of this chapter (Health Canada, 2001):

- to focus on the health of populations

---

2. People can become "non-status" when their refugee claim is rejected, when they do not have official identity documents or when their student visa, visitor's visa or work permit expires.

- to address the determinants of health and their interactions
- to base decisions on evidence
- to increase upstream investments (i.e., investments in root causes of health outcomes)
- to apply multiple strategies
- to collaborate across sectors and levels
- to use mechanisms for public involvement
- to show accountability for health outcomes.

SOCIAL DETERMINANTS

Given that the population health approach emphasizes upstream investments, this chapter will focus on interacting social determinants—including gender, socio-economic status (SES), discrimination[3] and social support—operating throughout the lifespan to influence depression among immigrant and refugee women.

Conceptual Model

The literature raises a number of possibilities for pathways by which social determinants may affect depression, including material and psychosocial pathways. This chapter focuses on the chronic stress psychosocial pathway, which is explained in this section and outlined in Figure 1. The *stress model of mental illness* emphasizes the inequalities in opportunity arising from the organization of social statuses, including gender, class and race, that affect susceptibility to psychological breakdown (McDonough & Walters, 2001; Wheaton, 1999).

In the 1970s, Brown and Harris determined that acute, stressful life events and longer-term stressors play an important role in the precipitation of many first episodes of depression, and that exposure to stressful events dramatically increases the risk of a depressive episode in subsequent weeks or months (Denton et al., 2004; Fenta et al., 2004; Maughan, 2002). While life events are considered *acute stressors*, social determinants such as discrimination, decreased socio-economic status and decreased social support—are inequalities in opportunity associated with migration that act as *chronic stressors* to influence the onset and recurrence of depression (Beiser, 1999; Kleinman, 1988; Maughan, 2002). In addition, they can be particularly destructive stressors given that they threaten a central part of a person's identity (Cassidy et al., 2004; Thoits, 1991).

The *transactional model of stress* suggests that self-esteem mediates the association of such stressors to depression. When individuals evaluate a negative event as stressful,

3. For the purposes of this chapter, *discrimination* is defined as "the process by which a member, or members, of a socially defined group is, or are, treated differently (especially unfairly) because of his/her/their membership of that group … This unfair treatment arises from 'socially derived beliefs each [group] holds about the other' and 'patterns of dominance and oppression, viewed as expressions of a struggle for power and privilege.' People and institutions who discriminate adversely accordingly restrict, by judgement and action, the lives of those against whom they discriminate" (Krieger, 2001, p. 693). "Discrimination" is used instead of "racism" in order to encompass discrimination based on a combination of factors, including race, gender, migration status and religion.

they perceive their self-image to be threatened. This threat may affect their self-esteem, which then affects their level of psychological distress (Cassidy et al., 2004). Perceived control, representing "individuals' generalized perceptions of how much influence they have over their circumstances and life course" (Bullers, 2000, p. 100), has also been examined as a mediator in the relationship between social determinants and depression (Bullers, 2000; Kleinman, 1988; Taylor & Seeman, 1999). There is strong empirical support for this relationship in a variety of contexts (Bullers, 2000; Taylor & Seeman, 1999). Sociological research suggests that perceived control is an indicator of an individual's access to resources, whereby individuals of higher social position (e.g., people with higher SES, men) have greater influence over their employment, education, housing, health care, etc. (Bullers, 2000). Higher perceived control is associated with better mental health (Taylor & Seeman, 1999). The combination of high expectations for control and low opportunities to exercise control results in the highest levels of reactivity, comprised of increasing cardiovascular and/or neuroendocrine[4] activity and lowering of immune function (Taylor & Seeman, 1999).

This chapter proposes a model of depression causation, where self-esteem and perceived control are combined to represent disempowerment due to the important links between them. The extent to which a person feels powerful influences his or her sense of self-esteem (Turner et al., 1999). Disempowerment is proposed to mediate the association between the chronic stressors of discrimination, lowered SES and lowered social support, and depression. In addition, discrimination may affect depression via its economic consequences (e.g., underemployment resulting in lowered SES), as indicated in Figure 4-1.

FIGURE 4-1

Conceptual Model of Social Determinants of Depression

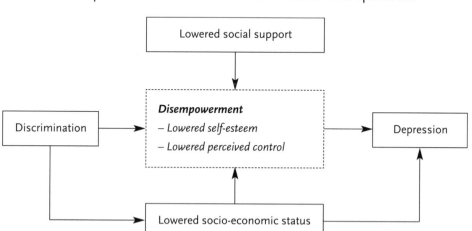

4. The National Cancer Institute (www.cancer.gov/Templates/db_alpha.aspx?CdrID=45803) defines neuroendocrine as "having to do with the interactions between the nervous system and the endocrine system. Neuroendocrine describes certain cells that release hormones into the blood in response to stimulation of the nervous system."

Gender plays a significant role in these relationships. Women more frequently suffer the consequences of relationships of power, control and inequity in their lives (Moss, 2002). Thus, women tend to have lower self-esteem and lower perceived control than men (Bullers, 2000; Turner et al., 1999). In most countries, women have lower socio-economic status than men (Moss, 2002). Evidence also indicates that men and women give and receive different levels of social support, need different types of support, seek support in different ways, and are thus differentially affected by social support (Heaney & Israel, 1997; Moss, 2002; Mulvihill et al., 2001; Turner et al., 1999). In addition, women are also more frequently responsible for offering support to immediate and extended family and friends (Bullers, 2000) and may not receive the support they need (Fischer et al., 2004; Moss, 2002; Watkins & Whaley, 2000).

Epidemiology of Depression

To understand inequities in depression, it is important to start by examining the epidemiology of depression. Mood disorders are one of the most common mental illnesses in the general population, making depression a particularly important measure of mental health (Health Canada, 2002). Canadian studies indicate that 7.9 to 8.6 per cent of adults living in the community have met the criteria for diagnosis of major depression at some time in their lives (Health Canada, 2002). Of Canadians aged 12 and over, 7.9 per cent report symptoms indicating at least one experience with major depression in a 12-month period (Ali, 2002). Studies consistently report higher rates of depression among women than men, with female-to-male ratios averaging 2:1 (Health Canada, 2002; Maughan, 2002; Nolen-Hoeksema, 1995; Stewart et al., 2003; Ussher, 2000; World Health Organization [WHO], n.d.).

There is some evidence that refugees have particularly high rates of depression (Kleinman, 1988). In their analysis of the 1996–97 Canadian National Population Health Survey (NPHS), Wu et al. (2003) did not find a significant difference between rates of depression among immigrants and the Canadian-born population. They did find varying rates of depression between different ethnic communities, with varying effects of socio-economic status on rates of depression between them (Wu et al., 2003).

Visible minorities were found to have better mental health profiles than non–visible minorities regardless of socio-economic and social support disparities, but this analysis is limited in its informativeness as it did not incorporate length of time in Canada, migration status or gender in its comparison of depression rates between ethnic communities (Wu et al., 2003).

One analysis, which did incorporate length of time in Canada, found that immigrants who arrived in Canada less than 10 years ago had lower rates of depression than the Canadian-born population, while those who arrived 10 to 14 years ago or more than 20 years ago did not have significantly different rates of depression from the Canadian-born population (Ali, 2002). The report does not, however, distinguish between immigrants and refugees, or men and women, a gross oversight given the distinctions between these subgroups of immigrants and the well-known higher rates of depression among women (Ussher, 2000; Kessler, 2000; Nolen-Hoeksema, 1995; WHO, n.d.). In addition, the analysis is limited by the cross-sectional nature of the data. Longitudinal data is needed in order to determine whether depression rates rise with length of time in Canada.

Considering the impact of depression on the lives of immigrant and refugee women highlights the significance of prevalence and incidence rates along with the need for prevention. Depression has a significant impact on the lives of immigrant and refugee women, impairing their ability to cope with the daily challenges of resettlement, including meeting their basic needs (Health Canada, 2002). The World Health Organization (WHO) cites major depression as the leading cause of years of life lived with disability (YLDS) and the fourth leading cause of disability-adjusted life years (DALYS) in the world (Health Canada, 2002). Low-income ethnic minority and immigrant women suffer a greater burden from depression because they are less likely to benefit from prevention and to seek or receive appropriate care or treatment due to language and cultural barriers, lack of adequate information and lack of appropriate services (Beiser, 2005; Miranda et al., 2003). In addition, for immigrant and refugee women with families, depression affects their ability to care for their children and families, and thereby affects family functioning (Beiser et al., 1989).

Gender Differences in the Etiology of Depression

In trying to understand what is behind the differences in prevalence and incidence rates of depression between men and women across cultures, it is important to examine the evidence of gender differences in the etiology of depression.

The etiology of depression involves a complex interaction of genetic, biological, psychosocial and social factors (Maughan, 2002; Stewart et al., 2003). This chapter focuses on addressing social determinants of depression among immigrant and refugee women, so will examine social support, discrimination and socio-economic status, as well as the pathways by which they affect depression.

SOCIAL FACTORS

Social determinants, such as lowered social support, discrimination and lowered socio-economic status, act as chronic stressors to influence depression among immigrant and refugee women, as proposed by the conceptual model outlined in Figure 4-1 (Beiser, 1999; Kleinman, 1988; Maughan, 2002). The following sections review the evidence supporting this model by first summarizing literature on each of the three determinants and then focusing on the evidence linking them to depression via the disempowerment pathway.

Social Support

There are two main aspects of social support that influence its impact on mental health:

- structural support—existence and quantity of social relationships (e.g., marital status, group membership, number of friends) and interconnectedness of a person's social network
- functional support—the degree to which interpersonal relationships serve particular functions (e.g., emotional support, instrumental support, informational support, affirmational support5) (Sherbourne & Stewart, 1991).

Social support is usually considered a protective factor that buffers the negative impact of stressors on mental health. In the context of migration, however, there is a substantial loss of social support. Sometimes loss or separation from immediate family members, including partners and/or children, occurs during the process of migration. The loss of immediate family, extended family and community, combined with the value placed on independence over interdependence in Canada, leads to a feeling of great isolation in many women (Mawani, 2001). This is especially challenging during resettlement, when the need for emotional and affirmational support is especially acute, and when immigrant and refugee women are often significant providers of support to their families and communities.

STRUCTURAL SUPPORT

Research indicates that the impact of marital status on depression differs by gender. Some research indicates that marital status is a protective factor for men (Beiser et al., 1993). For women, however, the risk of depression is greatest for those who are married, lower for those who are widowed and divorced and lowest among those who are single (Maughan, 2002; Nolen-Hoeksema, 1995; Ussher, 2000). Single mothers and young married women caring for young children tend to be at particularly high risk for depression (Maughan, 2002). Marriage can provide social and economic support to women, but it can also increase stress experienced by women due to increased caregiving responsibilities and power imbalances in relationships (Alegria & Canino, 2000; Spitzer, 2005). The quality of marital relationships, including the timing, consistency and reliability of support they provide, is important to consider (WHO, 2000).

Marital relationships are certainly affected by migration. Spouses/partners often migrate at different times and are thereby separated for months or even years. This can lead to the breakdown of communication and relationships (Rousseau et al., 2001). Additional research suggests that postmigration stressors affect the gender dynamics in marital relationships, increasing the potential for marital conflict (Hyman et al., 2004). Further research is needed to examine the association of marital conflict, separation and breakdown with depression in immigrant and refugee women.

In terms of group membership, immediate and extended family, like-ethnic community, religious community, neighbourhood and mainstream society are all groups that immigrant and refugee women may belong to and turn to for support.

---

5. Affirmational or appraisal support refers to the "provision of information that is useful for self-evaluation purposes, that is, constructive feedback, affirmation, and social comparison" (Heaney & Israel, 1997, p. 180).

Expectations of the support that may be received from these groups are influenced by the support those communities provided in the women's country of origin.

The presence of a significant, established like-ethnic community in the city where an immigrant resides has been found to have a positive effect on immigrant mental health (Fenta et al., 2004; Beiser, 1999). The like-ethnic community is said to provide some material advantages (e.g., help in finding jobs) and a sense of belonging, cultural identity and historical continuity, which have particular relevance for mental health (Fenta et al., 2004). Also, the more established a particular ethnic community is, the more likely that ethnospecific services (including first-language services) are available.

The literature is particularly limited in its analysis of gender differences in the effect of like-ethnic community support. If women are expected to give more support than they receive, having an established like-ethnic community in the community they resettle in may be draining rather than protective for women.

FUNCTIONAL SUPPORT

Research focusing on the social support experiences of immigrants and refugees in Canada has identified the following key issues: lack of informal support, lack of awareness of available formal support and discomfort seeking formal support (Mawani, 2001). Affirmational support from others who have successfully adapted and emotional support from family, friends and other members of their communities are critical to immigrants' settlement processes during a time when they are separated from family and friends in their countries of origin (Simich et al., 2003).

PATHWAYS FROM SOCIAL SUPPORT TO DEPRESSION

Research has found that receiving social support contributes to more stable and positive self-esteem (Turner et al., 1999). Suffering a loss of support or experiencing a lack of needed support can thereby contribute to lowered self-esteem. Immigrants and refugees have described feeling downtrodden and helpless with a sense of desperation, disappointment and despair when they did not receive support they needed (Simich et al., 2004). When a lack of formal social support limits their access to the housing, education and employment that they feel entitled to, it may lower their self-esteem and perceived control (Simich et al., 2004).

Pregnancy and the postpartum period are points in the life course when immigrant and refugee women are in particular need of social support. Lack of support may be especially disempowering for women who would have received much social support from family and community members in their country of origin during these times (Zelkowitz et al., 2004).

Discrimination

With the changing demographic profile of immigrants to Canada, and the incongruence between their increasing levels of education and decreasing economic returns, discrimination is a factor that is being increasingly discussed (Dunn & Dyck, 2000; McIsaac, 2003; Omidvar & Richmond, 2003; Ruddick, 2003). In the 1990s, 73 per cent of recent immigrants were "visible minorities" (up from 68 per cent in the 1980s and

52 per cent in the 1970s) and by 2016, visible minorities are projected to account for one-fifth of Canadian citizens (McIsaac, 2003). Analysis of 2001 census data also demonstrates a remarkable growth in Islam, Hinduism, Sikhism and Buddhism, consistent with changing immigration patterns toward increased immigration from Asia and the Middle East (Statistics Canada, 2001).

Despite these demographic changes, epidemiological research on discrimination as a determinant of mental health is in its infancy (Health Canada, 1999; Noh et al., 1999; Krieger, 2000). Much of the research that has been done is American, with simplistic racial divisions (Noh et al., 1999) and no differentiation between newcomers and visible minorities who may have been in the country for generations (Dunn & Dyck, 2000). In addition, most of the research is focused on racial discrimination, with only a few including gender discrimination in their analyses (Krieger, 2000; Hyman, 2001) and fewer still including discrimination based on age, immigration status, religion, nationality or sexual orientation. Combined analyses of the various forms of discrimination are important because individuals may face discrimination of multiple forms simultaneously (Krieger, 2000). Gender differences in experiences and impact of discrimination also need to be examined (Cassidy et al., 2004).

Some cross-sectional studies have shown a link between discrimination and depression (Kaspar & Noh, 2001; Noh et al., 1999; Beiser, 1999), but they have used different and often simplistic measures of discrimination that do not differentiate between levels, sources and types of discrimination.

Recent findings from Canada's Ethnic Diversity Survey reveal that the most common experiences of discrimination took place at work or when applying for a job or promotion (Statistics Canada, 2003). Beiser and Hou (2001) examined the relationship between unemployment and depression and found that, for men in particular, unemployment was a strong risk factor for depression. They did not, however, specifically examine the role of perceptions of employment discrimination in the association.

PATHWAYS FROM DISCRIMINATION TO DEPRESSION
Discrimination may affect depression via material or psychosocial pathways. Discrimination may operate through lowered SES—resulting from barriers to employment, education and housing—to affect depression (Krieger, 2000). Discrimination may also be mediated by disempowerment (lowered self-esteem and perceived control) to affect depression (Kaspar & Noh, 2001), as proposed in Figure 1. Low self-esteem is significantly associated with a greater risk of depressive symptoms (Turner et al., 1999). One study offers partial support for the role of self-esteem as a mediator between perceived ethnic discrimination and depression (Cassidy et al., 2004). This pathway is especially critical given the inequities in distribution of opportunity, respect and power (Turner et al., 1999) resulting from discrimination.

Socio-Economic Status
Some work has been done to differentiate social class from socio-economic status (SES) in theory and research. *Social class* is defined as "a social relation linked to the production of goods and services (e.g., owner, self-employed, worker; manager, supervisor,

non-managerial employee)" (Muntaner et al., 2004, p. 56). *Socio-economic status* is defined as "the location of persons along a continuum of economic, political or cultural attributes (e.g., income, educational achievement, occupational prestige)" (Muntaner et al., 2004, p. 53). Literature examining the association of social class and depression, particularly that among immigrants and refugees, is limited. Research has tended to focus more on the association of socio-economic status to depression.

An inverse relationship between socio-economic status and ill-health has been recognized and measured in different ways for hundreds of years (Adler et al., 1994; Singh-Manoux et al., 2002). The three most common measures of SES are income, education and occupation; and in the general population of most countries, a relationship between SES and health is evident with any of these measures (Adler et al., 1994). In addition, a socio-economic gradient, where the relationship between SES and health is present at every level of SES, has been shown to exist for almost all health outcomes in countries all over the world (Adler et al., 1994; Blane, 2001; Lynch & Kaplan, 2000; Mustard, 1996; Winkleby et al., 1992).

This is true for mental health outcomes including depression (Lorant et al., 2003). There is an increased risk of depression among people with lower income (Kleinman, 1988). As income increases linearly, the risk of depression decreases (Lorant et al., 2003). Such a relationship has also been demonstrated among Canadian immigrants (Ali, 2002).

This is particularly disconcerting given the challenges immigrants and refugees face in gaining employment that corresponds to their skills and qualifications. Despite the fact that their average level of education was higher than that of any previous cohort and even higher than that of Canadian-born individuals, in the 1990s, immigrants were not as successful in finding employment as their predecessors (Human Resources Development Canada [HRDC], 2001; Omidvar & Richmond, 2003; McIsaac, 2003; Ruddick, 2003). The most recent Canadian census data (Statistics Canada, 2001) also indicates that higher education was positively associated with higher income for Canadian-born individuals. Individuals with a university degree made up 60 per cent of those in the top income category (McIsaac, 2003). This association between education and income did not apply to immigrants, even for those with a university degree and knowledge of an official language (McIsaac, 2003). There was an overrepresentation of university-educated immigrants in low-skill and low-income jobs; and in occupations of all skill levels, recent immigrants earned less than Canadian-born individuals (McIsaac, 2003). Recent immigrants to Canada also report higher unemployment rates than Canadian-born individuals (Kinnon, 1999).

There are significant differences between the labour market participation rates of recent immigrant men and women. By 2001, in all major immigrant-receiving centres, the income gap between immigrants and Canadian-born individuals narrowed for recent immigrant men. In contrast, the gap widened for recent immigrant women (almost doubled since 1991). Immigrant women did not achieve the same level of participation in the labour force as men, but they performed better than their male counterparts in terms of earnings. The reasons for these differences are unclear (McIsaac, 2003).

In this context, temporary unemployment or underemployment may be expected by all immigrants, including refugees, while long-term unemployment or underemployment may not be expected and thereby may have a more significant negative impact on mental health, including depression (Kinnon, 1999; Williams & Berry, 1991).

PATHWAYS FROM SOCIO-ECONOMIC STATUS TO DEPRESSION
Lack of recognition of credentials understandably leads to low perceived control and lowered self-esteem, both of which are associated with a higher risk of depression. Research has identified stress, loss of self-esteem, stigma, powerlessness, lack of hope and fatalism as potential mechanisms by which poverty affects negative health outcomes (Turner et al., 1999; Cattell, 2001). These mechanisms are very relevant for recent immigrants to Canada, whose income is substantially reduced by lack of recognition of their credentials, especially if they perceive this lack of recognition as a proxy for discrimination.

Recommendations

This section outlines recommendations based on the evidence reviewed and summarized in this chapter, in the hopes that mental health practitioners will carefully consider the recommendations in their work.

As advocated by a population health approach, collaboration with community-based agencies, along with outreach to and dialogue with immigrant and refugee women are the foundations for service provision; these will be discussed first as overarching strategies. Then more specific recommendations will be presented, focused on addressing different points in the pathways from social determinants to depression. These recommendations aim to prevent onset of depression, shorten episode duration and prevent recurrence of depression among immigrant and refugee women.

OVERARCHING STRATEGIES

Partnerships and Collaboration
- Use the knowledge and expertise of community-based settlement and ethno-specific agencies as an important resource and consultation base.

> *Case study:* The Asian tsunami in December 2004 gave rise to the development of the Local Distress Relief Network, comprised of mental health professionals, Tamil community settlement service providers, mental health researchers, school board representatives, policy-makers, etc., in response to emergent Tamil community mental health needs in Toronto. The network collaborated on a number of activities, including the development of print resources for Tamil

community members and teachers, and a workshop to discuss culturally appropriate models of distress relief (Simich et al., 2006). After the
tsunami, Tamil ethnospecific and settlement agencies were inundated
with requests for support from community members. These agencies
could not meet all the needs because of limited human resources,
particularly limited staff trained to provide mental health services. At
the same time, mainstream mental health services were not seeing the
rise in Tamil clients they expected. Tamil agencies and mainstream
mental health services collaborated in order to bridge this gap.

Outreach
- Use community-based agencies and settlement services as a resource for
  outreach to immigrant and refugee women.
- Partner with settlement services and ethnospecific agencies where immigrant
  and refugee women may go to meet other needs (e.g., inadequate social support,
  low SES, discrimination) that may put them at risk for depression.

> *Case study:* Toronto community health centres (CHCs) connect with
> settlement and ethnospecific agencies and services (e.g., the Language
> Instruction for Newcomers to Canada [LINC] program and other ESL
> classes, faith communities) to promote awareness of the services they
> offer. They develop formal and informal referral arrangements to
> strengthen these connections (Hoen & Hayward, 2005).

Dialogue
- Continue to ask clients about their contexts and experiences as well as their
  perspectives of solutions, during the planning and delivery of programs and
  services.

Nothing can replace ongoing dialogue with clients and client groups, especially
given the heterogeneity of migrants. It is critical to give clients the opportunity to tell
their stories and share information on what strategies may work for them in their
context. This in itself is empowering and can counteract some of the disempowerment
immigrants and refugees experience in their settlement process.

> *Case study:* Toronto CHCs involve newcomers in planning their pro-
> grams to ensure responsive programs and boost participants' self-esteem
> (Hoen & Hayward, 2005). St. Joseph's Women's Health Centre uses the
> guidance of a community advisory panel made up of former clients and
> women currently living in their catchment area.

> *Case study:* The Sherbourne Health Centre and the St. Joseph's
> Women's Health Centre provide client-centred programming, includ-
> ing individual and group therapy, that encourages participants to share
> their stories and perspectives. Some clients may find the incorporation

of music, art and/or crafts particularly helpful in their therapy, depending on their particular cultural contexts (Hoen & Hayward, 2005; S. Roberts, personal communication, February 13, 2006).

ADDRESSING THE PATHWAYS TO DEPRESSION

Screening
- Incorporate the interrelationships of clients' socio-economic status, social support and experience of discrimination when assessing risk and/or screening for depression.

Immigrant and refugee clients who identify discrimination as a factor in their diminished socio-economic status are likely to be at greater risk of depression than those who do not. Clients without adequate informal support, particularly affirmational and emotional support, may be at even greater risk.

Empowering
- Advocate for policy and systemic change at different levels to address discrimination—inherent in some formal support systems and services—that disempowers women.

  Example: Partner with federal, provincial and local umbrella organizations that focus on advocacy—such as the Ontario Council of Agencies Serving Immigrants, the Council of Agencies Serving South Asians, the Chinese Canadian National Council, the African Canadian Social Development Council, the Hispanic Development Council and the Toronto Women's Network—to strengthen advocacy campaigns.

  Example: Join existing coalitions such as the Status Campaign, made up of individuals and organizations advocating for the regularization of all non-status immigrants living in Canada.

- Incorporate translation and interpretation into service provision.

Consider translation and interpretation by trained interpreters as a mode of empowering people who are disempowered by discrimination, lowered SES and lack of social support. Providing translation and interpretation helps people feel included in the society they live in, and is not simply a method of improving access to care.

The importance of incorporating translation and interpretation into service provision cannot be underestimated. It is especially critical when offering support/service to those who may feel more comfortable using their first language when in distress. Women may also feel more comfortable discussing the complex circumstances and emotions related to their experiences of discrimination, lowered SES and lack of social support in their first language.

Case study: Access Alliance Multicultural Community Health Centre trains and employs cultural interpreters on a fee-for-service basis.

Case study: The Centre for Addiction and Mental Health has cultural interpreters available at all times and at no cost to CAMH clients, if requested by CAMH service providers.

(For more information on translation and interpretation, and CAMH's fundamental change in approach to the delivery of interpreter services, see Chapter 6.)

- Give clients the opportunity to discuss their experiences of discrimination, reduced SES and lack of social support along with their feelings associated with those experiences.

The emotional support gained from individual therapy and a combination of affirmational and emotional support gained from workshops and group sessions could empower women by helping them to regain their self-esteem and perceived control to deal with their situations.

Addressing Discrimination

- Hear and validate women's experiences with discrimination and acknowledge the injustice inherent in their experiences.

Recognize discrimination as something that profoundly affects women's self-esteem. If practitioners feel threatened by people expressing experiences of discrimination, they should do the work necessary to deal with those feelings, so that they do not minimize women's experiences.

- Provide women with strategies and support for addressing discrimination, recognizing the challenges inherent in doing so.

Work with clients to develop strategies for responding to discrimination, acknowledging that different styles of coping work for different people and within different cultural contexts.

- Empower clients by helping them to understand and recognize their rights within the context of the Canadian Charter of Rights and Freedoms.

Example: Partner with agencies such as the Centre for Equality Rights in Accommodation, the Ontario Human Rights Commission and Legal Aid to ensure that clients are informed of their rights and that their rights are upheld.

Addressing Socio-Economic Status

- Provide support to help women to obtain evaluation and recognition of their foreign credentials.

Example: Refer women to World Education Services, a not-for-profit organization, partially funded by the Government of Ontario, that focuses on integration of individuals with foreign credentials into Canadian academic and professional environments.

Example: Refer women to one of twenty-four new bridge training programs funded by the Government of Ontario to help internationally trained professionals and tradespeople upgrade their professional language skills and training, prepare for qualifying exams and gain entry into their fields in Canada.

- Address reduced ses by providing support and encouragement to help women use their resourcefulness to increase their household income and/or meet their needs in other ways.

  Example: Refer women to services that provide basic needs such as food and clothing, or provide such support in-house if possible (e.g., St. Joseph's Women's Health Centre provides a clothing exchange to their clients).

  Example: Provide women with or refer them to self-employment skills training, to help them launch small businesses such as catering, home child care and tailoring services.

Addressing Social Support
- Provide immigrant and refugee women with space and programs to help them rebuild the social networks that they have lost in the process of migration and resettlement.

  Example: Provide programs that enable women to connect with others who share their experiences and/or interests (e.g., parenting groups, community kitchens, sewing groups and knitting circles).

Conclusion

Discrimination, lowered ses and inadequate social support experienced by immigrant and refugee women can all be disempowering through their effects on self-esteem and perceived control, particularly when they are experienced in combination with each other, and thus affect women's risk for depression.

Research that tests the pathways from social determinants to depression in immigrant and refugee women is limited. Further research is needed to better understand the complexity of the interrelationships between various social determinants of depression and the potential pathways by which social determinants operate in relation to each other to affect depression in immigrant and refugee women.

In the meantime, organizations and service providers can prevent the onset of depression, shorten episode duration and prevent recurrence of depression among immigrant and refugee women, by working to minimize their risk of experiencing discrimination, lowered SES and lowered social support and/or the disempowerment resulting from them. Given the limited evidence on social determinants of depression for immigrant and refugee women in Canada, which in turn limits the potential for evidence-based interventions, evaluation of interventions to add to this evidence base are another important contribution that practitioners can make to reducing the risk and consequences of depression for a group already facing significant challenges.

References

Adler, N.E., Boyce, T., Chesney, M.A., Cohen, S., Folkman, S., Kahn, R.L. et al. (1994). Socioeconomic status and health: The challenge of the gradient. *American Psychologist, 49* (1), 15–24.

Alegria, M. & Canino, G. (2000). Women and depression. In L. Sherr & J. St. Lawrence (Eds.), *Women, Health and the Mind*. West Sussex, UK: John Wiley and Sons, Ltd.

Ali, J. (2002). Mental health of Canada's immigrants. How healthy are Canadians? Annual report 2002. *Supplement to Health Reports, 13* (Catalogue No. 82-003, pp. 1–11). Ottawa: Statistics Canada. Available: www.statcan.ca/english/freepub/82-003-SIE/2002001/pdf/82-003-SIE2002006.pdf. Accessed January 5, 2008.

Beiser, M. (1999). *Strangers at the Gate: The Boat People's First Ten Years in Canada*. Toronto: University of Toronto Press.

Beiser, M. (2003). Why should researchers care about culture? *Canadian Journal of Psychiatry, 48* (3), 154–160.

Beiser, M. (2005). The health of immigrants and refugees in Canada. *Canadian Journal of Public Health, 96* (Suppl. 2), S30–S44.

Beiser, M. & Hou, F. (2001). Language acquisition, unemployment and depressive disorder among Southeast Asian refugees: A 10-year study. *Social Science and Medicine, 53* (10), 1321–1334.

Beiser, M., Johnson, P.J. & Turner, R.J. (1993). Unemployment, underemployment and depressive affect among Southeast Asian refugees. *Psychological Medicine, 23* (3), 731–743.

Beiser, M., Turner, R.J. & Ganesan, S. (1989). Catastrophic stress and factors affecting its consequences among Southeast Asian refugees. *Social Science and Medicine, 28* (3), 183–195.

Blane, D. (2001). Commentary: Socioeconomic health differentials. *International Journal of Epidemiology, 30* (2), 292–293.

Bullers, S. (2000). The mediating role of perceived control in the relationship between social ties and depressive symptoms. *Women and Health, 31* (2–3), 97–116.

Cassidy, C., O'Connor, R.C., Howe, C. & Warden, D. (2004). Perceived discrimination and psychological distress: The role of personal and ethnic self-esteem. *Journal of Counseling Psychology, 51* (3), 329–339.

Cattell, V. (2001). Poor people, poor places, and poor health: The mediating role of social networks and social capital. *Social Science and Medicine, 52* (10), 1501–1516.

Commission on Social Determinants of Health. (2005). Towards a Conceptual Framework for Analysis and Action on the Social Determinants of Health—Draft. May 5, 2005 version, pp. 1–35.

Denton, M., Prus, S. & Walters, V. (2004). Gender differences in health: A Canadian study of the psychosocial, structural and behavioural determinants of health. *Social Science and Medicine, 58* (12), 2585–2600.

Dunn, J. & Dyck, I. (2000). Social determinants of health in Canada's immigrant population: Results from the National Population Health Survey. *Social Science and Medicine, 51* (11), 1573–1593.

Fenta, H., Hyman, I. & Noh, S. (2004). Determinants of depression among Ethiopian immigrants and refugees in Toronto. *Journal of Nervous and Mental Disease, 192* (5), 363–372.

Fischer, A.H., Rodriguez Mosquera, P.M., van Vianen, A.E.M. & Manstead, A.S.R. (2004). Gender and culture differences in emotion. *Emotion, 4* (1), 87–94.

Health Canada. (1999). *Canadian Research on Immigration and Health.* Ottawa: Minister of Public Works and Government Services.

Health Canada. (2001). *The Population Health Template: Key Elements and Actions That Define a Population Health Approach.* Ottawa: Health Canada Population and Public Health Branch.

Health Canada. (2002). *A Report on Mental Illnesses in Canada.* Ottawa: Health Canada Editorial Board Mental Illnesses in Canada.

Heaney, C.A. & Israel, B.A. (1997). Social networks and social support. In K. Glanz, F.M. Lewis & B.K. Rimer (Eds.), *Health Behavior and Health Education: Theory, Research and Practice* (2nd ed.; pp. 179–205). San Francisco, CA: Jossey-Bass.

Hoen, B. & Hayward, K. (2005). *CHC Mental Health Services for Newcomers: A Guide Reflecting the Experience of Toronto Community Health Centres.* Toronto: Access Alliance Multicultural Community Health Centre.

Human Resources Development Canada. (2001). Recent immigrants have experienced unusual economic difficulties. *Applied Research Bulletin, 7* (1), 7–8. Available: www.sdc.gc.ca/en/cs/sp/sdc/pkrf/publications/nlscy/uey/2001-002381/v7n1_e.pdf. Accessed January 8, 2008.

Hyman, I. (2001). *Immigration and Health.* Health Policy Working Paper Series. Ottawa: Minister of Public Works and Government Services.

Hyman, I., Guruge, S., Mason, R., Gould, J., Stuckless, N., Tang, T. et al. (2004). Post-migration changes in gender relations among Ethiopian couples living in Canada. *Canadian Journal of Nursing Research, 36* (4), 74–89.

Kaspar, V. & Noh, S. (2001, November). *Discrimination and Identity: An Overview of Theoretical and Empirical Research.* Ethnocultural, Racial, Religious, and Linguistic Diversity and Identity Seminar, Halifax, NS.

Kessler, R.C. (2000). Gender differences in major depression: Epidemiological findings. In E. Frank (Ed.), *Gender and Its Effect on Psychopathology* (pp. 61–84). Washington, DC: American Psychiatric Press.

Khandor, E., McDonald, J., Nyers, P. & Wright, C. (2004). *The Regularization of Non-Status Immigrants in Canada, 1960–2004: Past Policies, Current Perspectives, Active Campaigns.* Toronto: STATUS Campaign. Available: www.ocasi.org/status/Regularization_booklet.pdf. Accessed January 15, 2008.

Kinnon, D. (1999). *Canadian Research on Immigration and Health: An Overview.* Ottawa: Minister of Public Works and Government Services.

Kirmayer, L.J. (2001). Cultural variations in the clinical presentation of depression and anxiety: Implications for diagnosis and treatment. *Journal of Clinical Psychiatry, 62* (Suppl. 13), 221–227.

Kirmayer, L.J. & Groleau, D. (2001). Affective disorders in cultural context. *Cultural Psychiatry: International Perspectives, 24* (3), 465–478.

Kleinman, A. (1988). *Rethinking Psychiatry*. New York: The Free Press.

Krieger, N. (2000). Discrimination and health. In L. Berkman & I. Kawachi (Eds.), *Social Epidemiology* (pp. 36–75). Oxford: Oxford University Press.

Krieger, N. (2001). A glossary for social epidemiology. *Journal of Epidemiology and Community Health, 55* (10), 693–700.

Langford, C.P.H., Bowsher, J., Maloney, J.P. & Lillis, P.P. (1997). Social support: A conceptual analysis. *Journal of Advanced Nursing, 25* (1), 95–100.

Lorant, V., Deliege, D., Eaton, W., Robert, A., Philippot, P. & Ansseau, M. (2003). Socioeconomic inequalities in depression: A meta-analysis. *American Journal of Epidemiology, 157* (2), 98–112.

Lynch, J. & Kaplan, G. (2000). Socioeconomic position. In L. Berkman & I. Kawachi (Eds.), *Social Epidemiology* (pp. 13–35). New York: Oxford University Press.

Maughan B. (2002). Depression and psychological distress: A life course perspective. In D. Kuh & R. Hardy (Eds.), *A Life Course Approach to Women's Health*. New York: Oxford University Press.

Mawani, F.N. (2001). Sharing Attachment Across Cultures: Learning from Immigrants and Refugees. Ottawa: Health Canada.

McDonough, P. & Walters, V. (2001). Gender and health: Reassessing patterns and explanations. *Social Science and Medicine, 52* (4), 547–559.

McIsaac, E. (2003). Immigrants in Canadian cities: Census 2002—What do the data tell us? *Policy Options, 24* (5), 58–63.

Miranda, J., Chung, J.Y., Green, B.L., Krupnick, J., Siddique, J., Revicki, D.A. et al. (2003). Treating depression in predominantly low-income young minority women: A randomized controlled trial. *Journal of the American Medical Association, 290* (1), 57–65.

Moss, N.E. (2002). Gender equity and socioeconomic inequality: A framework for the patterning of women's health. *Social Science and Medicine, 54* (2), 649–661.

Mulvihill, M.A., Mailloux, L. & Atkin, W. (2001). *Advancing Policy and Research Responses to Immigrant and Refugee Women's Health in Canada*. Winnipeg, MB: Centres of Excellence for Women's Health.

Muntaner, C., Eaton, W.W., Miech, R. & O'Campo, P. (2004). Socioeconomic position and major mental disorders. *Epidemiologic Reviews, 26* (1), 53–62.

Mustard, J.F. (1996). Health and social capital. In D. Blane, E. Brunner & R. Wilkinson (Eds.), *Health and Social Organization: Towards a Health Policy for the 21st Century* (pp. 303–313). New York: Routledge.

Noh, S., Beiser, M., Kaspar, V., Hou, F. & Rummens, J. (1999). Perceived racial discrimination, depression, and coping: A study of Southeast Asian refugees in Canada. *Journal of Health and Social Behavior, 40* (3), 193–207.

Noh, S., Speechley, M., Kaspar, V. & Wu, Z. (1992). Depression in Korean immigrants in Canada: I. Method of the study and prevalence of depression. *Journal of Nervous and Mental Disease, 180* (9), 573–577.

Nolen-Hoeksema, S. (1995). Epidemiology and theories of gender differences in unipolar depression. In M.V. Seeman (Ed.), *Gender and Psychopathology* (pp. 63–87). Washington, DC: American Psychiatric Press.

Omidvar, R. & Richmond, T. (2003). *Immigrant Settlement and Social Inclusion in Canada*. Perspectives on Social Inclusion: Working Paper Series. Toronto: Laidlaw Foundation.

Public Health Agency of Canada. (2002). *Population Health Approach*. Available: www.phac-aspc.gc.ca/ph-sp/phdd/approach/index.html. Accessed January 5, 2008.

Rodgers, B. (2002). Commentary on "Depression and psychological distress: a life course perspective." In D. Kuh & R. Hardy (Eds.), *A Life Course Approach to Women's Health*. New York: Oxford University Press.

Rousseau, C., Mekki-Berrada, A. & Moreau, S. (2001). Trauma and extended separation from family among Latin American and African refugees in Montreal. *Psychiatry, 64* (1), 40–59.

Rousseau, C. & Drapeau, A. (2004). Premigration exposure to political violence among independent immigrants and its association with emotional distress. *Journal of Nervous and Mental Disease, 192* (12), 852–856.

Ruddick, E. (2003, March). *Immigrant Economic Performance: A New Paradigm in a Changing Labour Market*. Paper presented at the 6th National Metropolis Conference, Edmonton, AB.

Salokangas, R.K.R., Vaahtera, K., Pacriev, S., Sohlman, B. & Lehtinen, V. (2002). Gender differences in depressive symptoms: An artefact caused by measurement instruments? *Journal of Affective Disorders, 68* (2–3), 215–220.

Sherbourne, C.D. & Stewart, A.L. (1991). The MOS social support survey. *Social Science and Medicine, 32* (6), 705–714.

Simich, L., Beiser, M. & Mawani, F.N. (2003). Social support and the significance of shared experience in refugee migration and resettlement. *Western Journal of Nursing Research, 25* (7), 872–891.

Simich, L., Mawani, F., Wu, F. & Noor, A. (2004). *Meanings of Social Support, Coping, and Help-Seeking Strategies among Immigrants and Refugees in Toronto*. CERIS Working Paper Series, No. 31. Available: www.ceris.metropolis.net/Virtual%20Library/health/2004%20CWPs/CWP31_Simich%20etal.pdf. Accessed January 5, 2008.

Simich, L., Rummens, J.A., Andermann, L. & Lo, T. (2006). *Mental Health in Public-Health Policy and Practice: Providing Culturally Appropriate Services in Acute and Post-Emergency Situations*. CERIS Working Paper Series, No. 43. Available: http://ceris.metropolis.net/annual%20reports/05_06Report/Appendix111.pdf. Accessed January 15, 2008

Singh-Manoux, A., Clarke, P. & Marmot, M. (2002). Multiple measures of socio-economic position and psychosocial health: Proximal and distal measures. *International Journal of Epidemiology, 31* (6), 1192–1199.

Spitzer, D.L. (2005). Engendering health disparities. *Canadian Journal of Public Health, 96* (Suppl. 2), S78–96.

Statistics Canada. (2001). Selected Income Characteristics (35), Immigrant Status and Place of Birth of Respondent (21B), Age Groups (6), Sex (3) and Immigrant Status and Period of Immigration (11) for Population, for Canada, Provinces, Territories and Census Metropolitan Areas, 2001 Census—20% Sample Data. Ottawa: Author. Catalogue No. 97F0009XCB01043. Available: www12.statcan.ca/english/census01/products/standard/themes/RetrieveProductTable.cfm?Temporal=2001&PID=68538&APATH=3&GID=517770&METH=1&PTYPE=55496&THEME=43&FOCUS=0&AID=0&PLACENAME=0&PROVINCE=0&SEARCH=0&GC=99&GK=NA&VID=0&FL=0&RL=0&FREE=0. Accessed January 5, 2008.

Statistics Canada. (2003). *Ethnic Diversity Survey: Portrait of a Multicultural Society*. Ottawa: Minister of Industry. Catalogue No. 89-593-XIE. Available: www.statcan.ca/english/freepub/89-593-XIE/89-593-XIE2003001.pdf. Accessed January 5, 2008.

Stewart, D.E., Gucciardi, E. & Grace, S.L. (2003). Depression. In *Women's Health Surveillance Report: A Multi-dimensional Look at the Health of Canadian Women*. Ottawa: Canadian Institute for Health Information. Available: http://secure.cihi.ca/cihiweb/dispPage.jsp?cw_page=PG_29_E&cw_topic=29. Accessed January 8, 2008.

Taylor, S.E. & Seeman, T.E. (1999). Psychosocial resources and the SES-health relationship. *Annals of the New York Academy of Sciences, 896* (1), 210–225.

Thoits, P.A. (1991). On merging identity theory and stress research. *Social Psychology Quarterly, 54* (2), 101–112.

Turner, R.J., Lloyd, D.A. & Roszell, P. (1999). Personal resources and the social distribution of depression. *American Journal of Community Psychology, 27* (5), 643–672.

Ussher, J.M. (2000). Women and mental illness. In L. Sherr and J. St. Lawrence (Eds.), *Women, Health and the Mind*. West Sussex, UK: John Wiley & Sons, Ltd.

Watkins, P.L. & Whaley, D. (2000). Gender role stressors and women's health. In R.M. Eisler & M. Hersen (Eds.), *Handbook of Gender, Culture, and Health* (pp. 43–46). Mahwah, NJ: Lawrence Erlbaum Associates.

Wheaton, B. (1999). Social stress. In C.S. Aneshensel & J.C. Phelan (Eds.), *Handbook of the Sociology of Mental Health*. New York: Kluwer Academic/Plenum Publishers.

Williams, C.L. & Berry, J.W. (1991). Primary prevention of acculturative stress among refugees: Application of psychological theory and practice. *American Psychologist, 46* (6), 632–641.

Winkleby, M.A., Jatulis, D.E., Frank, E. & Formann, S.P. (1992). Socioeconomic status and health: How education, income, and occupation contribute to risk factors for cardiovascular disease. *American Journal of Public Health, 82* (6), 816–820.

World Health Organization. (n.d.). *Gender Disparities in Mental Health*. Geneva: WHO, Department of Mental Health and Substance Dependence. Available: www.who.int/entity/mental_health/media/en/242.pdf. Accessed January 5, 2008.

World Health Organization. (2000). *Women's Mental Health: An Evidence Based Review*. Geneva: WHO, Department of Mental Health and Substance Dependence. Available: http://whqlibdoc.who.int/hq/2000/WHO_MDS_MDP_00.1.pdf. Accessed January 5, 2008.

Wu, Z., Noh, S., Kaspar, V. & Schimmele, C.M. (2003). Race, ethnicity, and depression in Canadian society. *Journal of Health and Social Behavior, 44* (3), 426–441.

Zelkowitz, P., Schinazi, J., Katofsky, L., Saucier, J.F., Valenzuela, M., Westreich, R. et al. (2004). Factors associated with depression in pregnant immigrant women. *Transcultural Psychiatry, 41* (4), 445–464.

Chapter 5

Recognizing Spirituality as a Vital Component in Mental Health Care

ENID COLLINS

In the last few decades, people in western societies have increasingly turned to eastern-based philosophies to find answers to healing that have been missing in our mainstream medical practices. People are now adopting holistic approaches[1] that integrate body, mind and spirit as a way to find meaning in their lives, promote health and wellness and slow the aging process. Mainstream health care practitioners—including doctors, psychiatrists, nurses and psychologists—have also acknowledged connections between mind, body and spirit. (Chopra, 1993; Dossey, 1991, 1996.) However, *spirituality*—with its focus on the spirit or soul rather than the physical or psychological—still plays a marginal role in mainstream medical and mental health practice (Cherry, 1999; Helman, 2000). Newcomers to Canada—many of whom arrive from countries where spirituality is assumed to be an integral part of health and healing—are met with a health care system that often doesn't even acknowledge the role of the spiritual.

Since the 19th century, allopathic medicine (medicine that treats disease conventionally, i.e., with remedies such as drugs producing opposite effects to the symptoms) has been the main focus of medical practice in western countries. Allopathic medicine, with its scientific rationales for the causes and cures of illness, and its use of bio-medical

---

1. Holistic approaches include homoeopathy, naturopathy, Ayurveda, traditional Chinese medicine, energy therapy, chiropractic, yoga and meditation. Healing systems such as Ayurveda and traditional Chinese medicine, which emphasize wholeness of mind, body and spirit, have existed in India and China for centuries (Ng, 2002; Shroff, 2000). Chinese medicine has roots that date back to the 1300s and Ayurvedic medicine existed in India for over five thousand years. The influences of colonialism eroded these and other indigenous systems of healing.

technology to treat illness and disease, has privileged drugs and surgical interventions as the primary, accepted methods of treating disease.

An allopathic approach to medicine supports reductionism, an approach that views the body as separate parts that can be treated individually. Specialization in medicine is organized on this premise (Helman, 2000; Rosenberg, 2002; Shroff, 2000). The resulting separation of body, mind and spirit contributes to the marginalization of spirituality in healing modalities. Because the mental health system usually operates within the medical model, expressions of spirituality—often an integral part of the lives of immigrant and refugee women—have also been marginalized. This chapter invites mental health practitioners to consider practice approaches that recognize spirituality as central to holistic care for immigrant and refugee women in Canada.

Rituals that Celebrate and Support Women

Throughout human history, holistic healing practices were carried out by women whose knowledge had been passed down from one generation to the next through various forms of oral communication, such as folklore, dances, chants and parables. These different types of communication gave voice to diverse forms of spiritual expression that are part of diverse cultural identities. They are present in cultural traditions of Aboriginal People in Canada as well as in some African cultures (Elabor-Idemudia, 2002; Rosenberg, 2002). Health and wholeness were associated with harmony in nature; natural substances from plants and animals were often used to treat various illnesses. Women in some matriarchal cultures were revered as givers of life. Various rituals associated with pregnancy, childbirth and initiation of an infant into a social group are strongly linked to spiritual expressions. Rituals are important parts of all human societies. They contribute to the maintenance, celebration and renewal of social groups. In societies around the world, rituals surrounding events that mark significant life transitions include spiritual symbols and celebration. Women are usually at the centre of these celebrations (Helman, 2000; Rosenberg, 2002).

Women express spirituality, including religious beliefs, through various language constructs that come from their cultural contexts. For example, some women may use dialects, metaphors and proverbs that are unique to their culture. In some cultures, stories that connect women to important life events may be learned through oral traditions that are passed from one generation to another (Elabor-Idemudia, 2002; Rosenberg, 2002). Language provides the vehicle for "expressions of inner longings and meaningful interpretation of the world and a person's experience in it" (Swinton, 2001, p. 148). Women's friendships, circles of healing and religious rituals are additional ways that women express spirituality. For example, in western societies, including Canada, rituals such as baby and wedding showers, are demonstrations of the support that women friendships represent.

Women supporting other women during significant life transitions are part of cultures around the world. Celebrations and ceremonies usually bring together extended family, friends and community. For example, blessings of infants and naming ceremonies are important events that can take on spiritual meaning. For many cultural groups, a religious component is part of these rituals. (In Chapter 16, Paola Ardiles, Cindy-Lee Dennis and Lori Ross discuss the role of rituals in caring for a new mother during the postpartum period, especially during the first 30 to 40 days following childbirth.) Some cultural groups, such as Latin Americans, may require the mother and infant to wear various religious charms or amulets to protect them against the *evil eye* (Helman, 2000)—strong glances cast by an envious person that can result in mental illness. For immigrant and refugee women who are separated from their family and community, the opportunity to participate in rituals around life transitions and to share a spiritual connection may be lost during the initial phase of uprooting and resettlement in a new country. This loss may add another layer of stress that could contribute to mental health problems.

As newcomer women resettle and rebuild their lives in Canada, they may seek to join various faith communities that also provide spiritual resources and material support. However, some groups may also create obstacles to women if gender oppression continues in these faith-based groups, which might, in turn, negatively affect the mental and physical health of immigrant and refugee women. Gender oppression can negatively affect women's lives in many ways; for example, rigidly defined gender roles may constrain creative expression of their spirituality and result in women being excluded from positions of leadership in faith-based groups.

Religion versus Spirituality

There is a tendency to equate spirituality with religion. However, despite some commonalities, there are significant differences between these concepts.

Religion includes numerous organized systems, each of which has its own unique set of doctrines, rituals, structures and beliefs and operates within a strong institutional context. Followers of various religions are expected to adhere to tenets of their faith. Among the most common world religions, monotheistic religions such as Christianity, Islam and Judaism advocate achieving spirituality through a divine power, a single god (Levin, 2001). Patriarchy is an institutionalized feature of religions worldwide. Many women participate in religious communities, yet they are often barred from positions of leadership and power. Most religions base their support for adherence to rigid gender roles on various scriptures. However, Smith (2000) analyzed how some sections of Christian scripture that are used to justify subordination of women could also be used to affirm and support women in developing leadership roles within Christian communities.

Spirituality is a broader concept than religion that cannot be defined by any one model. It encompasses the relationship of the individual to the wider universe. Some descriptors of spirituality found in literature include love; hope; purpose; meaning of life; meaningful relationships; as well as connections with the wider universe, the sacred and the divine, a higher being and the environment. Elkins describes the elements of spirituality this way:

> Spirituality refer[s] to . . . the breath of life. It involves opening up our hearts and cultivating our capacity to experience awe, reverence and gratitude. It is the ability to see the sacred in the ordinary, to feel the poignancy of life, to know the passion of existence and to give ourselves over to that which is greater than ourselves. Its aim: to bring about compassion. Its effect: good physical and mental health. (Elkins, 1999, p. 46)

Women express their spirituality in numerous ways. They may form spiritual connections that include networks, prayer groups, yoga, meditation and art. For some groups, such as black people, who for generations experienced racial discrimination, spiritual expression has included "singing, dancing, mourning, affirming, worshipping, contemplating, reflecting, shouting, praying, preaching and testifying" (Martin & Martin, 2002, p. 1).

For many people, participation in organized religion enables them to express and celebrate their spirituality. Others find many ways beyond religion to express spirituality.

Research Linking Spirituality to Positive Health Outcomes

Since the 1970s, research that links religion, spirituality and health has grown (Dossey, 1991; Levin, 2001), and research designs have also become more rigorous. Among the various elements of spirituality, religious aspects are the most frequently researched. This could be related to the notion that spirituality has traditionally been associated with religion. As well, it has been easier to describe and develop measures for some religious practices (Harrison & Condon, 2004).

For example, activities such as praying, attending and actively participating in the church, synagogue, temple or mosque, as well as religious support are among the variables included in research on religion and health. Levin (2001), an epidemiologist whose work focuses on religion, spirituality and health, reviewed more than 300 studies investigating links between various aspects of religion and heart and circulatory conditions such as hardening of the arteries, heart attacks, high blood pressure and other conditions, including arthritis and cancer. Cumulatively, research findings demonstrate positive outcomes associated with religious participation in people who have various diseases (Cherry, 1999; Dossey, 1996; Levin, 2001).

Based on the findings of a randomized and double-blinded clinical trial at the School of Medicine at University of California, San Francisco, Byrd (1988) noted significant positive outcomes between religious interventions and heart disease among 400 patients. Patients in the experimental group were given relevant medical treatment for their cardiac condition and, in addition, were assigned to prayer groups where they were prayed for by Catholics and Protestants drawn from across the United States. Each person in the group was prayed for by five to seven people. Patients in the control group received only medical treatment appropriate to their condition. Patients in the group that was not prayed for developed more complications than those in the group that received prayers. Three times as many patients in the not-prayed-for group developed fluid in their lungs, and five times as many patients in that group required antibiotics compared with those in the group that was prayed for (Byrd, 1988; Harrison & Condon, 2004; Levin, 2001).

Harris and colleagues' (1999) study at the Mid America Heart Institute in Kansas City, Missouri, used a similar design with the intent to replicate the Byrd study. The researchers randomly divided more than 900 patients into two groups: a prayer group and a control group. The patients in the prayer group were assigned to teams of people who were asked to pray for them daily for four weeks. Patients in the group that was prayed for did better in their overall clinical symptoms than those in the group that was not prayed for (Harris et al., 1999; Harrison & Condon, 2004; Swinton, 2001).

Despite strong evidence linking aspects of religion and spirituality to positive health outcomes, how these effects occur is not well understood. Several authors (Dossey, 1996; Levin, 2001; Swinton, 2001) suggest that spirituality leads to increased self-esteem, a sense of well-being, meaning and purpose in life, increased social support in both tangible and intangible ways, and a sense of community and lessened isolation. From my observations, worship and outreach programs offered to immigrant and refugee women in faith communities include inviting them to supportive activities such as seasonal celebrations that introduce them to customary Canadian rituals; providing them with needed goods such as clothing, furniture and shelter; and offering English-language skills. Those who access these programs are frequently women who are raising young children.

Research Linking Spirituality to Mental Health

Although most studies focus on various aspects of religious affiliation and physical health problems, some researchers are now investigating the role of spirituality, especially its links to mental health (Dossey, 1991, 1996; Swinton, 2001). For example, a recent Canadian study examined effects of home-based spirituality education in people with mood disturbances (Moritz et al., 2006). Research conducted by Moritz and colleagues (2006) between 2001 and 2002 at the University of Calgary, in conjunction with the Canadian Institute of Natural and Integrative Medicine (CINIM), examined the effects of an eight-week home-based spirituality education program on its ability to improve mood and quality of life for patients with mood disturbances. The researchers conducted a randomized clinical trial with 165 people with mood disorders who were randomly assigned to one of three groups: (1) a home-based spirituality education program, which was developed by CINIM; (2) a mindful meditation program; and (3) no treatment. All participants continued to take medications that were previously prescribed. Group 1 underwent an audiotaped education program over an eight-week period that covered concepts about the role of spirituality in their lives. Group 2 attended an eight-week program where participants practised mindful meditation with an instructor. They were also asked to practice mindful meditation at home daily for eight weeks, and were given an audio-taped program that they could listen to before their daily practice. Group 3 received no treatment, but at the end of the 12-week study they were given the home-based spirituality education program.

Evaluation of mood disturbances was measured by a tool consisting of several items that described anger, depressed mood, confusion, fatigue, tension and vigour. Quality of life was measured by another tool, which included several items that described dimensions of physical, social and mental health. Data were analyzed using quantitative methods. The researchers reported that at the end of eight weeks and 12 weeks, Group 1, the group that had received the home-based spirituality education program, demonstrated marked improvement in mood and quality of life.

Schreiber and her colleagues (2000) studied the experiences of a group of West Indian women in Toronto. Findings of their study demonstrated that these women used a social process called "being strong." Reliance on their belief in God was part of the strategy that gave them strength to deal with depression.

In his book *Spirituality and Mental Health Care: Rediscovering a Forgotten Dimension* (2001), Swinton reported the findings of a study on the link between spirituality and depression:

> As one reflects on the nature of depression, it becomes clear that it is a profoundly spiritual experience that cannot be understood and dealt with through drugs and therapy alone. Its central features of profound hopelessness, loss of meaning in life, perceived loss of relationship with God or a higher power, low self-esteem and general sense of purposelessness, all indicate a level of spiritual distress. (pp. 95–96)

The three women and three men participants in Swinton's qualitative study indicated that spirituality:

- provided a meaningful framework that helped people to cope with depression
- offered meaningful answers when the participants lost hope and questioned everything that seemed inexplicable
- gave people strength to hang on when life seemed like an abyss
- provided participants with a source of hope to deal with pain and suicidal thoughts, even when life seemed desolate
- strengthened people's resolve when social connections were weakened and they felt "isolated, lonely and unable to find a foothold back into relationships and community" (Swinton, 2001, p. 118).

Spirituality in the Post-Migration Context

Gender roles are embedded in the social, political, economic and religious fabric of society. For example, in some cultures women work in the agricultural sector, planting and reaping harvest while caring for children and families. Ceremonies to mark harvest gathering, or even to celebrate environmental changes such as giving thanks for rain after prolonged droughts, take on some form of spiritual expression. These sorts of celebrations bring solidarity to communities. Traditional agricultural methods were commonly used in some African societies until they were eroded by colonial influences. Women played important roles in the economy by making decisions about agriculture, such as what crops to plant and consume (Elabor-Idemudia, 2002).

Experiences of immigrant and refugee women are shaped by multiple and changing identities that reflect history, culture, gender, race, religion, education, language and other factors. The processes of uprooting and resettlement disrupt some identities and create major stresses for these women. For many immigrant and refugee women, loss of familiar ways of expressing spirituality, compounded by lack of employment opportunities and downward mobility, disrupt the ability to meet physical needs such as housing and may lead to impaired physical and mental health. Separation of parents and children can be especially traumatic. (See Chapter 10 on the challenges faced by Caribbean women and their children who are separated and then reunite during the immigration process.)

Opportunities to celebrate significant milestones such as birthdays and graduations and to mark other important events with, for example, funeral rituals involving whole communities are lost to these women. The separation can be so deeply felt that it is not uncommon for family members to return the remains of loved ones who have lived in Canada for many years to their home countries to be interred. The funeral ceremonies in the home country provide opportunities for extended family and community members (even those who have been separated for prolonged periods) to celebrate as well as to bring closure to the grieving process. For women who are not able to participate in celebrations, separation leads to increased anxiety and ultimately to further social isolation as they grow apart from family and familiar community.

In addition, some refugee women may have witnessed or experienced violence including rape or torture or observed the murder of loved ones, and may not have had the chance to grieve with family and community. Sudden separation from families and communities robs women of supports in expressing spirituality while going through grieving and healing experiences. (While Chapter 14 addresses trauma work with Latin American women, the clinical discussion is relevant to women from any culture.)

GENDER AND FAITH COMMUNITIES

For women from many cultural groups who maintain religious affiliations, faith communities form a major part of their identity, even though institutionalized gender oppression may exist within these communities (Stuckey, 1998). Women who are faithful to their religious traditions may accept these realities without question or may not see viable opportunities to challenge such practices. As women begin to adjust to a new society, some may find new ways to exercise agency by challenging long-standing patriarchal traditions that have impeded their spiritual expression. For example, immigrant women members of the Muslim Canadian Congress challenge gender inequality in their faith community by leading mixed-gender prayers (Teotonio, 2005).

Participation in faith communities provides connections and enables women to build new friendships as they settle in Canada. They look inward to the community for support, such as finding appropriate friends for their children and eventually marriage partners. Mosques become gathering places where many activities, including social group meetings for women and youth take place (Elmi, 1999; Rosenberg, 1999). Among women who represent newcomer groups, such as Somalis and Palestinians, these connections to community provide positive spaces where women express their spiritual connections, which might lessen the stresses of uprooting and separation (Isrealite et al., 1999). However, some women who are not landed immigrants may attend faith communities but may not feel comfortable disclosing their immigration status; as a result, they may be marginalized within the faith group. Divisions among cultural groups related to ethnic, language or religious differences may add another layer of stress.

Many health maintenance practices of women immigrants and refugees are culturally based and include a wide range of beliefs about how people conduct their lives including eating habits, dress, prayer and rituals to stay well or regain health when they become ill. In some societies, ritual wearing of amulets, charms and religious medals to bring good luck or ward off bad luck or ill health are part of everyday practice. People with mental or physical illnesses may seek indigenous healers who are part of the local community (Helman, 2000). In Chapter 9, the authors describe how Sudanese women have different cultural definitions and meanings of mental health, and they urge mental health professionals to incorporate indigenous beliefs and practices into their work.

PERCEPTIONS OF MENTAL ILLNESS: VARIATIONS BETWEEN CLIENTS AND PRACTITIONERS

Mental health practitioners may not be aware of immigrant and refugee women's unique experiences. This lack of understanding may lead to inaccurate diagnosis and treatment. For example, a practitioner may be unwilling to explore a woman's perception that her illness is caused by a curse or the evil eye. In addition, a woman may have difficulty speaking in English and expressing the cultural meanings of her experience.

Psychiatrists may prescribe psychotropic drugs or other treatment for women's symptoms without considering their beliefs and life experiences. While women may respond differently to psychotropic drugs than men, research hasn't sufficiently explored these differences. And drug companies use advertisements to promote the use of psychotropic drugs as a solution to women's problems (Helman, 1992; Shroff, 2000).

Integrating Spirituality into Mental Health Care

How can mental health practitioners work with immigrant and refugee women to develop strategies that include women's spirituality as an integral part of their practice? How can mental health practitioners promote holistic healing? Answers to these questions are complex and require critical examination of how mental health services are structured and implemented. Practitioners need to develop new ways of thinking and framing practice beyond the medical model.

A THEORETICAL FRAMEWORK

Jean Watson provides an excellent framework for integrating spirituality in care. She writes for a nursing audience, but the concepts she discusses are relevant for other mental health practitioners. Watson views people as having dimensions of mind, body and spirit, which, in healthy states, are in harmony (as cited in Rafael, 2000). Watson believes that illness occurs as a result of conscious or unconscious disharmony among the three. In other words, people are able to consciously change their situation. She stresses three components, which are integral to interactions between the person and the nurse:

- The lived experiences of the person and nurse or other caregiver are critical when both come together in a caring moment.
- Unique dimensions of mind, body and spirit make up the wholeness of the person.
- People have multiple ways of knowing. These include four distinct ways: empirical (knowledge based), aesthetic (creative ideas such as music, art, dance), metaphysical (connections with a higher being) and humanistic (connections with other human beings).

Watson advocates that practitioners engage in transpersonal caring, in which they try to understand the worldview of clients and consider the meanings of their life events (as cited in Rafael, 2000).

Mental health practitioners should consider holistic approaches that view the body, mind and spirit as an integrated whole, and that acknowledge spirituality as central in the healing process. Women who seek wholeness and transformation through spirituality should have a plan of care that includes the practices that they value in promoting healing. They must be seen as agents in control of their health who engage in healing practices that influence their whole life.

Mental health practitioners who are not already committed to holistic practices need to develop new lenses through which they may attempt to understand the experiences of immigrant and refugee women. They may need to go beyond their personal and professional perspectives, which may mean suspending their perceptions of cultural and professional privilege. Swinton (2001) states that mental health caregivers need to develop therapeutic understanding in their work. They need to "cross 'over'" (p. 141) into the clients' experience and communicate understanding and empathy.

PRACTICAL STRATEGIES FOR MENTAL HEALTH PRACTITIONERS

Self-awareness

- Consider practice from a philosophical standpoint whereby self-awareness underlies every encounter. Some self-reflective questions to consider asking are: What are my own views on spirituality? How do my views influence decisions in my practice?
- Consider situations that might lead to moral and ethical dilemmas—when values are in conflict either on a personal, interpersonal or societal level. Questions that practitioners might ask are: What issues create moral and ethical dilemmas in my practice? Which of my personal values are challenged?
- Ask critical questions, such as: How comfortable am I working with women from various sexual orientations and cultural and religious groups? Do I consider their behaviours quaint or bizarre? What biases get in the way of providing care?
- Acquire knowledge concerning physical, cultural and spiritual dimensions of women's experiences by asking women about their spirituality, and about their beliefs about illness, such as: What do you think is the cause of your illness? What do you do to stay healthy? What are your beliefs about the meaning of life? Do you participate in a religious/faith community?

Advocacy

- Support a common goal to develop holistic strategies that honour women's experiences as holistic and that include physical, mental and spiritual aspects.
- Honour women's values and beliefs and challenge actions of colleagues that may devalue or negate women's experiences.
- Challenge institutional practices, policies and procedures that create barriers to spiritual expression and work to provide a safe space where women can express and affirm unique spiritual expression.

Knowledge

- Acknowledge various formal and informal ways of knowing (including knowledge gained through cumulative life experiences). Explore unique ways of knowing and expressing spirituality. Ask women what might help them to connect to their spirituality, such as their previous practices around music, prayer, poems, imagery, meditation, dance, and rituals and practices.
- Establish a climate in which a woman can develop the trust needed for her to feel comfortable sharing her experience. Use open statements, such as, "Tell me about any experiences that are meaningful for you." Be alert for cues that she is ready to talk about such experiences.
- Recognize that women's experiences are derived from intersections of cultural, historical, social, political, racialized and gendered positions, which change as they deal with new situations.

Communication

- Be vigilant about language used in encounters with clients. Do not lump clients together as disease entities and refer to them with labels such as "schizophrenics" or "bipolars." Identify them as people first, for example, "women living with schizophrenia."
- Recognize legitimate roadblocks to women's sharing; for example, a woman who has experienced torture may not be open to talking with a health professional about some past experiences. (Chapter 12 addresses the difficulty some women have in disclosing stories of persecution when seeking refugee status.)
- Use resource people such as interpreters wisely. In some cultures, mental health problems may be stigmatized, such that women may not feel comfortable telling their story through certain individuals. The interpreters may not translate a woman's words accurately, to protect the woman from what may be perceived as dangerous information. The interpreter may also want to present the cultural group in a positive light when translating information related to issues that are stigmatized. (For more information on translation and interpretation, see Chapter 6 on the community interpreter.)
- Recognize and acknowledge points of vulnerability. For example, some women who speak with a distinct accent or are not fluent in English may feel uncomfortable expressing themselves for fear of ridicule.

Agency

- People have the ability to make decisions and take action on their own behalf. Explore with women their strengths, and affirm past and present accomplishments. (See Chapter 14 on trauma work with Latin American women in Canada.)
- Help women use and build on their strengths. Strategies include helping women to develop realistic goals and plans to reach their goals.
- Encourage women to find their voice, and to talk about their values and beliefs about their health and illness. Facilitating statements are helpful, such as:

"What are your thoughts about your health situation?" Some women come to a point where they use their own experience to become advocates and mentors for other women.

Community
- Encourage women to align with communities that are empowering. For example, some communities provide positive mentoring and support where women may learn life skills and find role models for themselves and their children. However, as noted in Chapter 12 on trauma among refugee women and Chapter 7 on services for immigrant women, communities where persistent conflict exists can create added stress for women.

Conclusion

In this chapter, I have argued that spirituality is an integral part of the experiences of many immigrant and refugee women in Canada. Most women who are uprooted suffer hardships. Refugee women's lives are further complicated by forced migration often due to war, violence and/or persecution. Multiple stressors take their toll on women, causing many to seek mental health care from a system that is usually based on the medical model and in which expressions of spirituality are marginalized. Most women demonstrate fortitude and resilience and go on to successfully adapt to life in the new country. Women who are immigrants and refugees experience various hardships associated with uprooting and resettlement. However, every woman has unique experiences, and mental health practitioners need to be mindful of each woman's vulnerabilities as well as strengths and incorporate spirituality as central to holistic approaches in mental health care for immigrant and refugee women.

References

Byrd, R.C. (1988). Positive therapeutic effects of intercessory prayer in a coronary care unit population. *Southern Medical Journal, 81* (7), 826–829.

Cherry, R. (1999). *Healing Prayer: God's Divine Intervention in Medicine, Faith and Prayer.* Caramel, NY: Guideposts.

Chopra, D. (1993). *Ageless Body, Timeless Mind: The Quantum Alternative to Growing Old.* New York: Three Rivers Press.

Dossey, L. (1991). *Meaning and Medicine: A Doctor's Tales of Breakthrough and Healing.* New York: Bantam Books.

Dossey, L. (1996). *Prayer Is Good Medicine.* San Francisco: Harper Collins.

Elabor-Idemudia, P.E. (2002). The retention of knowledge of folkways as a basis of resistance. In G. Dei, B. Hall & D. Rosenberg (Eds.), *Indigenous Knowledges in Global Contexts: Multiple Readings of Our Worlds* (pp. 102–119). Toronto: University of Toronto Press.

Elkins, D.N. (1999, September/October). Spirituality: It's what's missing in mental health. *Psychology Today*, pp. 45–48.

Elmi, A.S. (1999, September). *A Study on the Mental Health Needs of the Somali Community in Toronto.* Toronto: York Community Services & Rexdale Community Health Centre. Available: http://ceris.metropolis.net/Virtual%20Library/health/elmi1.pdf. Accessed January 15, 2008.

Harris, W.S., Gowda, M., Kolb, J.W., Strychacz, C.P., Vacek, J.L. Jones, P.G. et al. (1999). A randomized, controlled trial of the effects of intercessory prayer on outcomes in patients admitted to the coronary care unit. *Archives of Internal Medicine, 159* (19), 2273–2278.

Harrison, A. & Condon, M. (2004). Spiritual wellness and illness. In M. Condon, *Women's Health: Body, Mind and Spirit—An Integrated Approach to Wellness and Illness* (pp. 562–576). Upper Saddle River, NJ: Prentice Hall.

Helman, C. (1992). *Culture, Health and Illness* (2nd ed.). London: Butterworth-Heinemann.

Helman, C. (2000). *Culture, Health and Illness* (4th ed.). London: Butterworth-Heinemann.

Israelite, N., Herman, A., Alim, F., Mohamed, H., Khan, Y. & Caruso, L. (1999). Waiting for "Sharciga": Resettlement and the roles of Somali women. *Canadian Woman Studies: Immigrant and Refugee Women, 19* (3), 80–86.

Levin, J. (2001). *God, Faith and Health: Exploring the Spirituality-Healing Connection.* New York: John Wiley & Sons.

Martin, E.P. & Martin, J.M. (2002). *Spirituality and the Black Helping Tradition in Social Work.* Washington, DC: NASW Press.

Moritz, S., Quan, H., Rickhi, B., Liu, M., Angen, M., Vintila, R. et al. (2006). A home study–based spirituality education program decreases emotional distress and increases quality of life: A randomized, controlled trial. *Alternative Therapies, 12* (6), 26–35.

Ng, R. (2002). Toward an embodied pedagogy: Exploring health and the body through Chinese medicine. In G. Dei, B. Hall & D. Rosenberg (Eds.), *Indigenous Knowledges in Global Contexts: Multiple Readings of Our Worlds* (pp. 168–183). Toronto: University of Toronto Press.

Psychiatry Forum Needs Black Survivors. (2005, March 31). *Share.* Available: www.sharenews.com/2005_Archives/3-31-05-home.html, under the heading "Family." Accessed January 5, 2008.

Raphael, A.R. (2000). Watson's philosophy, science, and theory of human caring as a conceptual framework for guiding community health nursing practice. *Advances in Nursing Science, 23* (2), 34–49.

Rosenberg, C.E. (1999). Diversity and community: Palestinian women in Toronto. *Canadian Woman Studies: Immigrant and Refugee Women, 19* (3), 75–79.

Rosenberg, D.C. (2002). Toward indigenous wholeness: Feminist praxis in transformative learning on health and the environment. In G. Dei, B. Hall & D. Rosenberg (Eds.), *Indigenous Knowledges in Global Contexts: Multiple Readings of Our Worlds* (pp. 137–154). Toronto: University of Toronto Press.

Schreiber, R., Stern, P.N. & Wilson, C. (2000). Being strong: How Black West-Indian Canadian women manage depression and its stigma. *Journal of Nursing Scholarship, 32* (1), 39–45.

Shroff, F.M. (2000). Forget reform: We need a revolution! Better health for Canadian women through holistic care. In D.L. Gustafson (Ed.), *Care and Consequences: The Impact of Health Care Reform* (pp. 271–294). Halifax, NS: Fernwood.

Smith, M.B. (2000). *Gender or Giftedness: A Challenge to Rethink the Basis for Leadership within the Christian Community—A Study on the Role of Women Prepared for the Commission on Women's Concerns of the World Evangelical Fellowship.* Markham, ON: Evangelical Fellowship of Canada. Available: www.evangelicalfellowship.ca/resources/resource_viewer.asp?Resource_ID=51. Accessed January 5, 2008.

Stuckey, J.H. (1998). *Feminist Spirituality: An Introduction to Feminist Theology in Judaism, Christianity, Islam and Feminist Goddess Worship.* Toronto: York University, Centre for Feminist Research.

Swinton, J. (2001). *Spirituality and Mental Health Care: Rediscovering a "Forgotten" Dimension.* London: Jessica Kingsley.

Teotonio, I. (2005, April 23). Woman leads mixed-gender prayers for city Muslims. *Toronto Star,* p. A19. Available: www.muslimcanadiancongress.ca/20050423.pdf. Accessed January 5, 2008.

Chapter 6

The Community Interpreter
A Critical Link between Clients
and Service Providers[1]

DIANA ABRAHAM AND STELLA RAHMAN

Transnational migration is coloured by a myriad of circumstances that challenge, and demonstrate the resiliency of, individuals and families as they strive to deal with the emotional demands of adjusting to a strange new land. At the same time, service providers in the multidisciplinary field of mental health are also challenged as they try to understand and work with women from an increasingly diverse range of social locations, countries of origin, and ethno-racial and linguistic backgrounds. The population of women with limited proficiency in Canada's official languages is not limited to newly arrived immigrants. Indeed, many Aboriginal Peoples, who are fluent in one or more of their indigenous languages, have limited proficiency in English and French (Health Canada, 1998). Likewise, a number of women who are citizens and long-term residents of Canada are fluent in their mother tongue but have limited capacity in either of Canada's official languages (Health Canada & Interdepartmental Committee on Aging and Seniors Issues, 2002).

In this chapter, we address issues that come into play when clients and service providers in the mental health field do not share a common language. We provide a model for best practices when working with clients who have limited proficiency in English and French (LE/FP).[2] And we suggest actions for service providers and others in

1. Thank you to Marco Fiola, PhD, and Dorene Weston, MBA, of Full Circle Consulting, who provided valuable feedback on the drafting of this chapter.
2. We suggest that the term "limited English/French proficiency" (LE/FP) more accurately represents the reality of immigrant clients than does the term "non-English/non-French speakers."

the mental health field who are committed to providing quality care to female clients who have limited proficiency in Canada's official languages. This chapter:

- provides an overview of the current statistics on the number of females who are Aboriginal, Canadian citizens, newcomers and long-term residents who have limited proficiency in English and French
- addresses how language barriers affect program participants' access to services, inhibit the abilities of service providers to work with LE/FP program participants and contribute to the financial costs of services
- focuses on how the trained community interpreter is a critical link to the process of overcoming language barriers, provides an overview of the basic skills required to be a community interpreter and outlines the role and competencies of community interpreters in the health care sector
- addresses the role and code of ethics guiding community interpreters in mental health settings, and the paradigm shift (fundamental change in approach) that occurred when interpreter services were delivered at the Centre for Addiction and Mental Health in Toronto
- suggests guidelines for working with interpreters to deliver mental health care to LE/FP clients
- addresses how the lack of a public policy of language barriers contributes to social inequity, and suggests the need to push for the recognition of limited proficiency in the official languages as grounds for discrimination in the *Canadian Human Rights Act.*

Statistical Overview

Table 6-1, which is based on the most recently available Canadian census data (Statistics Canada, 2002), provides a snapshot of the total number of females who, in the terminology of Statistics Canada, have no knowledge of French or English.[3]

These statistics reflect the well-known demographic with respect to the provinces of British Columbia, Ontario and Quebec—and, in particular, the cities of Vancouver, Toronto and Montreal—as they are the primary settlement areas of immigrants and refugees to Canada. However, these statistics also indicate that while the numbers may be lower in other provinces, there are still female members of these key immigrant-settlement communities who have limited proficiency in the official languages and who may need services in the mental health sector. That these numbers are growing is evident in the narrative accompanying the census data, which noted that "Canada is becoming more and more a multilingual society in the wake of growing numbers of immigrants whose mother tongue is neither English nor French" (Statistics Canada, 2002).

---

3. For a breakdown of this data by territory and province, go to the Statistics Canada website at
    www12.statcan.ca/english/census01/Products/standard/themes/DataProducts.cfm?S=1&T=41&ALEVEL=2&FREE=0.

TABLE 6-1

Knowledge of Official Languages, 2001 Counts for Females

LOCATION	KNOWLEDGE OF OFFICIAL LANGUAGES				
	ENGLISH ONLY	FRENCH ONLY	ENGLISH AND FRENCH	NEITHER ENGLISH NOR FRENCH	TOTAL
Canada	10,048,410	2,125,875	2,628,760	271,705	15,074,760
Newfoundland and Labrador	246,105	80	12,450	365	258,995
Prince Edward Island	59,145	35	9,110	45	68,330
Nova Scotia	411,430	425	50,040	555	462,455
New Brunswick	205,255	35,530	126,200	235	367,220
Quebec	169,005	2,063,040	1,365,990	35,860	3,633,895
Ontario	4,868,410	23,950	721,590	142,455	5,756,400
Manitoba	497,950	655	56,520	5,675	560,800
Saskatchewan	458,955	165	27,250	1,760	488,125
Alberta	1,338,865	990	109,105	19,540	1,468,510
British Columbia	1,753,760	960	146,880	63,195	1,964,790
Yukon Territory	12,580	10	1,595	30	14,225
Northwest Territories	16,270	20	1,595	215	18,110
Nunavut	10,680	15	440	1,765	12,895

Source: Adapted with permission from Statistics Canada publication *Language Composition of Canada: Highlight Tables 2001 Census, Catalogue 97F0024XIE2001003*. Released date: December 10, 2002. www.statcan.ca/bsolc/english/bsolc?catno=97F0024XIE2001003.

Language Barriers to Mental Health Services

The 2001 Longitudinal Survey of Immigrants to Canada (Statistics Canada & Citizenship and Immigration Canada, 2003) found that 15 per cent (or 4,400) of the immigrants who participated in the survey cited language as a barrier to access to health care services in general.

Empirical Canadian research into the ways the presence of language barriers inhibits the access and delivery of health care services to LE/FP patient populations is limited.[4] One investigation of this area is Bowen's (2001) literature review *Language Barriers in Access to Health Care*. Although not specific to the mental health sector, Bowen's investigation signalled that language, rather than cultural beliefs and practices of patients, may be the most significant barrier to initial contact with health services. While the evidence is limited, there is also some suggestion that LE/FP may result in high use of specialist and diagnostic services (Bowen, 2001). Furthermore, LE/FP client populations are thought to have reduced access to mental health and counselling-related services. Bowen's literature review also suggests that delays in seeking care and lack of understanding of diagnoses

4. Flores et al. (2003) has written one of the few empirical studies on the consequences of interpreter errors.

and compliance with treatment may also be due to language barriers. Of particular concern are the ways in which language barriers may compromise the quality of care. Improperly trained interpreters may not appropriately follow a code of ethics around confidentiality, and also not take the necessary steps to obtain patient consent. Furthermore, patients who do not speak the same language as their health care providers consistently report lower satisfaction than those who share the same language as their provider. This last finding in Bowen was validated in the research component of the Strengthening Access to Primary Health Care project sponsored by the Toronto-based Healthcare Interpretation Network, in which one service provider observed that clients with limited official language proficiency are:

> often unable to say everything they would like to, or ask the questions they have in mind. They can't advocate for themselves, and they can't adequately navigate through the health care system. As a result, the quality of care they receive suffers. (Abraham & Neilson, 2004)

EFFECTS ON SERVICE PROVIDERS, RESEARCH PARTICIPATION AND COSTS

In addition to the direct effects on patient access and care, Bowen (2001) indicates that language barriers also have a number of other effects on the treatment and care of language minorities. These include effects on research participation of language minorities, effects on health care providers, and costs to the health system. The Bowen findings suggest that language barriers make it difficult for providers to meet professional standards of care and increase providers' exposure to the risk of liability. Furthermore, both clinical and health services research tend to under-represent ethnic minorities, especially those who are not proficient in an official language. Bowen asserts that the consequence of excluding certain ethnic groups from biomedical research may mean that study results cannot be generalized to the entire population, and that less is known about the risk factors, disease prevalence and treatment responses of specific ethnocultural groups. Bowen's literature review also provides some evidence that language barriers may increase health care costs: delays in seeking care and misunderstandings of treatment recommendations may result in greater use of services and negative health outcomes.

Bridging the Language Barrier: The Community Interpreter

In her essay, "The Professionalisation of Community Interpreting," Holly Mikkelson (n.d.) quotes the definition found in the announcement of the First International Conference on Community Interpreting—The Critical Link: Interpreters in the Community:

> Community Interpreting enables people who are not fluent speakers of the official language(s) of the country to communicate with the providers of public services so as to facilitate full and equal access to legal, health, education, government, and social services.

Mikkelson continues:

> Thus, community interpreting is distinguished from other types of interpreting, such as conference or escort interpreting, in that the services are provided to the residents of the community in which the interpreting takes place, not to conference delegates, diplomats, or professionals traveling abroad to conduct business.

As per the above definition, examples of the type of locations where community interpreters practise include mental health and legal aid services, public welfare and housing programs, and teacher/parent meetings in local schools.

REVIEW OF THE THEORY, PRACTICE AND SKILLS OF COMMUNITY INTERPRETERS

Language interpreting is a process of translating words from the source language (the speaker's language) into the target language (the language of the person being addressed by the speaker). Interpreting, which appears to be relatively simple, is, as illustrated in the following outline of the tasks (Abraham & Weston, 2002) and types of interpreting, an enormously complex skill.

The interpreter's work begins by actively listening to what the speaker says. Active listening means that the interpreter must listen to what is being said and try to understand what the speaker is trying to convey. If the wording needs to be adjusted or changed, the interpreter must change the words into something that will be understood in the target language. Take, for example, the question "Do you have siblings with the same problem?" In some languages, the notion of "sister" and "brother" is much broader than what is generally recognized in Western cultures, and includes other members of the same community who are members of the same age group. The interpreter must be able to detect any possible risk of misunderstandings and adjust his or her interpretation to get the information sought by the speaker in the source language.[5]

- The interpreter has to remember the client's words in the source language, and mentally rearrange the message in a way to convey the same meaning in the target language.
- The next step is to verbalize the message into the target language. This is the stage when the interpreter puts into words or expresses the original utterance in the language of the receiver of the message.

5. Example provided by Marco A. Fiola, C.Tr., C.Term., PhD, Department of French and Spanish, Ryerson University, Toronto.

- Spoken language interpreters who have been trained will also have mastered the skill of note taking to help them retain and mentally transpose the message. These notes are short forms of words, names, numbers and specific treatments or medications. For example, "z" can be short for asleep, "zing" can be short for sleeping and "J" can be short for happy. The notes will only be meaningful to the writer and, unless there is a legal reason for not doing so, they are destroyed at the end of the interpretation assignment.

TYPES OF INTERPRETING

Depending on the circumstances, the interpreter may provide any of the following types of interpretation during the assignment.

Consecutive or dialogue interpreting

Consecutive or dialogue interpreting occurs when the messages are being consecutively transmitted between two people. Person 1 utters a message (usually one or two sentences), the interpreter interprets the message, Person 2 responds to Person 1, and the interpreter interprets this response, and so on. (Think of a two-way conversation with the third person repeating the dialogue between the speakers.)

Simultaneous interpreting

Simultaneous interpreting occurs in situations where the interpreter is called on to interpret the message while the speaker is still speaking. For example, there may be situations in a mental health setting, where the service provider would like monolingual Vietnamese parents of an English-speaking adolescent girl, who is the client, to understand what she is saying to the girl. In this case, the interpreter would be present to simultaneously interpret the English conversation between the service provider and her adolescent client into Vietnamese.

In a mental health setting, simultaneous interpreting may also be a preferred mode of interpreting, especially when the client is upset or psychologically/mentally challenged, and speaks in long, sometimes illogical or irrational, utterances.

Telephone interpreting

Telephone interpreting occurs when the speakers are communicating via the telephone. In these situations, the interpretation may be done either simultaneously or consecutively. As there are no non-verbal cues, interpreters are challenged to interpret the messages based on their comprehension of the message as it is delivered over the telephone. Unless it is absolutely essential, telephone interpreting is not recommended for interventions that are related to the mental health of the client.

Sight translation

Sight translation is the oral translation of a written text from one language into another. This means the interpreter has to have the ability to read a text in one language and repeat

TABLE 6-2

Core Competencies for Interpreters in the Health Care Sector

KNOWLEDGE	SKILLS
• Has knowledge of the Canadian health care system, health care terminology and areas of medical specialization • Is aware of his or her personal values and attitudes and the impact these may have on the interpretation process • Understands the potential impact of cultural, emotional and linguistic factors on interpersonal communication • Has a clear understanding of his or her own language capabilities and limitations and will only accept assignments for which he or she is qualified • Is aware of the impact of non-verbal cues on communication and therefore on the interpretation process • Is aware of liability and risk issues related to interpreting in the health care sector • Recognizes the need and takes action to debrief after emotionally charged assignments with both the service provider and the person responsible for the interpreter service	• Is fluent in two languages and can use them without one language influencing the form of the other (as mentioned, the interpreter must use active listening to detect any risk of misunderstanding and adjust his or her interpretation to get the information sought) • Is able to interpret messages into and from both languages without additions, deletions or distortions to the meaning • Is able to maintain composure and provide accurate interpretation in sensitive and emotionally charged situations • Recognizes an appropriate moment to interrupt if he or she needs clarification, or is having trouble concentrating, and does so in a diplomatic manner • Speaks audibly and clearly

Source: Adapted from Abraham et al. (2004) *Handbook for Trainers* with permission from Healthcare Interpretation Network, Toronto.

it aloud in the second language. In a mental health setting, this may mean that the interpreter has to read a consent form in English and repeat the text in Spanish.

INTERPRETER COMPETENCIES

The ability to master the skills outlined above and to interpret confidently depends on the interpreter having a number of competencies. The above list, which is adapted from *A Handbook for Trainers: Language Interpreting in the Healthcare Sector* (Abraham et al., 2004), reflects current thinking in Ontario on the types of competencies required by community interpreters in the health care sector.[6]

6. For a full listing of the competencies that are expected of interpreters in the health care sector, see Section 1, Framework for the Delivery of Interpretation Services in the Health Care Sector (pp. 11–15), in *A Handbook for Trainers: Language Interpreting in the Healthcare Sector* (Abraham et al., 2004).

The Community Interpreter in a Mental Health Setting

Since there are currently no formal procedures for the accreditation of community interpreters in Canada, and there are no provincial or national standards to guide this practice, the definition of their role in a mental health setting is in many respects determined by the context in which the services are delivered. As a result of this unregulated situation, a Google search on this matter will reveal a range of understandings of the role and responsibilities of the community interpreter. For the purpose of this discussion, we provide examples of the role statement and the code of ethics that are provided in *A Handbook for Trainers: Language Interpreting in the Healthcare Sector*. This manual states that the role of the interpreter in a mental health setting is "to deliver, as faithfully as possible, messages transmitted between patients, family members, and service providers who do not share a common language" (Abraham et al., 2004).

Based on the example provided in the training manual, the code of ethics that guides the professional practice of interpreters in the health care sector instructs on:

- upholding the confidentiality of any information learned and/or transmitted during the performance of interpretation, unless the interpreter has the express approval of all parties or when required by law
- respecting all persons involved in the interpreting engagement
- maintaining the fidelity (precision) of the messages conveyed between the speakers in the assignment
- addressing situations where conflicts of interest may arise.

THE INTERPRETER IN A MENTAL HEALTH SETTING

There are currently no comprehensive standards to guide the practice of community interpreters in Ontario, or, as far as we are aware, across Canada, and there are no formal procedures to accredit their practice. This lack of an accreditation process means that there are no common standards to guide either the practice of community interpreters or the training programs that are available. In Ontario, a number of not-for-profit, community-based interpreter services offer 100-hour training programs that provide the basic skills for the practice of community interpreting and interpreting in the health care sector. The scope of these training programs does not encompass the training of interpreters with the advanced level of skills necessary for interpreting in psychological testing and counselling or psychotherapy where the patients may be delusional. If an interpreter is required to work with service providers in any of the aforementioned situations, it is the responsibility of the service provider to ensure that the interpreter is competent to work on such an assignment. In the next section of this chapter, we outline a number of approaches that service providers might use to assess the abilities of interpreters who are assigned to work with them.

A number of these training programs insist that a prerequisite for training is the successful completion of a test to assess the individual's level of fluency in English and a second language, and their aptitude for interpreting. At the end of 2005, these tests, which were developed with the funding support of the Ontario Ministry of Citizenship and Immigration, were limited to the following languages: Albanian, Amharic, Arabic, Bengali, Bulgarian, Burmese, Cambodian, Cantonese, Czech, Dari, Dinka, Dutch, Farsi, Finnish, French, German, Greek, Gujarati, Hebrew, Hindi, Hungarian, Italian, Japanese, Korean, Kurdish (Kurmandji), Kurdish (Sorani), Low German, Nuer, Ojibwe, Ojicree, Mandarin, Pashto, Polish, Portuguese, Punjabi, Romanian, Russian, Serbo-Croatian, Somali, Spanish, Tagalog, Tamil, Tigrigna, Turkish, Twi, Ukrainian, Urdu and Vietnamese.

This means that the language fluency of interpreters who speak English and languages not included in this list will not have been assessed in the same way, and possibly not to the same degree.

CULTURAL INTERPRETATION SERVICES AT THE CENTRE FOR ADDICTION AND MENTAL HEALTH: A PARADIGM SHIFT

As recently as five years ago, the service providers associated with the Centre for Addiction and Mental Health (CAMH) depended on an essentially ad hoc interpreter program, which often included calling on staff who spoke English plus another language. In April 2001, senior management decided that CAMH would give priority to a client-centred model that would integrate the delivery of quality services to all members of its diverse client population. Thus, a commitment was made to the allocation of a centralized budget to support the annual costs of the Cultural Interpretation Services (CIS).

By using the term "cultural interpretation," CAMH refers to its commitment to client-centred care, which requires that a health care provider recognize the client's culture, the health care provider's culture and how both impact the health care provider–client relationship. Individual assessments are necessary to identify relevant cultural factors within the context of each situation for each client. An individual's culture is influenced by factors such as race, gender, religion, ethnicity, socioeconomic status, sexual orientation and life experience (College of Nurses of Ontario, 2005).

When interpreters are assigned, CIS will ensure that this cultural sensitivity is adhered to. For example, a South Asian woman from a Muslim background may feel more comfortable with a female interpreter rather than a male interpreter because of religious issues. Similarly, a man being assessed at the Sexual Behaviour Clinic may feel more comfortable with a male interpreter rather than a female interpreter because of the sexually explicit language that is used during the assessments.

Although it is still debatable whether or not the interpreter's role is that of a cultural expert/broker, it is a general expectation that the interpreter will be knowledgeable about his or her own cultural community and may provide general information to help the service provider understand the community.

This key change in the delivery of interpreter services has resulted in services that are offered by freelance interpreters who, at a minimum:

- have completed the language and skills assessment tests in the languages that are currently available[7]
- have completed the 100-hour basic interpreter skills training program delivered by local community-based agencies and/or are on the rosters of the Ontario Ministry of the Attorney General and the Immigration and Refugee Board
- have completed mandatory CAMH training on diversity, and addiction and mental health issues.

Interpreters, including American Sign Language interpreters, are available at all times and at no cost to CAMH clients, if requested by CAMH service providers. If interpreters are not available to be on site for acute emergencies, service providers may use a telephone interpretation service. CIS also offers translation (written) services in many languages—also at the request of CAMH service providers. These services are provided by translation agencies that have certified translators working for them.

The CAMH service provides interpreters to help with clinical encounters, community visits, phone calls and appointments at various government offices, such as the Ontario Ministry of Community and Social Services. The success of this initiative is evident in the marked increase in the demand for the service. Requests for interpreters have steadily gone up from 14 requests per month in the beginning of 2001 to approximately 140 requests per month in late 2005.[8]

This paradigm shift in the CAMH approach to the delivery of interpreter services demonstrates that the establishment of a carefully managed interpreter service—which is responsible for recruitment, screening and contracting with the interpreters and for delivery of timely services—depends on an organizational commitment to the funding to support the program. Feedback from CAMH service providers accessing the CIS indicates that the provision of language access services results in cost savings to both the health system and the larger society.

Guidelines for Working with Interpreters

We believe that all service providers in the mental health care field should provide the highest quality service possible to all of their clients with whom they do not share a common language. However, because, as indicated above, there are few community interpreters who are specialized in the mental health field, and because not all mental health services have the funding to purchase the service of those community interpreters who have been trained in the programs that are currently available, practitioners have no other choice but to work with individuals who have varying degrees of fluency in two languages and who may have not received any interpreter training.

---

7. For languages where tests are still not available, a personal interview is held to judge the language competency in English and the experience of working as interpreters is also taken into consideration.

8. For more information on the Cultural Interpretation Services at CAMH, you may contact Stella Rahman, clinical services consultant, by phone at 416 535 8501 or by e-mail at stella_rahman@camh.net.

It is within this context that we have borrowed and built on the work of Garcia-Peltoniemi and Egli (1988)[9] and offer the following guidelines for working with interpreters in the mental health sector. Garcia-Peltoniemi and Egli recognize that the formal training of professionals in the mental health sector has often not included opportunities to learn about, and to be trained in, the approaches to working with interpreters in the performance of tasks such as diagnostic interviews, counselling, psychotherapy, medication education or psychological testing. They also acknowledge that the demand to work with an interpreter may add to the "dimension of complexity to the activities performed by mental health professionals."

Service providers must recognize that the same professional standards and rules of conduct apply in situations where an interpreter is required as in situations where an interpreter is not required. Having untrained people providing mental health services carries clear risks and should be avoided if at all possible. This includes using family members or friends as interpreters: they may not have the necessary level of fluency in the two languages, they may lack the appropriate training, and their lack of impartiality may interfere with the assessment or treatment process and this too should be avoided. Finally, it is in the best interest of service providers to ensure that whenever possible they work with skilled interpreters who follow professional standards and a code of ethics.

The following guidelines are intended for service providers working with interpreters.

BEFORE THE SESSION

1. Determine the interpreter's level of language fluency, sensitivity to working in a mental health setting and general comfort with the task(s) to be performed.

2. Ensure that the interpreter is prepared to work in a situation that may be emotionally demanding or in which he or she may find the language and behaviour offensive.

3. Verify that the interpreter is a good match with your client. Consider age, gender, country of origin, cultural background, personal maturity, etc. (Interpreters who have completed the community-based training programs in Ontario will ask the client whether he or she is comfortable with the interpreter when they introduce themselves to the client.)

4. Ensure a common understanding of the role and responsibilities of the interpreter throughout the assignment. Again, although this may be less necessary when working with a trained interpreter, it doesn't hurt to validate your understanding.

---

9. Further information on the work of Garcia-Peltoniemi and Egli and on training resources can be found at www.cce.umn.edu/creditcourses/pti/services/refugee.html.

Activities in this situation may include:
- clarifying confidentiality and ethical guidelines that apply in professional relationships with clients
- verifying that the interpreter will not screen the client's comments for fear of offending the service provider, or because they may reflect poorly on the client or the ethnocultural community
- instructing the interpreter to ask for clarification immediately should he or she not understand either the service provider or the client
- alerting the interpreter to the potential for client utterances that may be distorted in their meaning
- ensuring that the interpreter understands that his or her function is to enable communication between the service provider and the client in as direct a manner as possible.

5. Provide the interpreter with information relevant to the purpose of the session. Include any information on potential areas of difficulty.

DURING THE SESSION

1. Speak directly to the client (e.g., "How are you feeling today?" not "How is she feeling today?"). If interpreters are untrained, you will need to instruct them to interpret the client's words in a direct manner. They should not begin with "He says" or "she says." Interpreters should interpret as the individual speaks (e.g., "I am not feeling well today.").

2. Keep sentences brief and concise, and avoid chained questions (e.g., "Do you smoke?" not "Do you smoke or drink alcohol?").

3. Do not engage in a side conversation with the interpreter. Be aware that the task of the trained interpreter is to interpret everything said in the intervention. Likewise, if an interpreter has to ask the service provider for clarification, this should be interpreted for the client.

AFTER THE SESSION

1. If the session has been emotionally charged, allow time for the interpreter to talk about it with you. Remember it is not the role of the interpreter to provide any explanations of the behaviour of the client.

WHEN A TRAINED INTERPRETER IS UNAVAILABLE

The important role that trained interpreters play in providing mental health services has not been broadly recognized, and funding for such services is limited. Therefore, it may not always be possible to purchase the services of a trained interpreter. At times service providers may depend on a family member or a community volunteer to interpret for the client. In this case, service providers have a role to play in ensuring that volunteer interpreters adhere to the above guidelines. Agencies sending trained and screened interpreters may request feedback from service providers on how well interpreters adhere to the guidelines.

Public Policy Change

To date there has been limited attention to the issue of linguistic barriers to the access to mental health services by women who have limited proficiency in Canada's official languages. The studies that have been done tend to be generalized to the LE/FP population. However, given the number of LE/FP females identified in the 2001 census, and the range of social-, economic-, familial-, employment- and educational-related experiences that may lead women to seek the services provided in the mental health sector, we know that the inability to communicate in one of Canada's official languages is a major barrier in their ability to benefit from the services to which they are entitled.

In previous sections, we spoke about the lack of comprehensive standards to guide the practice of spoken language interpreters in Ontario, and the absence of formal procedures to accredit their practice. We also alluded to the ways in which the lack of funding to support the delivery of interpreter services results in the reliance on family members and volunteers who may not have the objectivity and skills required for accurate interpretation.

This inequity in the social environment will continue as long as:

- there is no public policy that recognizes the right of equal access to services by people who have limited proficiency in English or French
- there are insufficient budget allocations to public-sector institutions—health care, social welfare, education and legal services
- there are no standards to govern the practice of spoken language community interpreters in Ontario.

The *Canadian Human Rights Act* (1985) states:

> The purpose of this Act is to extend the laws in Canada to give effect, within the purview of matters coming within the legislative authority of Parliament, to the principle that all individuals should have an opportunity equal with other individuals to make for themselves the lives that they are able and wish to have and to have their needs accommodated, consistent with their duties and obligations as members of society, without being hindered in or prevented from doing so by discriminatory practices based on race, national or ethnic origin, colour, religion,

age, sex, sexual orientation, marital status, family status, disability or conviction for an offence for which a pardon has been granted.

How might the picture look if "language" were added to the grounds for discrimination? In other words, if there were a public policy that acknowledges that while the majority of Aboriginal people, immigrants and refugees to Canada will strive to speak the official languages, there will be those Aboriginals, newcomer and long-term residents who will be discriminated against because of their limited proficiency in the official languages.

An understanding of what "pushes" public policy can be found in the example of sign language interpreting. The *Canadian Human Rights Act* (1985) identifies disability as a ground for discrimination and individuals requiring sign language interpreters are covered by the existing act. This entitlement was reinforced by the 1997 Eldridge decision by the Supreme Court of Canada, which stated that the failure to provide sign language interpretation where it is needed for effective communication in the delivery of health care services violates the rights of people who are hearing impaired. The Eldridge ruling states that governments cannot escape their constitutional obligations to provide equal access to public services. There is no equivalent ruling for language interpreting and there are few public records of the impact of misinterpretation on the lives of those who have limited proficiency in English or French.

In Ontario, a model for such collective action may be found in the work of the Healthcare Interpretation Network (HIN), which advocates for the recognition of the need for trained language interpreters in the delivery of health care services. In spite of the work of HIN, and some health care services' commitment to equity in the treatment of their clients, research has shown that expediency often takes priority and health care providers continue to call on volunteers and family members, including children, to act as interpreters.

Conclusion

In this chapter, we explained how linguistic barriers affect the delivery of health care services to LE/FP clients, and discussed how trained community interpreters might be the critical link to ensuring the delivery of quality services to female clients who have limited proficiency in Canada's official languages. We provided the basis for understanding the need for a concentrated effort on the part of all actors—service providers in the social, legal and health care services, advocates for social justice and equity, and the government of Canada—to push for legislative and policy change. Hopefully, it will not take a loss of life due to misinterpreted communication between client and service provider to address this social inequity and trigger a public policy change.

References

Abraham, D., Cabral, N. & Tancredi, A. (Eds.). (2004). *A Handbook for Trainers: Language Interpreting in the Healthcare Sector*. Toronto: Healthcare Interpretation Network.

Abraham, D. & Nielson, K. (2004). *Strengthening Access to Primary Health Care: Preliminary Research Findings*. Unpublished report, Healthcare Interpretation Network and Critical Link Canada, Toronto.

Abraham, D. & Weston, D. (2002). *Training Curriculum for Interpreters Associated with the Services Funded by the Violence against Women Prevention Initiatives and the Domestic Violence Justice Strategy, Citizenship Development Branch, Ministry of Citizenship*. Unpublished curriculum. Overview of the Constituent Tasks is adapted from Dr. Roda Roberts, Pedagogical Institute on Interpretation, Toronto, February 21–24, 1994.

Bowen, S. (2001). *Language Barriers in Access to Health Care*. Ottawa: Health Canada. Available: www.hc-sc.gc.ca/hcs-sss/pubs/care-soins/2001-lang-acces/index_e.html. Accessed January 5, 2008.

Canadian Human Rights Act, R.S. 1985, c. H-6. Available: http://lois.justice.gc.ca/en/H-6/. Accessed January 5, 2008.

College of Nurses of Ontario. (2005). *Practice Guideline: Culturally Sensitive Care*. Toronto: Author. Available: www.cno.org/docs/prac/41040_CulturallySens.pdf. Accessed January 5, 2008.

Eldridge v. *Attorney General of British Columbia*, [1997] 3 S.C.R. Available: http://csc.lexum. umontreal.ca/en/1997/1997rcs3-624/1997rcs3-624.html. Accessed January 15, 2008.

Flores, G., Laws, M.B., Mayo, S.J., Zuckerman, B., Abreu, M., Medina, L. et al. (2003). Errors in medical interpretation and their potential clinical consequences in pediatric encounters. *Pediatrics, 111* (1), 6–14. Available: http://pediatrics.aappublications.org/cgi/reprint/111/1/6.pdf#search=%22 Errors%20in%20medical%20interpretation%20and%20their%20potential%20clinical%20conseque nces%20in%20pediatric%20encounters%22. Accessed January 5, 2008.

Garcia-Peltoniemi, R.E. & Egli, E. (1988). Guidelines for working with interpreters. In L. Benhamida, B. Downing, E. Egli & Z. Yao, *Refugee Mental Health: Interpreting in Refugee Mental Health Settings* [Video workbook]. University of Minnesota Refugee Assistance Program, Mental Health Technical Assistance Program.

Health Canada. (1998). *Reaching Out: A Guide to Communicating with Aboriginal Seniors* (Catalogue No. H88-3/20-1998E). Ottawa: Minister of Public Works and Government Services Canada. Available: www.hc-sc.gc.ca/seniors-aines/pubs/communicating_aboriginal/pdf/reachingout_e.pdf. Accessed January 5, 2008.

Health Canada & Interdepartmental Committee on Aging and Seniors Issues. (2002). *Canada's Aging Population* (Catalogue No. H39-608/2002E). Ottawa: Minister of Public Works and Government Services Canada. Available: www.hc-sc.gc.ca/seniors-aines/pubs/fed_paper/pdfs/fed pager_e.pdf. Accessed January 5, 2008.

Mikkelson, H. (n.d.). *The Professionalisation of Community Interpreting*. Monterey, CA: Monterey Institute of International Studies. Available: www.acebo.com/papers/profslzn.htm. Accessed January 5, 2008.

Statistics Canada. (2002). *2001 Census: Analysis Series. Profile of Languages in Canada: English, French and Many Others*. Available: www12.statcan.ca/english/census01/Products/Analytic/companion/lang/ pdf/96F0030XIE2001005.pdf. Accessed January 5, 2008.

Statistics Canada and Citizenship Immigration Canada. (2003). *Longitudinal Survey of Immigrants to Canada: Initial Results from the First Wave of Interviews*. Available: http://policyresearch.gc.ca/ doclib/OECD_ElizabethRuddick_E.pdf. Accessed January 5, 2008.

Chapter 7

Services for Women

Access, Equity and Quality

ENID COLLINS, YOGENDRA B. SHAKYA, SEPALI GURUGE
AND EDWARD JASON SANTOS

The Canadian government's introduction of a multiculturalism policy in 1971 heralded major changes in services for immigrants and refugees, and, more broadly, in ethno-racial relationships. An infrastructure of non-profit agencies, or Immigrant Serving Organizations (ISOs), was established to facilitate the settlement of newcomers to Canada (Holder, 1998). Since then, there has been a significant increase in the number of agencies and categories of services that support new immigrants and refugees to deal with post-migration and settlement issues.

This chapter highlights the close connections between immigration and settlement services and mental health for newcomer women. It examines the range and types of immigration, settlement and mental health promotion services available for newcomer women and discusses the barriers and challenges that newcomer women face in accessing these services. In particular, it discusses the challenges that newcomer women face in navigating a complex matrix of services.

Because the immigration and settlement process can be a major health stressor, mental health services need to be seamlessly integrated within settlement services, and vice versa. Community agencies play a dynamic role in supporting women through the processes associated with their settlement in Canada: mental health professionals can draw on frameworks used by such agencies that situate women in the familial (micro), neighbourhood and community (meso), and societal (macro) contexts. Community agencies are adopting innovative program designs and collaborative strategies to meet the diverse settlement and mental health service needs of newcomer women. We present profiles of three of these.

Matrix of Services

With the growing number of immigrants to Canada, particularly in major cities, even agencies that provide generic services are increasingly pressed to cater their staffing and services to reflect the needs of immigrants (e.g., by hiring staff from immigrant communities, by hosting Language Instructions for Newcomers to Canada [LINC] classes, and by providing interpretation and settlement support). Many different types of settlement-focused agencies have been created. They have been referred to by many different names; for example, there are "settlement agencies," "ethno-specific agencies" and "immigrant-serving agencies." However, most of the categories used to refer to these agencies are quite simplistic and fail to capture the complex and dynamic ways that service agencies operate. Rather than a single typology, we have found the following *nested typology*,[1] based on four inter-related criteria—government affiliation, target community, scale of organization and type of services—to be useful in understanding the matrix of agencies and services for immigrants and refugees.

The first important basis for differentiating agencies is the level of government affiliation or support. Agencies can be fully government sanctioned, quasi-governmental or non-governmental. Quasi-governmental agencies include arms-length government agencies and/or agencies that receive most of their core funding from the government. (Community health centres, family service agencies and many settlement service agencies fall under this category.) Non-governmental agencies receive little or no core funding or support from the government and may be non-profit or private/for-profit. The number of non-profit agencies serving immigrant or ethno-racial communities (e.g., immigrant associations, legal aid services of specific immigrant communities) has grown significantly in the last decade, as have private/for-profit agencies offering services for immigrant communities (e.g., immigration lawyers/consultants' offices, employment agencies focused on immigrants). Some of these private/for-profit agencies have been known to charge exorbitant prices.

The second category for differentiating agencies is based on the target community. Agencies may serve the general population or may focus on specific communities. Among those that take a targeted approach, the focus community may vary by ethno-racial background, age (e.g., youth, seniors), gender, neighbourhood or populations with specific characteristics/needs (e.g., teen moms, people who are homeless, people living with HIV/AIDS). Agencies focused on specific ethno-racial communities are referred to as "ethno-racial agencies"; those serving immigrants in general are known as "immigrant-serving agencies" or "settlement agencies"; and those serving the general population are referred to as "community agencies" (although the term "community agency" is also used for small-scale agencies).

---

1. A "nested typology" recognizes that categories may be embedded with each other, rather than being discrete entities. For a discussion of different types of typologies, see Doty, D. H. and Glick, W.H. (1994). Typologies as a Unique Form of Theory Building: Toward Improved Understanding and Modeling. *The Academy of Management Review*, 19 (2), 230–251.

The scale of an organization is another criterion for differentiating agencies. Agencies can be large-scale, such as those with branches across the nation; they can be medium; or small-scale.

Agencies also differ by the number and type of services offered. While they may focus on offering a single service (e.g., employment support or housing), a growing number provide many services, and are thus referred to as "multi-service agencies." Even agencies mandated to deliver a specific service may offer a set of related services. For example, an agency focused on housing or health may provide other related services such as community development, capacity-building and public education activities that promote better housing and health.

The model, range and quality of service delivery can vary significantly based on the specific institutional features of the agency. Thus, the types and model of service delivery at a large, national-scale governmental agency may be significantly different from a quasi-governmental multi-service agency focused on family health, and even more dissimilar from that of a small non-governmental, non-profit immigrant association established by local leaders from a small immigrant community. Policy-makers, funding agencies, service providers and service users can benefit from a better understanding of the diversity and changing nature of the institutional make-up of agencies. For example, policy-makers, funding agencies or service providers trying to promote better collaboration between agencies first need to get a strong grasp of the institutional capacity, operational structure, scale, service areas and target communities of the different agencies concerned. Similarly, a newcomer family will be able to chart the service matrix more easily if they understand the differences in the agencies in their community.

While the nested typology presented here is useful for analytical purposes, in reality, agencies and the services they offer are complex, dynamic and evolving. Indeed, our attempt at proposing a multiply nested typology rather than a single typology is partly to highlight that agencies are complex, dynamic institutions that defy oversimplified, static classifications. The four-parameter typology we've described needs to be used with the following caveats. First, agencies can be differentiated by other parameters (e.g., by whether they belong to a network or whether they charge fees). Second, some parameters of the typology are ambiguous, evolving concepts. For example, people's understanding of what "small-scale" or "large-scale" means may differ, just as the terms "community" and "community agencies" are often interpreted differently. And many agencies that see themselves as non-governmental agencies may, in fact, be much more closely tied to government funding or directives than they realize.

If navigating the matrix of agencies and services can be confusing for Canadian-born or long-time permanent residents, it is even more confusing for newcomers. In fact, as we discuss later in more detail, getting relevant information about different services and navigating these services can be very stressful for newcomers, particularly if they aren't well co-ordinated and information about these services is not accessible.

The Role of Settlement Services and Ethno-Racial Agencies

The federal government allocates a considerable amount of financial resources to help newcomers adapt to and settle in Canada. However, these allocations have varied over the years. In general, financial resources are channeled through three groups of programs (Lim et al., 2005):

1. *Language Instructions for Newcomers to Canada (LINC):* The LINC program is intended to assure that adult newcomers have access to training in one of Canada's official languages soon after their arrival. Newcomers' language skills are assessed when they enroll in a LINC program to determine their level of language competency and training needs.

2. *Immigrant Settlement and Adaptation Programs (ISAP):* ISAP provides funding to organizations that assist newcomers to settle and integrate into communities by offering a range of services such as:
   • reception, which includes providing information kits to newcomers on arrival at ports of entry
   • referrals, which link newcomers to resources in the community (e.g., education and health and social services)
   • orientation, which includes familiarizing newcomers with services in their community (e.g., banking, daycare, public transportation, school registration)
   • interpretation and translation, which includes interpreting Canadian culture and symbols.

3. *Host Programs:* Funding under this category is allocated to various organizations to recruit and train volunteers who help newcomers to adapt, settle and integrate into Canadian life. Organizations that are eligible for funding include various provincial/territorial and municipal governments and non-governmental groups as well as businesses and community groups (Lim et al., 2005).

Most newcomers settle in major cities, such as Toronto, Vancouver and Montreal. Table 7-1 on page 123 offers a breakdown of funding sources in the Greater Toronto Area. While the data for these tables were collected between 2003–2004, major changes in the funding structure are anticipated. The 2006 federal budget included a commitment of over 1.3 billion dollars over a five-year period to assist provinces and territories in the resettlement of new immigrants. Because Ontario receives the largest numbers of immigrants annually, it will therefore receive a significant increase in funding for its settlement services.

Across Canada, the number and types of resources that support immigrants and refugees vary from province to province as well as between and within urban, suburban and rural areas. In Ontario, Newcomer Settlement Programs provide operational funding to agencies to offer direct services such as assessment, information and orientation, and general assistance for settlement in the early phase following newcomers' arrival. Indirect services that are funded include training for settlement workers and volunteers.

Table 7-2 describes key settlement services in the GTA.

TABLE 7-1

Sources of Funding to Settlement-Service Agency Locations in the Greater Toronto Area (2004)

	CITY OF TORONTO	DURHAM REGION	HALTON REGION	PEEL REGION	YORK REGION	TOTAL
Federal	136	4	3	25	21	189
Citizenship and Immigration Canada						
Host Program	2	1		1	3	7
Immigrant Settlement and Adaptation Program (ISAP)	57			8	6	71
Language Instruction for Newcomers to Canada (LINC)	57	1	2	16	6	82
Heritage Canada			1			1
Human Resources Development Canada (HRDC)	20	2			6	28
Provincial	55	1		5	15	76
Ministry of Citizenship and Immigration (MCI)	21	1		3	6	31
Ministry of Community and Social Services (MCSS)	13				3	16
Ministry of Health (MOH)	12			1	3	16
Ministry of Justice				1		1
Ministry of Training, Colleges and Universities (MTCU)	9				3	12
Regional/local	21	1		6	3	31
Foundations	44		1	5	6	56
Canadian Race Relations				1		1
Maytree	18			2		20
Trillium	26		1	2	6	35
Other	216	2	1	21	18	258
Charities					3	3
Community Access Program (CAP)	1					1
Job Search Workshop (JSW)	38	2		7	6	53
Legal Aid Ontario (LAO)	11					11
Ontario Women's Directorate (OWD)	1					1
Resettlement Assistance Program (RAP)	8					8
Settlement Education Partnership Toronto (SEPT)	7					7
Settlement Workers in Schools (SWIS)				1	3	4
Toronto District School Board (TDSB)	1					1
United Way (UW)	149		1	13	6	169

Source: Reprinted with premission. Lim, A., Lo, L., Siemiatycki, M. & Doucet, M. (2005). Newcomer services in the Greater Toronto Area: An exploration of the range of funding sources of settlement services. *Working Paper No. 35.* Toronto: Centre of Excellence for Research on Immigration and Settlement.

TABLE 7-2

Description of Key Settlement Services in the GTA (2004)

SERVICES	DESCRIPTION
Advocacy	• Defending newcomers' rights and entitlements concerning various issues such as housing and employment.
Counseling and Support Groups	• Counseling for children, youth, adults, family, married couples, and groups.
	• Support groups for groups such as seniors, youth, women, men, children, newcomers, single parents, victims of torture, and domestic violence.
Education	• Information regarding schooling for children, youth, and adults; tutoring services/groups and skill building workshops.
Emergency food services	• Food banks and community kitchens.
Employment	• Assistance with resumé writing, computer access, job searching, job skills training and vocational training.
English as a second language (ESL)	• For all ages and levels of competency.
Form filling	• Assistance with all application forms including government forms such as employment insurance, social insurance number, benefits, OHIP, immigration and citizenship, and social assistance. Other forms include school applications.
Health/Medical	• Includes health promotion and awareness programs, educational workshops regarding nutrition and basic health, and information about medical services in the community.
Housing	• Finding immediate housing, applying for subsidized housing, and assisting with basic information about such issues as rent, tenant rights, and landlord obligations.
Information and referral	• Provide links between newcomers and available services in their communities, such as legal, housing, employment, childcare, education, and health.
Legal	• Assistance with immigration applications, refugee claims, tenant issues, court appearances, and any other issues that require legal advice and referral.
Orientation	• Addressing immediate needs for settlement such as buying groceries, public transportation, shelter, orientation to Canadian life and Canadian culture.
Recreation and leisure	• Programs for all ages in a wide range of areas such as sports teams, swimming, cooking classes, art classes, and gardening.
Translation	• Translation of documents such as application and registration forms.
Interpretation	• Interpretation may include such issues as cultural contexts, Canadian systems, and documents.

Source: Reprinted with permission. Lim, A., Lo, L., Siemiatycki, M. & Doucet, M. (2005). Newcomer Services in the Greater Toronto Area: An exploration of the range of funding sources of settlement services. *Working Paper No. 35.* Toronto: Centre of Excellence for Research on Immigration and Settlement.

ETHNO-RACIAL AGENCIES

Ethno-racial agencies are usually formed in response to the specific needs identified by particular ethno-racial communities. They form part of a receiving community where newcomers may experience familiar culture and language. Through their formal and informal links to linguistic and kinship communities, these agencies provide a holistic approach to services, taking into account the physical, social and spiritual dimensions of newcomer women's lives.

The agencies try to provide services that are culturally and linguistically appropriate and responsive to women's needs in a just and equitable manner.

Some criteria for defining ethno-racial agencies include:
- focusing on specific ethno-racial groups and the issues of concern to them
- offering a range of programs and services to help newcomers orient to Canadian society, including language interpretation, and help in accessing services related to health, education and housing
- providing services mainly through volunteer staff, though professional staff may be recruited from within ethno-racial groups
- having funding support mainly from within the community, though other fundraising initiatives may be directed to mainstream agencies outside the community.

Ethno-racial agencies play a major role in enhancing both the strengths of the community, as well as the strengths of individual women. They may provide help with navigating governmental bureaucracy by, for example, facilitating access to immigration, legal, health, social and education systems.

Some newcomers may find employment and housing within the community, where they gain some initial work experience that may help them to become launched in the Canadian workforce. With ethno-racial agencies' support, some people gain skills that enable them to contribute to the growth of their community in areas such as financial, social and business initiatives. Ethno-racial agencies can help women and their families establish themselves in Canada (Holder, 1998) by addressing such needs as language interpretation, child care, English language skills development, counselling, advocacy and support for the family, and support around discrimination and domestic violence. Some ethno-racial agencies' exclusive mandate is to address the specific needs of women. For example, the Afghan Women's Counselling and Integration Community Support Organization in Toronto recognizes that women have special and distinct needs; therefore, it provides a range of programs addressing Afghan women's concerns and needs.

In spite of the critical role that ethno-racial agencies play they often experience significant financial problems. To obtain ongoing funding, these agencies may have to tailor their goals and activities to meet the mandate of their potential funders, which may or may not be compatible with the vision of the agency or the needs of the individuals within the communities (Ng, 1988).

Another concern for ethno-racial agencies relates to addressing certain issues that may be stigmatized within the community or that members may respond to differently. For example, women who may need to access services as a result of intimate partner violence, sexual abuse and mental illness may be reluctant to seek help from agencies within their community because of concerns about confidentiality and/or fear of retribution. Ethnic or religious conflicts may also surface when women from different countries who speak the same language come together in ethno-racial agencies. (For example, in Chapter 14, author Eva Saphir points out that Latin American women immigrants to Canada come from different regional and cultural backgrounds and do not see themselves as necessarily belonging to one community. Saphir highlights that each wave of Spanish-speaking people arriving in Canada considers new arrivals as belonging to a different group, while others might see these groups as homogeneous.)

Barriers and Challenges to Accessing Services for Newcomer Women

Many agencies across Canada provide services to newcomer immigrants and refugees; however, metropolitan areas—where most newcomers settle—tend to have a higher concentration of these agencies. Research into settlement services for new immigrants is relatively new. Among the emerging body of research studies, a comprehensive survey of services for newcomers in the Greater Toronto Area (GTA) was conducted by Lim et al. (2005). Their report, entitled *"Newcomer Services in the Greater Toronto Area: An Exploration of the Range of Funding Sources of Settlement Services"* is based on a survey of services in the GTA including Durham, York, Peel, Halton and Toronto, which is the most popular area for receiving new immigrants to Canada. The authors noted that newcomer services increased significantly in certain areas of the city of Toronto, including North York, Scarborough, Markham, Mississauga, Brampton, York Region and Peel. They list 238 settlement-service agencies across the GTA. Of this number, 20 agencies had more than one branch in the GTA and 116 were listed as ethno-specific based on their names. Lim et al. (2005) note that there are many agencies that address multiple areas of newcomer settlement issues; however, only some address women's issues specifically. Resources include support groups for women at risk and those experiencing domestic violence, crisis intervention services, pre- and post-natal counselling, parenting classes, and housing and legal issues.

While the number of agencies and services for immigrants and refugees has increased, the quantitative increase may not directly translate into qualitative improvements in access and equity of services for newcomers, particularly for newcomer women (Lim et al., 2005). This may be due to several factors. The agencies and services may be unevenly distributed, often concentrating in central locations rather than in areas where there is greatest need. Indeed, many neighbourhoods in Toronto with high newcomer populations (including Crescent Town, Oakridge, Thorncliffe Park, Agincourt, Lawrence Heights and Black Creek) remain highly underserved. Newcomers can find travelling to distant agencies for essential settlement and health services to be cumbersome, stressful and costly.

Even when agencies and services are nearby, newcomers may face other barriers to accessing the services because of difficulties in communicating and being understood. Agencies need to make concerted efforts in overcoming linguistic barriers since a large proportion of newcomers may have little or no knowledge of English or French when they arrive. Some newcomers, particularly refugees growing up in refugee camps, may have low literacy levels or have had their education interrupted because of conflicts and civil wars.

Newcomers may also face socio-economic barriers in accessing services. For example, those struggling to survive on multiple low-paying jobs may not be able to get time off work to access even vital health services. Not being able to secure affordable child care or lack of available information about such services may also preclude many newcomers, particularly women, from benefitting from other settlement services, such as language classes or job training programs.

Navigating a matrix of services in different locations can become onerous for newcomers. For instance, when women with children require settlement services, they are expected to approach different agencies to meet the diverse needs of the whole family and navigate a maze of agencies. Often women are not given information on how the services are organized and co-ordinated, so they may not readily access services that are appropriate to their situation. Guruge (2006) describes these difficulties as they relate to women who have experienced intimate partner violence: lack of information about available services, lack of linguistically and culturally appropriate services, lack of accessibility and portability, non-seamlessness of the services and various discriminatory practices present in such services.

Funding and other institutional constraints may preclude community and ethno-racial agencies from providing multiple services in one setting. Some community and ethno-racial agencies have developed innovative partnerships with each other to provide more co-ordinated services (e.g., partnership between shelters for people who are homeless and settlement agencies in response to the growing number of immigrants using homeless shelters, collaboration between health centres and interpretation service agencies, and collaboration between legal clinics and ethno-racial agencies).

Service design informed by research also becomes important for these agencies to provide services that more closely reflect the needs of the clientele and to situate the services in high needs areas. A growing number of community and ethno-racial agencies (including Women's Health in Women's Hands Community Health Centre, the Ontario Women's Health Network, Planned Parenthood Toronto, the Regent Park Community Health Centre and Access Alliance Multicultural Community Health Centre) have begun to do community-based research as a way to engage in evidence-based service design. For example, Access Alliance Multicultural Community Health Centre is conducting a research project on the mental health of government-assisted refugees (GARs) from Afghanistan, Burma and Sudan in order to develop culturally sensitive mental health services for its GAR clients. Similarly, based on their research on social determinants of HIV/AIDS risk among African and Caribbean women, Women's Health in Women's Hands Community Health Centre has developed several HIV/AIDS educational materials and prevention services for African and Caribbean women. The research has also led to African and Caribbean women's voices and issues being included in mainstream HIV/AIDS prevention programs.

Services for newcomers should not be relegated exclusively to "immigrant-serving agencies," "settlement agencies" or "ethno-racial agencies." Rather, all agencies should reconfigure their institutional policies, staffing and services to meet the needs of the rapidly growing and diverse immigrant and refugee populations. Furthermore, settlement services need to be seamlessly linked to mental health services. Separating from families in host countries, coming to a foreign land, finding jobs in an immigrant-unfriendly labour market, navigating the complex matrix of services, and feeling excluded, alienated or discriminated against can have a significant impact on the mental health of newcomers. Agencies serving newcomers need to recognize and address the mental health implications of immigration and settlement process; at the same time, mental health agencies need to reorient their services to better reach newcomers.

Mental Health and Settlement: Profiles of Three Agencies

This section highlights three key agencies that have begun to integrate mental health and settlement services in innovative ways. All resources that facilitate adaptation and settlement have a positive effect on newcomers' mental health. For example, support in gaining employment, housing and education are all important to newcomers' resettlement as mental health problems can be related to the stresses arising out of the challenges in accessing any of these services. It is, therefore, critical that resources and mental health promotion strategies be available to help women deal with migration-related stresses.

At the same time, women need support in coping with pre-existing mental health issues that may be compounded by stresses associated with migration and resettlement. For some women, mental health problems developed long before migration. These issues may, for instance, be a response to gender oppression—so common in many countries of the world— or to torture and rape, a reality for some refugee women that may be related to their decision to flee their home countries. A number of strategies for working with women who experience rape and trauma are discussed in Chapter 12 on clinical issues surrounding working with refugee claimants, in Chapter 14 on trauma work with Latin American women and in Chapter 15 on intimate partner violence.

Several agencies address health and settlement needs of the newcomer women to Canada; however, only a handful of agencies provide mental health specific services. The following highlights three agencies whose primary focus is the mental health and illness needs of newcomers, and who have specific services for women. We have organized our discussion around the agencies' guiding principles and the strengths of the services they provide.

CANADIAN MENTAL HEALTH ASSOCIATION

The Canadian Mental Health Association (CMHA) is a national voluntary organization with branches across the country. It addresses all aspects of mental health and mental illness through collaborative partnerships with consumers and their families, communities and government bodies. CMHA's guiding principles are based on the recognition that people with mental health problems are resilient and can participate in managing mental health challenges. In its statement of values and beliefs, CMHA advocates for social justice, access to appropriate and adequate resources, and self-determination and community integration to the fullest extent possible.

The strengths of its services include its availability in communities across Canada. CMHA provides a range of resources to consumers, including educational books and videotapes, and facilities such as computer workstations. It also provides individual and group supports for clients and caregivers, as well as services and programs that respond to clients' physical and social needs (e.g., housing, employment and community-based treatments).

CMHA's collaboration with other agencies and services in offering programs demonstrates its recognition of mental health as integrally related to all facets of life. CMHA recognizes that basic necessities of life such as employment, housing, education and social supports are integral to an individual's mental health. The organization also emphasizes that individuals and families have unique mental health needs at various stages across the life span. For example, they support programs for children and families, youth, women and the elderly. CMHA also assumes a substantial role in advocating for positive mental health for all Canadians. For instance, it works to influence public policy by submitting briefs and reports to parliamentary standing committees to ensure that mental health issues are addressed at the federal level.

A number of unique services are available to women through CMHA branches in communities across Canada. For example, "Let's Discuss It / Multicultural Women's Wellness Program" in Toronto is available for women who are socially isolated, who experience cultural and linguistic barriers to building new social networks and/or who are at risk of developing mental health issues. This program is offered in partnership with several groups including the Afghan Women's Counselling and Integration Community Support Organization, Greek Orthodox Community and Counseling Services, the Jamaican Canadian Association and the South Asian Women's Centre.

Another unique feature of CMHA is its responsiveness to marginalized groups. An example is the Mental Health Court Support and Diversion Program, which helps people with serious mental illness who are charged with committing a criminal offence to get mental health and support services rather than going through the courts.

Mental health professionals can obtain further information about the services unique to newcomer women by calling CMHA directly or by accessing their website.

ACROSS BOUNDARIES

Across Boundaries is a community mental health centre that provides a range of supports and services to people of colour with mental health problems. It adopts a holistic approach, recognizing the interdependence of the spiritual, emotional, physical, social, cultural, linguistic, economic and broader environmental aspects that affect the mental health and well-being of people of colour.

Across Boundaries recognizes the significant impact of racism on mental health, and believes in empowering people on their "healing journey." It is one of the few agencies across the Greater Toronto Area that provides mental health services specifically to people of colour from diverse cultural and linguistic groups, with a particular focus on the connection between racism and mental health. While many people who use its services are newcomers, some consumers are long-time residents in Canada. Its consumers come from various countries including parts of South Asia, East Asia, Africa, the Caribbean and the Middle East. Many of these people receive services in their native language.

Consumers are encouraged to participate in the development and delivery of programs. Services offered include new initiatives that focus on skills building, social and recreational activities, support groups, alternative complementary therapies and programs that use creative expressions such as art therapy sessions.

Across Boundaries uses innovative strategies to involve people in promoting mental health and in coping with mental illness. Their theatre group, for example, uses participatory methods of teaching and learning. Participants are encouraged to develop their own ideas, to move beyond problems and to act in ways to solve problems. They engage in activities such as dance, singing and creative writing that facilitate creativity and self-expression. Among other outcomes, participants gain confidence and learn to take risks, such as speaking out in a group setting when they are ready.

As a leader in ethno-racial mental health, Across Boundaries provides opportunities for education in areas related to anti-racism and anti-oppression. Their resources include a collection of books, research reports and videotapes. They also hold lectures, workshops and conferences.

HONG FOOK MENTAL HEALTH ASSOCIATION

In response to the needs of the large and growing community of East and South East Asians in the GTA, Hong Fook Mental Health Association (HFMHA) was established in 1982 with support and funding from both voluntary sector organizations and government. In partnership with various communities, HFMHA increases public awareness and knowledge of mental illness by providing culturally and linguistically appropriate services, and by offering services not only to people who experience mental health problems but also to family members. It offers culturally competent consultations to other mental health service providers. Its programs and services include assessments, referrals, short and long-term counselling, case management and a range of services to families (e.g., education workshops, counselling and self-help and mutual support groups).

HFMHA collaborates with other service providers and funding agencies—including those in the mainstream mental health system—to develop models of service to address new or unmet needs within the community. Mental health promotion initiatives include community education, stress management workshops and providing language-specific materials to their target communities. They also encourage volunteerism by offering training programs to support volunteers to work with people with mental illness, including escorting them to activities in the community. Within service agencies such as HFMHA volunteer recognition is an integral part of their programs. Recognition of volunteers may take various forms such as awards for some aspects of their services or participation in planned social events.

HFMHA's initiatives should be used as a model for providing effective mental health services to immigrant communities. However, less established immigrant communities with less financial and community resources would likely experience challenges in building and maintaining such a model of service and service delivery.

Conclusion

In this chapter, we described existing services to help newcomers adapt to life in Canada, while also presenting challenges for women in accessing the kinds of support they need to resettle. Support was defined not only as direct mental health care, but services that address practical needs (e.g., around employment, housing), recognizing that these are also elements that affect people's well-being.

The following is a summary of three key recommendations we have for improving access, equity and quality of services for newcomers:

1. All agencies—not simply "immigrant-serving organizations" or ethno-racial agencies—need to re-organize their staffing, institutional policies and services to better meet the needs of newcomers. In cities such as Toronto where approximately two-thirds of the population growth is due to immigration, and where the ethno-racial composition of the city is changing significantly, all levels of government need to:

    - substantially increase funding for immigrant-serving organizations and ethno-racial agencies, so these agencies do not have to operate from the margins
    - mandate "mainstream" agencies to reconfigure their institutional capacity and services to better reflect the diverse needs of immigrant and refugee communities.

2. Service providers need to better collaborate with each other to improve equity, accessibility and quality of services. The chapter presented examples of how some agencies are working together to:

- make their services more reflective of newcomer needs and conditions; for example, a growing number of community agencies in Toronto are conducting community-based research and evaluation to ensure that their services are more in line with community needs (the growing interest in community-based research led to the establishment of the Toronto Community Based Research Network in February 2007)
- improve access and equity; for example, some organizations are collaborating with other agencies that provide interpretation services to overcome linguistic barriers; together, they are also establishing service co-ordinating committees to serve the "hard to reach" groups and avoid service overlaps
- provide multiple services in a single site, where appropriate, such that newcomers can access their diverse needs more easily.

3. Settlement services need to be integrated with mental health services in seamless and non-stigmatizing ways. An emerging body of research is highlighting that the immigration and settlement process can be a major health stressor. Thus, settlement agencies need to increasingly address mental health issues related to immigration and settlement, while mental health agencies need to reorient their services so as to better reflect the needs of diverse immigrant and refugee communities. This includes helping newcomers to find affordable housing, secure meaningful employment, overcome linguistic barriers, and navigate health care and other services. The chapter presented profiles of three agencies that have begun to link settlement services and mental health services in accessible, innovative ways.

References

Across Boundaries [website]. (nd). Available: www.acrossboundaries.ca. Accessed January 4, 2008.

Afghan Women's Counselling and Integration Community Support Organization [website]. (nd). Available: www.afghanwomen.org. Accessed January 4, 2008.

Canadian Mental Health Association [website]. (nd). Available: www.cmha.ca. Accessed January 4, 2008.

Guruge, S. (2006). *The Influence of Gender, Racial, Social, and Economic Inequalities on the Production of and Responses to Intimate Partner Violence in the Post-Migration Context.* Doctoral dissertation, University of Toronto.

Hong Fook Mental Health Association [website]. (nd). Available: www.hongfook.ca. Accessed January 4, 2008.

Holder, S.B. (1998). The Role of Immigrant Serving Organizations in the Canadian Welfare State: A Case Study. Unpublished doctoral dissertation. Available: http://ceris.metropolis.net/Virtual%20 Library/community/holder1/holder1chpt1.htm. Accessed January 4, 2008.

Lim, A., Lo, L., Siemiatycki, M. & Doucet, M. (2005). Newcomer Services in the Greater Toronto Area: An exploration of the range of funding sources of settlement services. *Working Paper No. 35.* Toronto: Centre of Excellence for Research on Immigration and Settlement.

Ng, R. (1988). *The Politics of Community Services.* Toronto: Garamond.

Part 4

Working with Specific Groups

Chapter 8

Newcomer Girls in Canada

Implications for Interventions by Mental Health Professionals

HELENE BERMAN AND YASMIN JIWANI

I know I once longed to be white.
How? you ask.
Let me tell you the ways.
. . . .
when I was growing up, I read magazines
and saw movies, blonde movie stars, white skin,
sensuous lips and to be elevated, to become
a woman, a desirable woman, I began to wear
imaginary pale skin.
. . . .

(Nellie Wong, "When I Was Growing Up,"
as cited in Ohye & Daniel, 1999)

Canada was once a nation inhabited primarily by Aboriginal people, and later by people from Europe and, to a lesser extent, Asia. Canada now receives newcomers from virtually every continent. Current Canadian policy is to admit between 220,000 to 245,000 new permanent residents each year (Citizenship and Immigration Canada [CIC], 2003). According to a Canadian Council on Social Development (CCSD) report (CCSD, 2000), about one-third of all newcomers are under the age of 25. Statistics from Citizenship and Immigration Canada's 2002 immigration overview indicate that about 21 per cent of all immigrants are females under the age of 15 (CIC, 2003).

In this chapter, we focus on racialized newcomer girls, paying particular attention to the different social forces that intersect and influence their identities. This chapter:

- briefly discusses key national and international documents that influence the lives of newcomer girls and their access to services, drawing attention to the manner in which girls have been largely overlooked as a group deserving of attention
- reviews the literature that has informed current understandings about newcomer girls and young women, and highlights the challenges these girls face in their efforts to negotiate an identity or sense of self; their struggles to fit in; and the ways that gender, ability and sexual orientation intersect and influence their lives
- makes recommendations for mental health professionals regarding possible intervention strategies that can be implemented both to facilitate these girls and young women's adaptation in Canadian society, as well as increase their resilience in dealing with the everyday violence of racism and sexism.

A Note on Racialization

In its simplest term, *racialization* refers to the process whereby groups are marked on the basis of some kind of real or supposed difference—whether this be skin colour, culture, religion, language or nationality (Miles & Brown, 2003). Racialization is thus a relationship based on power—the power to define, contain and neutralize an *other*. As used in this context, "other" is not a neutral category, but is understood as inferior, and the process of "othering" is a process whereby that inferior position is sustained. In the case of newcomer girls, the process of racialization thus differentiates and marks them as subordinate others. It renders them inferior through a process where markers such as language, religion, culture and colour are devalued. As immigrants, all newcomer girls are racialized. However, in this chapter, our focus is particularly on racialized girls of colour—those who are marked as racial others.

Newcomer Girls in National and International Contexts

Several national and international treaties, policies and conventions, on the surface, appear to ensure full rights and equalities for newcomer girls in Canada. Foremost among these is the *United Nations Convention on the Rights of the Child* (1989), which Canada has signed. According to this document, all children have the right to a life that includes more than physical survival. They have the right to intellectual, spiritual and moral development in a family and a society conducive to such growth; to protection from physical and mental harm; and to education, adequate health care, and time and space to play. The convention further stipulates that children are entitled to their own identity—not only to have a name and a nationality, but also to have privacy, dignity and a voice in decisions that concern their lives. Other United Nations documents that concern the rights of children and to which Canada is bound are the *Convention Relating to the Status of Refugees* (1951) and the *Convention on the Elimination of All Forms of Discrimination against Women* (1981).

While all of these have an impact on the rights of immigrant and refugee girls, none explicitly mention girls. These treaties afford protection against rights violations to which girls are particularly vulnerable, such as sexual exploitation and gender inequality in education and health care, yet girls' particular needs are included under the categories "children and youth." The *Beijing Declaration* and *Platform for Action* (1995) sought to rectify the situation by dealing specifically with "the girl child." Despite this initiative, most analyses have tended to assume a generic construction of the girl child. This gender-neutral construction has left the realities of girls' lives unnamed and invisible. Thus, how different groups of girls fare has been given little attention, except in those studies that specifically deal with particular populations.

Current Understandings

A review of the literature reveals a vast body of research about newcomer youth. First, many of the published studies and government reports use terms such as "newcomer," "immigrant" or "refugee." The inference is that any of these terms may be used to characterize a single, homogeneous group, and that all individuals within that group share common features. Such characterizations are usually devised according to some system of classification that is usually based on cultural identity or origins. While these categories may serve some practical purpose, the use of culture as the unit of analysis is problematic and implies a greater degree of homogeneity within cultural groups than is warranted. The net result is that differences within groups are concealed (Meleis, 1996). Aside from this, the use of culture as a unit of analysis fails to take into consideration the dynamic and evolving nature of culture as a lived reality, changing and responding to new contexts and pressures.

A second and related issue is the widespread use of generic phrases such as "children and youth" or "children and adolescence." This use of gender-neutral language effectively obscures differences between males and females. Most importantly, in a world that privileges men over women, seemingly neutral terms such as "child" or "youth" in reality refer to the "male child." Most importantly, this de-gendered language negates the ways that multiple sources of oppression—such as sexism, racism, classism, homophobia and ableism—intersect and shape girls' lives.

The third concern relates to the emphasis in the literature on "high-risk behaviours" and the corresponding focus on individual outcomes while broader social and historical contexts are either minimized or overlooked entirely. Using the language of "risk factors" and "protective factors" (Champion & Kelly, 2002; Christopherson & Jordan-Marsh, 2004), researchers have attended to individual outcomes, while neglecting to consider how individual experiences are affected by the broader social and political context of girls' lives. The net result is a decontextualized and ahistorical account of the lives of newcomer girls that highlights weaknesses and deficits while failing to celebrate strengths, resilience and agency.

NEGOTIATING SELVES

Adolescence is widely understood as that stage of life when the formation of a personal identity is a crucial developmental task. In general, this process entails the ability to make choices and clarify values and priorities, to achieve insight into one's abilities and potential, and to gain an understanding of oneself in relation to society. The capacity to accomplish these tasks is filtered through one's family and social experiences and relationships, and is shaped by social, political and historical patterns of power and domination. While the process of identity formation is difficult under the best of circumstances, for newcomer girls and young women, efforts to untangle the large questions of identity are particularly complex. Because race, gender and class are central to their identities, growing up in a world where racism, sexism and classism are pervasive features of everyday life makes the process of identity development a huge challenge. For newcomer girls who may encounter other forms of discrimination, including those based on sexual orientation, ability, weight, size or attractiveness, the struggle for a sense of self is daunting, often accompanied by very real fears of rejection and isolation.

Identity formation for newcomer girls is, thus, established through multiple contexts, in addition to their newcomer status. While gender is paramount among these, much of the theoretical literature on child development and identity formation comes from research conducted with boys, and may more aptly be considered theories of male child development (Berman et al., 2000; Gilligan, 1982; Miller, 1976). For example, in *Childhood and Society,* Erickson (1950) outlines a series of developmental crises. With the exception of infancy, each stage is characterized by increasing degrees of separation and individuation. For girls and young women, however, research has shown that interconnections and relationships are typically more important than they are for boys and young men (Gilligan, 1982). Girls generally place a high value on maintaining close family ties and relationships. Their struggle is not for separation from the family, but for a new and more adult role and voice within it. Applying Gilligan's model to the young female newcomer, the challenge may be more about how to embrace North American culture, without separating from her culture of origin.

Goodenow and Espin (1993) discussed the issue of ego identity formation and the associated complexities faced by newcomer adolescents living in the United States. Based on in-depth interviews with five adolescent females who were recent immigrants from Latin American countries, the authors described the efforts used by these young women to accommodate the values and influences of both the "old and the new" culture, and to thereby achieve what was described as a "healthy bicultural identity." Of particular interest was the participants' view that had they remained in their countries of origin, they would have faced pressure to marry and have children early. While most indicated that marriage and child-bearing were included in their long-term plans, they now felt that they had other options available to them, including career and travel. Regarding sexuality and perceived North American norms, the young women in this research were disinclined to embrace what they saw as "promiscuousness" among girls their age. According to Goodenow and Espin (1993), these participants were moving toward "successful bicultural adjustment," retaining some valued aspects of a "traditional Latina identity," while rejecting others.

Several researchers have examined the notion of bicultural identities, and described strategies used by adolescent newcomers that enabled them to sustain the values embraced within both their country of origin and their "adopted" countries (Anisef et al., 2003; James, 1997; Kim, 2004; Lopez & Contreras, 2005; Mann, 2004; Seat, 2003). Desai and Subramanian (2003) discussed this process in relation to South Asian immigrant youth in Toronto. Although their research included males and females, these investigators addressed the issue of gender and noted that, while the process of negotiating identities was a complex undertaking for all newcomers, girls faced particular challenges in their efforts to fit in. For many of the young women in this research, it seemed impossible to be accepted by both the dominant white group, as well as within their own cultural group. Some who had been in Canada longer were reluctant to befriend more recent newcomers for fear that they would jeopardize their own hard-fought-for status of acceptance. Not wanting to stand out or be noticed, or be perceived as "different," the South Asian youth adopted a "pseudo-white" status (Desai & Subramanian, p. 141), believing that this would afford some type of protection.

A similar idea was shared by Kim (2004). In this qualitative study with young Korean immigrants in the United States, Kim described how these youth negotiated social, cultural and generational boundaries. According to Kim, adolescent immigrants are "either bicultural, enjoying the richness of the two cultures, or live in existential limbo, being confused between the culture of origin and the newly adopted culture" (p. 519). The participants in this study perceived a gap between themselves and their parents as they adopted American norms and values. Those who reported greater communication with their parents reported more satisfaction with themselves. Similarly, Goodenow and Espin (1993) noted the importance of girls' relationships with their mothers as an important influence when choosing to retain their Hispanic identity.

While much of this literature suggests that adolescent newcomer girls are successful in developing bicultural identities, the emphasis on culture, adaptation and assimilation highlights several problematic assumptions. For one, adaptation and assimilation are often considered to be synonymous, implying that successful adaptation can only be achieved through the incorporation of dominant values, and that assimilating the norms and values of the dominant society is a positive indicator. Further, these processes are assumed to be linear—following a progression through time, that is, moving from a newcomer status to gradually developing bicultural identities, which are then seen as indicative of adjustment/adaptation or acculturation. However, as Bhatia and Ram point out,

> When we adhere to universal models of acculturation, we undervalue the asymmetrical relations of power and the inequities and injustices faced by certain immigrant groups as a result of their nationality, race or gender. Being othered or racialized is part of many non-European immigrants' acculturation experience, and these experiences are tightly knitted with their evolving conceptions of selfhood. These experiences are revealed both in everyday, routine intercultural encounters and in a government or a state's history of laws about nationality, citizenship and immigration. (2001, p. 8)

Hence, not only are power inequalities flattened in much of the discussion of adaptation through assimilation, but equally problematic is the notion that this kind of adaptation is positive. Acculturation increases the potential of internalizing the values and norms of the dominant society. This means that the values of the dominant society are also internalized along with the hierarchical preferences of that society. So if particular groups are consistently seen as inferior and devalued, then the internalization of these values also results in reproducing these very preferences within groups. For instance, Pyke and Dang (2003) found that young American adults of Korean and Vietnamese descent created a hierarchy within their own group differentiating between the FOB (fresh off the boat) newcomers and the "whitewashed" (those who were considered to be assimilated). Pyke and Dang argue that, "This process of intraethnic othering is an attempt to resist a racially stigmatized status; however, it does so by reproducing stereotypes and a belief in essential racial and ethnic differences between whites and Asians" (2003, p. 168). In other words, bicultural identity development itself rests on defining those that fall outside the categories of the dominant and ethnic group.

Debold et al. (1999) suggest that not acculturating implies a degree of protection from the harmful values of the dominant, host society. It ensures that girls are more in touch with their voices and thoughts (Gilligan & Brown, 1992), less affected by sexism, less susceptible to pressures to conform to the idealized body image and sexually compliant behaviour, and more likely to access alternative role models from within their own communities (Brown et al., 1999). However, not acculturating also puts girls of colour at risk for other kinds of violence mediated by exclusion and marginalization (Tsolidis, 1990). The pressure to fit in and belong is a key factor in the socialization of girls and young women. It is mediated by consumption practices that encourage girls and young women with the purchasing power to obtain the same kinds of clothes, makeup and other commodities as their peers (Twine, 1996). This is particularly difficult for newcomer girls given that poverty is a dominant issue in the lives of at least 30 per cent of the immigrant youth of colour (Anisef & Kilbride, 2000).

Struggling to Fit In

The struggle to fit in, to achieve a sense of belonging both socially and academically, is a common theme throughout the literature. In one of the few studies in Ontario related to the mental health of adolescent female newcomers, Khanlou and her colleagues (2002) conducted focus groups with female newcomer youth as well as their parents, educators, social workers and settlement workers at two Toronto high schools, both with a large percentage of newcomers. Findings revealed that—although many of these young women reported relatively high degrees of confidence and competence around academic achievement, relationships with family and friends, and general feelings about themselves—they continued to struggle in their efforts to fit into Canadian society.

A central aspect of this struggle related to language and the difficulties they encountered in their efforts to attain a comfortable level of English fluency. This finding is one that has been described elsewhere by many researchers (Anisef & Kilbride, 2000; CCSD, 2000; Janzen & Ochocka, 2003; Rumbaut, 1991). Unable to interact with ease in English, the girls in Khanlou's study were quite literally silenced, heightening their sense of alienation and isolation and adversely affecting their sense of academic and social success. In order to gain increased acceptance by their Canadian-born counterparts, some participants told of anglicizing their name, despite the fact that they preferred their ethnic name (Khanlou et al., 2002).

These actions may be understood as a means for newcomer girls to break down barriers between themselves and others. However, viewed in another way, such practices may be seen as predictable responses to racism and discrimination. Changing their names was a strategy used by the girls to try to make themselves more acceptable or, more aptly, less "different." On the other hand, referring to the rates of depression among various migrant populations, Bhugra (2004) found that "if fluency in English is taken as one proxy measure of acculturation, then it would appear that higher levels of acculturation may lead to higher levels of psychological morbidity" (p. 252). His findings reflect that the struggle to fit in, through the appropriation and use of the dominant language not to mention normative values, could result in greater dissatisfaction as individuals realize that they are not being accepted for who and what they are but rather who and what they appear to be.

The struggle to fit in is often depicted in the literature as a dichotomized, "either/or" choice for girls as they decide between adherence to the traditional cultural values and ways of being associated with their country of origin on the one hand, and those of their "adopted" country on the other hand. Missing from this portrayal is an analysis of how the former is devalued and rendered inferior, and how the cultural scripts and expectations from both worlds are based on widely embraced and deeply entrenched male-dominant values.

A more comprehensive analysis of newcomer girls' struggles to fit in is one that accounts for the centrality of racism and sexism, and that examines how these are sanctioned and sustained in ways that are often subtle and insidious. In research with racialized immigrant and refugee girls living in British Columbia, Jiwani et al. (2002) found that racism was the most common form of violence these girls experienced. Similarly, in a series of focus groups with racialized immigrant and refugee youth, racism was a common theme that emerged in all of the groups (CCSD, 2000). The younger participants in the focus groups spoke of poor treatment at school by both teachers and other students, while older participants told of difficulties in obtaining employment, and harassment by the police because of their physical appearance. At the level of the individual experience of newcomer girls, the interaction of racism and sexism creates an environment in which " . . . racialized girls are inferiorized and . . . [where] they internalize dominant values which embody a rejection of the self and their cultural communities" (Jiwani, 1999, p. 25).

Research has shown that the experiences of young women of colour are deeply informed by their experiences of racism and their understanding of race. This in itself creates a profoundly different set of experiences for young, visible minority women compared to those of young women who are not visible minorities (Wright, 1998, pp. 221, 228). On the one hand, they are confronted with the usual adolescent challenges of identity formation, but must meet these tasks in the context of two cultures, both of which devalue or sexualize women and girls. At the same time, they must deal with the racism of mainstream society and its many and varied manifestations. The result is an inability to identify, and therefore resist, all but the most blatant forms of racism or sexism. In essence, racialized newcomer girls face a tremendous struggle in their efforts to fit in, and the odds against them are enormous.

INTERSECTING REALITIES

Reviewing the research on newcomer girls underscores the need to expand our knowledge concerning the lives of diverse groups of newcomer girls and young women. This requires us to break down the linear frameworks that underlie much of the research literature. Young immigrant women are much more than "newcomer girls." Some are racialized girls of colour; some are lesbian, bisexual or transgendered; some live in impoverished socio-economic conditions; some have experienced violence prior to immigrating and others are experiencing violence in their new homes; and some may be differently abled. Or there may be any combination of these. Even within particular ethnocultural groups, there is enormous variation. For many, violence—either subtle or explicit—is a pervasive feature in their lives. These are areas that have received very little research attention. Most commonly, newcomer girls are discussed as a homogeneous group whose members all share features in common with one another by virtue of their newcomer status. This failure to acknowledge the multiple social identities that shape their lives does these young women a huge disservice and contributes to harmful and fundamentally flawed stereotypes.

For lesbian, bisexual or transgendered girls of colour, the taboo against homosexuality is reinforced by an alliance between male-dominant power in the dominant society and male-dominant structures within racialized communities (Bannerji, 2000; Jiwani, 2005). The normalization of heterosexuality, in conjunction with racism that may be insidious or explicit, leads to intense isolation and condemnation of these young women from the larger society and from within their own communities. (For a discussion of issues around counselling lesbian and bisexual women, see Chapter 11.)

In his study of homosexual youth from diverse cultural and racial backgrounds, Savin-Williams (1994) found that the youth were forced to choose between identifying themselves culturally or identifying themselves as homosexuals. It was difficult for them to assume a "bicultural" identity, as homosexual identity was considered taboo. The close-knit nature of racialized ethnic communities exerts a force here as families' reputations are considered to be contingent on the behaviour of their children. Hence, if children come out as gay, lesbian, bisexual or transgendered, then within the normative, taken-for-granted framework of heterosexuality that prevails both within these communities and within the larger societies, the impact is greater on the families vis-à-vis the community in which they reside. Indeed, as Li and Orleans (2001) suggest, on the basis of their in-depth interviews with young Asian lesbians, these women did not only have to deal with the process of coming out to themselves but also had to witness the process of coming out for their families. Ultimately, newcomer girls of colour who are lesbians, bisexual or transgendered struggle for acceptance both within their own community as well as within communities of other lesbian, bisexual and transgendered girls and women.

With respect to newcomer girls who are differently abled, the research is virtually nonexistent. This point was highlighted by Stienstra and Owen (2004) who observed that the few studies conducted in this area have been undertaken from the vantage point of service providers, focusing on the need for culturally appropriate services. Much research is still needed for us to understand the unique situations of newcomer girls with disabilities.

Even without research available, it is reasonable to assume that in a world that privileges able-bodied, white, male bodies, and where racism and sexism are pervasive features of everyday life, differently abled young newcomer females are likely to encounter considerable hardships. These are further compounded when we consider the dominant heterosexual orientation of communities as described above and the pressures on families for their children to marry and reproduce. In some respects, the stigma and isolation are similar to that experienced by newcomer families with lesbian daughters (Jiwani, 2005). However, the situation for newcomer girls with disabilities may be further complicated by the depiction of some disabilities, such as those that exist at birth (are congenital), as "legitimate" and others, such as HIV/AIDS or even chronic depression and other mental health issues, as "illegitimate." Seen as such, these issues are understood as signs of individual failure reflecting an inability or unwillingness to adjust to the new situation, and thus often attributed to the failure of the families involved for not adequately socializing the individuals who are affected. Again, these kinds of understandings are not unique to immigrant communities, rather they are pervasive within the larger host society. In the case of the immigrant community, it is the tendency to turn inward, the focus on cohesion within the community that forms a tightly bounded social structure whereby views, values and attitudes are shared and held in common and thus are experienced more intensely. Tyagi (1999) in her study of incest summarizes it best when she says:

> Communities of colour, particularly new immigrants and refugees, have subcultures that operate differently from the dominant culture, particularly if they are struggling to survive in a hostile or racist host environment. In order to deal with stresses inherent in discontinuity and change, communities turn naturally to known, familiar values, behaviours, and beliefs. Many turn further inwards to their sense of ethnic identity and accompanying values in an effort to enhance community belongingness. To do so however, it is axiomatic that (a) the subculture's own cultural values be constructed as good and therefore worthy of preservation; (b) problems, dissonant ideas be externalized as a disruptive, coming from the outside, i.e., the host-culture; (c) a mythology be created that the values from the source (the motherland, country of origin) are the standard and impervious to change; (d) the only method of ethnic identity preservation is to preserve that standard; and (e) these positions be legitimized and endorsed by community leadership. (p. 174)

Most of the research with newcomer girls in Canada has been conducted in large urban centres. Given that most newcomers settle in the major cities, this makes sense. However, there is also a population of newcomer girls living in rural settings. In one of the few studies concerning this group of newcomers, Miedema and Wachhotz (1998) reported that the lack of cultural relevance in most social service programs deterred newcomer women from seeking services. Fears of the police, concerns about deportation of themselves or their families and general suspicion of the legal system, as well as racism, further dissuade newcomer girls from seeking services (Blaney, 2005; Janovicek, 2000; Jiwani et al., 2002). In her work on newcomer girls in Victoria, Lee (2005, 2006) points to the exclusion that the girls experience living in a landscape that is filled with imperial English symbols and architecture and where cultural difference is relegated either to the margins or legitimized only in the form of exotic cuisine.

CITIZENSHIP, RACISM AND THE BURDEN OF BICULTURALISM

The circumstances that bring newcomer girls to Canada vary widely. Some arrive with their family in search of a better life. Others are forced to flee because of personal or political threats of persecution—they leave abruptly, breaking ties with their country, culture, traditions and families. Some have experienced racism and other forms of violence such as sexual abuse prior to coming to Canada. Regardless of the circumstances, all experience some degree of uprooting, loss and separation. Understanding the consequences of uprootedness in the lives of newcomer girls, and how ideas of citizenship, community and home are experienced by these young women is an important, though understudied, area.

Gonick (2000) discussed the notions of citizenship and "Canadian-ness" in the context of immigrant and refugee girls in Canada. Based on her research with girls of Vietnamese and Chinese backgrounds, Gonick mapped what it means to be Canadian, and sought to examine how this understanding is shaped by discourses of race, multi-culturalism and nation. According to Gonick, legal and geographical categories comprise important aspects of one's national identity, but these are by no means the only ones. Less commonly mentioned is the way in which national identity is structured by categories of racial and ethnic privilege. This idea is illustrated by one of the girls in her research who conceded that with the necessary legal documentation, she will become a Canadian citizen, but when asked if she will then be Canadian, she replied "No, I'm half Chinese and half Vietnamese" (p. 98). Thus, being Canadian is more than a legal designation and is a category that is reserved for "real" Canadians (see next paragraph). By contrast, Vietnamese or Chinese immigrants will always be "marked" by their racial and ethnic difference. These findings have also been echoed in other studies dealing with mixed-race and second-generation young women of colour (Aujla, 2000; Mahtani, 2002; Pratt, 2002).

Articulating a similar perspective, Kamala Viswesaran (as cited in Aujla, 2000) commented on the seeming innocence of the question, "Where do you come from?" so often directed toward racialized newcomers. As Jiwani (2006) noted, the subtext to this question is that the "real" Canadian is normatively constructed as a person who is white. Through the asking of such questions about origin and identity, their position as "different" or "other" becomes fixed, and full acceptance becomes an elusive and unattainable goal.

Espin (1995) and Yuval-Davis (1992) discussed the burden that young women must bear as upholders and managers of multicultural citizenship, as the group that ultimately determines what aspects of the "old" and the "new" cultures will be maintained or acquired, as well as if and how these will be blended. For the most part, this responsibility is restricted to the highly visible aspects of culture that are the most benign, namely food, clothing and dance. In this manner, young women become "symbols of acculturation" (Aapola et al., 2005). This construction of a young woman as the ideal "blended citizen" is a depoliticizing agenda that neutralizes concerns of racism, sexism or classism and establishes a young newcomer woman of color as a "depoliticized, entertaining Other" (p. 182). In other words, they are seen as more acceptable as "exotic" others who bring to the table novel cultural differences that are non-threatening and consumable. Indeed, Bourne et al. (1998) found similar sentiments being articulated by the young women of colour who participated in their study.

Efforts to outline patterns of acculturation success or failure among cultural groups are particularly problematic when we consider the astonishing degree of racial, ethnic, cultural, language, religious and class diversity encapsulated within such broad groupings such as "Asians" or "Latin Americans." As we see in the research, culture is commonly linked with family socialization patterns, identity formation, home/school culture conflict and religion, and rarely associated with class, socio-economic status, marginality and racism. Even when the presence of racism and/or sexism is acknowledged, with few exceptions, researchers rarely consider their effects.

Much of the acculturation/biculturalism discourse appears to be grounded in static ideas of cultural dissimilarity and discreteness. Such concepts limit our expectations of the world and restrict our ability to imagine alternatives. They do not recognize the new spaces of culture, language and identity formed in the context of displacement and difference, and are unable to recognize the resolutions and resistance of cultural practices that redirect frustration, anger and discord borne of encounters with ethnocentrism, racism, sexism, ableism and homophobia. In such a context of absence, discussions about resistance become paramount in redirecting attention to the newcomer girls' agency in forging a sense of identity that is resilient and celebratory.

Hooks has written about a type of resistance in her discussion about "back talk" and "talking back" (1990). Growing up in a southern black community, where children were meant to be seen and not heard, talking back was to invite punishment. To speak when one was not spoken to was a courageous act, an act of risking and daring. It was in this atmosphere that she listened to the voices of black women who "spoke in a language so rich, so poetic, that it felt to me like being shut off from life, smothered to death if one was not allowed to participate" (p. 337). It was in this world of woman talk that hooks learned what it meant to have a voice. In her words:

> Moving from silence into speech is for the oppressed, the colonized, the exploited, and those who stand and struggle side by side, a gesture of defiance that heals, that makes new life and new growth possible. It is that act of speech, of "talking back" that is no mere gesture of empty words, that is the expression of moving from object to subject, that is the liberated voice. (p. 340)

This tradition of silence is long. Anzaldua (1990) wrote about various expressions heard repeatedly throughout her own childhood in Puerto Rico, all reinforcing the social imperative for girls and women to remain silent. *En boca cerrada no entran moscas.* "Flies don't enter a closed mouth." *Ser habladora* refers to being a gossip and a liar, to talking too much. And *Muchachatistas bien criadas* means well-bred girls don't answer back.

Gilligan (1982) spoke of a type of resistance that comes from a feminist perspective and that can be seen as a strength, an indication of physical and emotional health or courage. Acts of resistance can range from speaking out, to avoiding substance abuse, to addressing conflict with a friend in order to stay connected, to making direct challenges within a patriarchal context (e.g., advocating against racism or sexism). The common thread is the maintenance of one's voice and speaking one's own truth, being part of a resonant relationship in which girls are able to speak freely and hear their voices clearly. These types of relationships are, in themselves, acts of resistance.

Key Issues and Strategies for Mental Health Professionals

> "Who is to say that robbing a people of its language is less violent than war?"
>
> (Ray Gwyn Smith, as cited in Ferguson et al., 1990, p. 203)

Adolescent girls who are newcomers to Canada are forced to negotiate many different terrains. In this section, we discuss approaches that may be useful to facilitate this process. However, rather than offering a toolkit of strategies that mental health professionals should adopt, we discuss some of the key issues that need to inform any meaningful engagement with young women who are newcomers to Canada. Moreover, while much of this discussion is directed toward mental health professionals, any comprehensive response cannot be undertaken by any single professional group but, rather, requires a collaborative effort on the part of the health, legal, educational and social service communities. The following are strategies that girls have identified as most helpful to them:

- developing strategies to confront systemic racism and sexism
- developing anti-racist curricula relevant to girls and young women
- creating meaningful cultural programs
- creating safe spaces for girls to talk about racism and violence
- encouraging strategies of resistance
- encouraging others to see equality as a societal necessity.

DEVELOP STRATEGIES TO CONFRONT SYSTEMIC RACISM AND SEXISM

Newcomers are taught that Canada is a humanitarian country where equality applies to all, regardless of race, gender or class. However, research with young women who are newcomers to Canada reveals that racism, supported and sustained in subtle and not-so-subtle ways, continues to be a central defining feature in their lives. While efforts that are geared toward enhancing self-esteem, or other individually oriented solutions may be useful, it is our view that by themselves such initiatives fail to challenge the root cause of the problem and are unlikely to result in significant, lasting change. More fruitful approaches are collective strategies that confront, question and challenge systemic forms of racism and the power dynamics that perpetuate social injustice and that incorporate institutional change.

DEVELOP ANTI-RACIST CURRICULA RELEVANT
TO GIRLS AND YOUNG WOMEN

Based on their research with South Asian youth in Canada, Desai and Subramanian (2003) have observed that awareness of one's status as "other" contributes to a sense of cultural pride, in part a response to the devalued position accorded racialized newcomer girls. Much of this is played out in the schools, where they spend a substantial amount of time. Thus, mental health professionals can work collaboratively with educators to develop anti-racist curricula and after-school activities that are meaningful and relevant to these girls and young women. For such programs to be successful, guidance counsellors, teachers and principals need to be sensitized to the subtle and explicit manifestations of racism and discrimination, and gain an understanding of how these are sustained within the school environment. School policies and practices that may contribute to the marginalization of newcomer girls need to be examined. One example is the tendency for newcomer girls to be excluded from advanced courses and streamed into English-as-a-second-language or remedial classes, or given aptitude tests that are culturally irrelevant to them. Although well-intentioned, the net result is increased feelings of "difference" and further isolation.

CREATE MEANINGFUL CULTURAL PROGRAMS

Mental health professionals can also play an important role in the creation of cultural programs to foster increased understanding and appreciation of different cultures. Such programs afford an opportunity to move the notion of "embracing diversity" beyond the level of song and dance, or the exotic allure of difference, and can contribute to a more multi-layered and complex appreciation of the dynamic nature of culture and the workings of race, class and gender in the school environment. However, it is equally important that mental health professionals not succumb to fixed and static notions of culture. Culture itself has to be understood as that complex of values, lifestyles, behaviours, attitudes and ways of being that are fluid and dynamic and that evolve in response to external and internal factors. Thus cultural programs need to begin with a questioning of culture itself and to include an analysis that accounts for the global impact of hybrid cultural forms that have emerged due to migration, the influence of the mass media and global economic links. Cultural programs that facilitate interaction between girls from different backgrounds would offer one avenue by which the notion of culture could be explored and the variations within cultural groups identified and affirmed. This would also help dismantle stereotypes.

CREATE SAFE SPACES FOR GIRLS TO TALK ABOUT RACISM AND VIOLENCE

Safe spaces, both within and outside of schools are needed where girls can talk openly, where their voices can be heard, and where they can learn about strategies to resist and counter racism and other forms of everyday violence. Resistance is often viewed negatively and refers to a tendency for people to balk at moving toward a goal or a propensity for them to block efforts to change. However, resistance may be thought of as a positive trait in that it may honour the experiences of newcomer girls and their ability to develop strategies to manage and overcome the feelings associated with racism, discrimination and exclusion.

ENCOURAGE STRATEGIES OF RESISTANCE

The role of resistance in the development of girls' self-esteem was discussed by Ward (1996) in relation to black girls in the United States. By instilling in these young women an ability to identify and analyze issues of power and authority embedded in relationships, they become increasingly able to critique messages about "colour-blind meritocracy" where upward mobility is open to all. Those who are not prepared to confront racism become vulnerable to self-deception and self-hatred. Further, the world then appears as chaotic, unpredictable, hostile and rejecting. Girls who learn about the workings of racism, gender, class and power are, in turn, empowered to address these in a forthright manner. In essence, healthy resistance fostered through a liberating truth-telling has a transformative quality.

At the same time, speaking the truth can have a cost. It is necessary to be *wisely resistant* (Robinson & Ward, 1991). By naming the political realities and discussing these difficulties, resistance strategies can be formulated and shared. However, a balance is needed between encouraging resistance and "mouthing off." Given the political climate and its harsh realities, it is necessary to teach a form of resistance that is responsible, respectful and safe.

ENCOURAGE OTHERS TO SEE EQUALITY AS A SOCIETAL NECESSITY

Most importantly, we need to foster a more equitable and just society, one in which the embracing of difference is not merely rhetoric designed to appease particular groups or orchestrated as a vacant celebration of diversity. Rather, such an equitable society requires a dismantling of the hierarchy of preference and privilege where skin colour, class, able-bodiedness and heterosexuality are the prerequisites of acceptance and belonging.

Conclusion

Responding to the needs and challenges faced by newcomer girls and young women requires that mental health professionals use approaches that are creative and flexible. There is no single strategy that fits all situations. Rather, mental health professionals will achieve greatest success if interventions are established and implemented in collaboration with the girls and women they are intended to serve. In a similar vein, the limited research pertaining to newcomer girls in Canada highlights the critical need for scholarly attention to this largely overlooked population. Establishing research partnerships that include girls and young women, consistent with participatory action research methodologies, enhances the likelihood that research will be relevant and meaningful. Most importantly, we need to go beyond unilinear notions of "the newcomer girl" and develop interventions that reflect the multiple and intersecting realities in the lives of newcomer girls and young women.

References

Aapola, S., Gonick, M. & Harris, A. (2005). *Young Femininity: Girlhood, Power and Social Change*. Houndmills, UK: Palgrave Macmillan.

Anisef, P. & Kilbride, K.M. (2000). *The Needs of Newcomer Youth and Emerging "Best Practices" to Meet Those Needs: Final Report*. Toronto: Joint Centre of Excellence for Research on Immigration and Settlement.

Anisef, P., Kilbride, K.M. & Khattar, R. (2003). The needs of newcomer youth and emerging "best practices" to meet those needs. In P. Anisef & K.M. Kilbride (Eds.), *Managing Two Worlds: The Experiences and Concerns of Immigrant Youth in Ontario* (pp. 196–234). Toronto: Canadian Scholars' Press.

Anzaldua, G. (1990). How to tame a wild tongue. In R. Ferguson, M. Gever, T. Minh-ha & C. West (Eds.). *Out There: Marginalization and Contemporary Cultures*. Cambridge, MA: MIT Press.

Aujla, A. (2000). Others in their own land: Second generation South Asian Canadian women, racism, and the persistence of colonial discourse. *Canadian Woman Studies, 20* (2), 41–47.

Bannerji, H. (2000). *The Dark Side of the Nation: Essays on Multiculturalism, Nationalism and Gender*. Toronto: Canadian Scholars' Press.

Berman, H., McKenna, K., Traher, C., Taylor, G. & MacQuarrie, B. (2000). Sexual harassment: Everyday violence in the lives of girls and women. *Advances in Nursing Science, 22* (4), 32–46.

Bhatia, S. & Ram, A. (2001). Rethinking "acculturation" in relation to diasporic cultures and postcolonial identities. *Human Development, 44* (1), 1–18.

Bhugra, D. (2004). Migration and mental health. *Acta Psychiatrica Scandinavica, 109* (4), 243–258.

Blaney, E. (2005). *Situating Girls' and Young Women's Experiences of Violence in Rural Areas*. Unpublished manuscript, Intersecting Sites of Violence in the Lives of Girls Research Project.

Bourne, P., McCoy, L. & Smith, D. (1998). Girls and schooling: Their own critique. *Resources for Feminist Research, 26* (1/2), 55–68.

Brown, L.M., Way, N. & Duff, J.L. (1999). The others in my I: Adolescent girls' friendships and peer relations. In N.G. Johnson, M.C. Roberts & J. Worrell (Eds.), *Beyond Appearance: A New Look at Adolescent Girls* (pp. 205–225). Washington, DC: American Psychological Association.

Canadian Council on Social Development. (2000). *Immigrant Youth in Canada.* Ottawa: Author.

Champion, J.D. & Kelly, P. (2002). Protective and risk behaviours of rural minority adolescent women. *Issues in Mental Health Nursing, 23* (3), 191–207.

Christopherson, T.M. & Jordan-Marsh, M. (2004). Culture and risk taking in adolescents' behaviours. *MCN: The American Journal of Maternal/Child Nursing, 29* (2), 100–105.

Citizenship and Immigration Canada. (2003). *Facts and Figures 2002: Immigration Overview.* Ottawa: Minister of Public Works and Government Services Canada.

Debold, E., Mikel Brown, L., Weseen, S. & Kearse Brookins, G. (1999). Cultivating hardiness zones for adolescent girls: A reconceptualization of resilience in relationships with caring adults. In N.G. Johnson, M.C. Roberts & J. Worrell (Eds.), *Beyond Appearance: A New Look at Adolescent Girls* (pp. 181–204). Washington, DC: American Psychological Association.

Desai, S. & Subramanian, S. (2003). Colour, culture, and dual consciousness: Issues identified by South Asian immigrant youth in the greater Toronto area. In P. Anisef & K.M. Kilbride (Eds.), *Managing Two Worlds: The Experiences and Concerns of Immigrant Youth in Ontario* (pp. 118–161). Toronto: Canadian Scholars' Press.

Erikson, E. (1950). *Childhood and Society.* New York: W.W. Norton and Company.

Espin, O. (1995). "Race," racism, and sexuality in the life narratives of immigrant women. *Feminism and Psychology, 5* (2), 223–238.

Ferguson, R., Gever, M., Minh-ha, T. & West, C. (Eds.). (1990). *Out There: Marginalization and Contemporary Cultures.* Cambridge, MA: MIT Press.

Gilligan C. (1982). *In a Different Voice: Psychological Theory and Women's Development.* Cambridge, MA: Harvard University Press.

Gilligan, C. & Brown, L.M. (1992). *Meeting at the Crossroads: Women's Psychology and Girls' Development.* New York: Ballantine Books.

Gonick, M. (2000). Canadian = blonde, English, white: Theorizing race, language, and nation. *Atlantis, 24* (2), 93–104.

Goodenow, C. & Espin, O.M. (1993). Identity choices in immigrant adolescent females. *Adolescence, 28* (109), 173–183.

hooks, b. (1990). Talking back. In R. Ferguson, M. Gever, T. Minh-ha & C. West (Eds) *Out There: Marginalization and Contemporary Cultures.* Cambridge, MA: MIT Press.

James, D.C.S. (1997). Coping with a new society. *The Journal of School Health, 67* (3), 98–102.

Janovicek, N. (2000). *On the Margins of a Fraying Social Safety Net: First Nations and Immigrant and Women's Access to BC Benefits.* Vancouver: FREDA Centre for Research on Violence against Women and Children.

Janzen, R. & Ochocka, J. (2003). Immigrant youth in Waterloo Region. In P. Anisef & K.M. Kilbride (Eds.), *Managing Two Worlds: The Experiences and Concerns of Immigrant Youth in Ontario* (pp. 37–68). Toronto: Canadian Scholars' Press.

Jiwani, Y. (1999). Erasing race: The story of Reena Virk. *Canadian Woman Studies, 19* (3), 178–184.

Jiwani, Y. (2005). *Intersecting Violence(s): Racialized Girls and Young Women of Colour.* Unpublished manuscript, The Alliance of Canadian Research Centres on Violence, London, ON.

Jiwani, Y. (2006). *Discourses of Denial: Mediations of Race, Gender and Violence.* Vancouver:

University of British Columbia Press.

Jiwani, Y., Janovicek, N. & Cameron, A. (2002). Erased realities: The violence of racism in the lives of immigrant and refugee girls of colour. In H. Berman & Y. Jiwani (Eds.), *In the Best Interests of the Girl Child* (pp. 47–88). London, ON: The Alliance of Canadian Research Centers on Violence.

Khanlou, N., Beiser, M., Cole, E., Freire, M., Hyman, I. & Kilbride, K.M. (2002). *Mental Health Promotion among Newcomer Female Youth: Post-Migration Experiences and Self-Esteem.* Ottawa: Status of Women Canada.

Kim, S. (2004). The experiences of young Korean immigrants: A grounded theory of negotiating social, cultural, and generational boundaries. *Issues in Mental Health Nursing, 25* (5), 517–537.

Lee, J. (2005). Talking about "us": Racialized girls, cultural citizenship and growing up under whiteness. In C.L. Biggs & P.J. Downe (Eds.), *Gendered Intersections: An Introduction to Women's and Gender Studies* (pp. 164–169). Halifax, NS: Fernwood Publishing.

Lee, J. (2006). Locality, participatory action research, and racialized girls' struggles for citizenship. In Y. Jiwani, C. Steenbergen & C. Mitchell (Eds.), *Girlhood: Redefining the Limits* (pp. 89–108). Montreal: Black Rose Books.

Li, L. & Orleans, M. (2001). Coming out discourses of Asian American lesbians. *Sexuality & Culture, 5* (2), 57–78.

Lopez, I.R. & Contreras, J.M. (2005). The best of both worlds: Biculturality, acculturation, and adjustment among young mainland Puerto Rican mothers. *Journal of Cross-Cultural Psychology, 36,* 192–208.

Mahtani, M. (2002). Interrogating the hyphen-nation: Canadian multicultural policy and "mixed race" identities. *Social Identities, 8* (1), 67–90.

Mann, M.A. (2004). Immigrant parents and their emigrant adolescents: The tension of inner and outer worlds. *The American Journal of Psychoanalysis, 64* (2), 143–153.

Meleis, A.I. (1996). Culturally competent scholarship: Substance and rigor. *Advances in Nursing Science, 19* (2), 1–16.

Miedema B. & Wachholz, S. (1998). *A Complex Web: Access to Justice for Abused Immigrant Women in New Brunswick.* Ottawa: Status of Women Canada.

Miles, R. & Brown, M. (2003). *Racism: Key Ideas Series.* London & New York: Routledge.

Miller, J.B. (1976). *Toward a new psychology of women.* Boston: Beacon Press.

Ohye, B.R. & Daniel, J.H. (1999). The "other" adolescent girls: Who are they? In N. Johnson, M. Roberts & J. Worell (Eds.), *Beyond Appearance: A New Look at Adolescent Girls* (pp. 115–130). Washington, DC: American Psychological Association.

Pratt, G. (2002). Between homes: Displacement and belonging for second generation Filipino-Canadian youths. *Research on Immigration and Integration in the Metropolis: Working Paper Series,* No. 02-13. Vancouver: Vancouver Centre of Excellence.

Pyke, K. & Dang, T. (2003). "FOB" and "whitewashed": Identity and internalized racism among second generation Asian Americans. *Qualitative Sociology, 26* (2), 147–172.

Robinson, T. & Ward, J.V. (1991). A belief in self far greater than anyone's disbelief: Cultivating healthy resistance among African American female adolescents. In C. Gilligan, A. Rogers & D. Tolman (Eds.), *Women, Girls and Psychotherapy: Reframing Resistance* (pp. 87–103). Binghamton, NY: Harrington Park Press.

Rumbaut, R. (1991). The agony of exile: A study of the migration and adaptation of Indochinese refugee adults and children. In F.L. Ahearn & J.L. Athey (Eds.), *Refugee Children: Theory, Research, and Services* (pp. 53–91). Baltimore: Johns Hopkins University Press.

Savin-Williams, R.C. (1994). Verbal and physical abuse as stressors in the lives of lesbian, gay male, and bisexual youths: Associations with school problems, running away, substance abuse, prostitution, and suicide. *Journal of Consulting and Clinical Psychology, 62* (2), 261–269.

Seat, R. (2003). Factors affecting the settlement and adaptation process of Canadian adolescent newcomers sixteen to nineteen years of age. In P. Anisef & K.M. Kilbride (Eds.), *Managing Two Worlds: The Experiences and Concerns of Immigrant Youth in Ontario* (pp. 162–195). Toronto: Canadian Scholars' Press.

Stienstra, D. & Owen, M. (2004). *Advancing the Inclusion of Persons with Disabilities: Gender, Qualitative, and Global Indicators.* Ottawa: Office for Disability Issues, Knowledge Development Unit.

Tsolidis, G. (1990). Ethnic minority girls and self-esteem. In J. Kenway & S. Willis (Eds.), *Hearts and Minds: Self-Esteem and the Schooling of Girls* (pp. 53–69). London: The Falmer Press.

Turner, V. (1969). *The Ritual Process.* Chicago: Aldine.

Twine, F.W. (1996). Brown skinned white girls: Class, culture and the construction of white identity in suburban communities. *Gender, Place and Culture, 3* (2), 205–224.

Tyagi, S.V. (1999). Tell it like it is: Incest disclosure and women of colour. *Canadian Woman Studies, 19* (3), 173–177.

United Nations. (1951). *Convention Relating to the Status of Refugees.* Geneva: UN Office of the High Commisioner for Human Rights. Available: www.unhchr.ch/html/menu3/b/o_c_ref.htm. Accessed January 5, 2008.

United Nations. (1981). *Convention on the Elimination of All Forms of Discrimination against Women.* Geneva: UN. Available: www.hrweb.org/legal/cdw.html. Accessed January 5, 2008.

United Nations. (1989). *Convention on the Rights of the Child.* Geneva: UN General Assembly. Available: www.unhchr.ch/html/menu3/b/k2crc.htm. Accessed January 5, 2008.

United Nations. (1995, September). *Beijing Declaration* and *Platform for Action.* Fourth World Conference on Women, Beijing, China. Geneva: UN Division for the Advancement of Women, Department of Economic and Social Affairs. Available: www.un.org/womenwatch/daw/beijing/index.html. Accessed January 5, 2008.

Ward, J.V. (1996). Raising resisters: The role of truth telling in the psychological development of African American girls. In B.R. Leadbeater & N. Way (Eds.), *Urban Girls: Resisting Stereotypes, Creating Identities* (pp. 85–99). New York: New York University Press.

Wright, M.A. (1998). *I'm Chocolate, You're Vanilla: Raising Healthy Black and Biracial Children in a Race-Conscious World.* San Francisco, CA: Jossey-Bass.

Yuval-Davis, N. (1992). *Nationalism, Racism, and Gender Relations.* The Hague: Institute of Social Studies.

Chapter 9

Women at the Centre of Changing Families

A Study of Sudanese Women's Resettlement Experiences

B. KHAMISA BAYA, LAURA SIMICH AND SARAH BUKHARI

Since 2000, Sudan has risen to sixth place among Canada's top 10 source countries for refugees (Citizenship and Immigration Canada, 2005). By 2004, the Sudanese community in the Greater Toronto Area had reached an estimated 15,000 to 20,000, owing to both voluntary and forced migration. The extended civil war in Sudan has led to more than two million deaths and the displacement of at least four million people, with about half a million seeking refuge in Kenya, Uganda, Ethiopia and Chad. Many Sudanese endured prolonged periods of displacement and deprivation in refugee camps and cities in neighbouring countries. The brunt of the two-decade war fell on women—especially those from the south and more recently those from the west—as many were compelled to assume sole responsibility for their families in the absence of their men who were either fighting, dead or displaced elsewhere (Hutchinson & Jok, 2002). Women have suffered extreme poverty, hunger, aerial bombardment, sexual violence and other trauma. (Chapter 14 discusses trauma work with Latin American women, but is also relevant to other populations.)

Sudanese war-affected refugees have been exposed to violence and traumatic incidents, with estimates of posttraumatic stress (PTS) prevalence in refugee camp populations ranging from 32 per cent (Pelzer, 1999) to 46 per cent (Karunakara, 2004). Other reports show that in camps where conditions are comparatively less harsh, Sudanese refugees demonstrate a remarkable sense of well-being (Hoeing, 2004), showing resilience and coping skills under favourable social conditions during resettlement (Goodman, 2004; Jeppsson & Hjern, 2005; Muecke, 1992).

The Sudanese community is characterized by internal ethnic and religious diversity (Abusharaf, 1997, 2002). Most Southern Sudanese are Christian and those from Northern Sudan tend to be Muslim. Dozens of languages, including English and Arabic, are spoken among Sudanese. Consequently, the categorization "Sudanese immigrants and refugees" captures a diverse and complex range of regional, social, ethnocultural and religious identities, experiences and realities, all of which have implications for how services are provided. Sudanese women in Canada mirror these diversities, and their settlement experiences are further compounded by the discriminatory and oppressive gender ideologies of Sudanese customary social structures, norms and expectations (Hale, 1997; Jok, 1998), as well as by the racial, gender and other social inequalities that affect women's mental health in North America (Chen et al., 2005; Denton et al., 2004; Galabuzi, 2004; Good et al., 2002; Williams & Williams-Morris, 2000).

In this chapter, we discuss findings from the first comprehensive community-based research undertaken from 2003 to 2004 with Sudanese in Canada. Our study took place in seven southern Ontario cities. We sought to understand settlement challenges and social determinants of health and to provide insights and recommendations for improving settlement services for Sudanese immigrants and refugees in Ontario. The study did not set out to specifically investigate Sudanese women's mental health, but it provided an important context for understanding settlement issues that affect women's mental health.

We situate this discussion within the context of the multiple and intersecting social identities of newcomer women to show how the intersection of these identities based on race, gender, culture and class is relevant in understanding newcomer Sudanese women's mental health issues. Such contextual knowledge is likely to be transferable to understanding social determinants of mental health for other refugee and immigrant women. We outline relevant social and health care practice-oriented guidelines for working with Sudanese women, who have specific challenges and strengths that may be shared by other recently arrived immigrant and refugee women in Canada today. We discuss the implications of discrimination and oppression on the mental health of Sudanese immigrant and refugee women, while also recognizing their strengths and self-help initiatives. The study's survey findings indicate that one of the most challenging areas of adaptation for Sudanese immigrants and refugees is in the family sphere, often the locus of essential social support for settlement and mental health. Due to the central role women play in Sudanese family units, we begin our discussion with a general outline of the Sudanese family context.

Background

SUDANESE FAMILY CONTEXT

Sudanese come from societies with traditions of communal responsibilities, where interdependent and extended family structures and mutual support are norms (Simich et al., 2004). Families are typically large, multi-generational and interdependent, and have, as in most African societies, strong loyalties (Kayango-Male & Onyango, 1984; Toubia, 1988). In refugee camps for internally displaced persons in Sudan, almost half of families have eight or more members and 65 per cent have six or more—including not only parents and children but also grandparents, adult siblings and cousins (Nogid, 2003).

The extended family is the single most important unit in Sudanese society, playing a pivotal role in all areas of social, economic and political life. It provides the individual with a strong sense of security and protection, as well as a nurturing environment of reciprocal rights and obligations. Each family shares a collective ancestry, a collective respect for elders and a collective obligation and responsibility for the welfare of other family members. Not surprisingly, therefore, even personal self-identity posits a collective self: family, clan and community are the principal sources of primary identification and attachment. It is to the extended family, rather than to the government, that a person first goes to seek help. The extended family customarily provides social services to its members and is responsible for the young, elderly and those with a physical or mental illness; this is especially a reality in rural areas where most Sudanese live. The weight of these social services, however, tends to fall predominantly on women (Bhaloo, 2005; Simich et al., 2004; Toubia, 1988). The familial relationship is not always limited to kin: its boundaries can expand to include close friends and neighbours as "family." The concept of extended family also tends to include the local community; "village" or "neighbourhood" often denotes relations of mutuality, co-operation and role flexibility (Bhaloo, 2005; Kafele & Khenti, 1999); hence, the famous African saying, "It takes a village to raise a child."

Understanding what "family" means and its central role to most Sudanese is critical in comprehending the deep and painful sense of loss and anguish Sudanese refugees feel and generally express at the dispersal of their family networks due to conflict and forced internal and external displacement (Rousseau et al., 2001). For Sudanese women—regardless of social and cultural differences—the key means of support is the family, which provides a source of primary identification and attachment. Not only are family members obligated to help in the mediation and resolution of family conflicts because of a shared responsibility in maintaining individual and collective family well-being, but family elders are particularly respected and relied on as trusted counsellors and mediators in the family (Bhaloo, 2005). The absence of family elders in Canada is, consequently, a major issue for many Sudanese families, especially for women who rely on elders' mediating role in the family. This loss is compounded by the fact that Sudanese immigrant and refugee women—consistent with their customary social welfare role back in Sudan—often feel responsible for their family's mental well-being as well as their own (Bhaloo, 2005).

The loss of a strong family network is particularly difficult for Sudanese women who, like women from other African cultures, rely less on their husbands as on the extended family to help with decision-making and work around the home. This is quite unlike the typical North American couple, who are more likely to share responsibility for decisions, and to both be income earners (Edward, 2004; Kayango-Male & Onyango, 1984; Siqwana-Ndulo, 1998). Significantly, the conjugal relationship is not necessarily the central supportive relationship for Sudanese women. Instead, women's emotional needs are often met predominantly through relationships to other women (Bernard, 1987; Bhaloo, 2005; Edward, 2004; Jok, 1998).

MENTAL HEALTH CONSIDERATIONS

To the best of our knowledge, there is no specific term for the concept "mental health" in Sudanese languages. Rather, mental health or mental well-being is defined in a culturally grounded, functional way; in other words, in terms of the person's ability to function in a healthy way in his or her environment. When this environment changes, as with migration, there are obvious challenges to coping.

Behavioural changes are the key way of identifying that someone needs attention. A woman who is mentally unwell may thus be described as "not herself," "sick" or "not well" (Bhaloo, 2005). In a small qualitative study of Sudanese women refugees' mental health in Hamilton, Ontario, Sudanese participants cautioned against the use of the term "mental health" because of its conflation with "insanity" and the stigma associated with that word (Bhaloo, 2005). This suggests that an appropriate working definition of mental health or well-being may have to be developed in partnership with the Sudanese community while at the same time deconstructing the stigma attached to the terms "mental health" and/or "mental illness."

Culture shapes perceptions of the causes of and responses to mental distress (Angel & Williams, 2000; Beiser, 2003; Brown et al., 1999; Karasz, 2005; Kirmayer, 1989; Scrimshaw, 2001; Sue, 2006; Young, 1982). Like many other African peoples (Janzen & Green, 2003), Sudanese have historically had indigenous systems of healing and medical practices for addressing physical and mental illness. The introduction of western biomedical systems in Sudan has not completely supplanted these systems and practices. This is especially the case in Southern Sudan where formal health care has been virtually non-existent for decades because of the civil war. Indigenous health practices include herbal medicines, special foods, manipulative treatments (e.g., bone-setting), healing and purification rituals and emotional therapies (e.g., trance and spirit possession). Indigenous African beliefs can strongly influence attitudes toward mental illness and help-seeking, but they may also result in reluctance or delays in seeking psychiatric care when needed (Gureje & Alem, 2000).

Sudanese immigrants tend to seek help for mental distress from both indigenous and biomedical practitioners; although, like other African cultural groups and newcomers in general, they rely on family, friends and other informal community supports first and foremost (Ahmed et al., 1999; Bhaloo, 2005; Ensik & Robertson, 1999). This may not just be due to their lack of experience with formal psychiatric services, but because informal sources are experienced as more therapeutic (Al-Krenawi & Graham, 1999; Loewy et al., 2002; Murthy, 1998). The therapeutic value of indigenous health practices such as trance and spirit possession rituals among Northern Sudanese women (Boddy, 1988, 1995) and use of expressive metaphors such as locating mental distress in the "heart" (Frode, 1998) suggest that collaborating with Sudanese who can act as cultural interpreters and peer support service providers may strengthen formal health care providers' responses. (For more on cultural interpretation, see Chapter 6.)

Theoretical Frameworks

Our community-based study was guided by an integrative theoretical framework, which structured our understanding of the interacting risks and protective factors affecting mental health in the context of settlement in Canada (Beiser, 2005; Thurston & Vissandjée, 2005). Adopting a holistic framework of practice premised on critical race feminism is appropriate in working with Sudanese immigrant and refugee women, because critical race feminism recognizes the relationship between individual problems (the personal) and structural inequalities (the political). *Critical race feminism* examines, within a multidisciplinary context, the intersection of women's social identities—premised on race, ethnicity, gender, class and other "isms"—and how these multiple identities shape women's lives. It rejects the idea that there is one authentic female or minority "voice," and resists *essentializing* (in other words, reducing the definition of someone's identity to one characteristic, such as race or ethnicity) or generalizing the experiences of women of colour. That is to say, it rejects the notion of an essential or monolithic experience for women of colour. Instead, critical race feminism calls for a deeper understanding of the lives of women of colour based on the multiple nature of their identities and their various and multilayered experiences of multiple discriminations (Wing, 1997).

Critical medical anthropology, which situates a person living with a mental distress or a health problem within larger social structures (Lock & Scheper-Hughes, 1996), guided our qualitative interpretation. Elements of participatory community-based research also helped to ground our study and analysis of intersecting socio-cultural determinants of health (Guruge & Khanlou, 2004). *Community-based research* (CBR) is "a collaborative approach to research that equitably involves all partners in the research process and recognizes the unique strengths that each brings. CBR begins with a research topic of importance to the community with the aim of combining knowledge and action for social change to improve community health and eliminate health disparities" (Minkler & Wallerstein, 2004).

The Study

Our community-based study (Simich et al., 2004) included both quantitative and qualitative components and involved 220 structured, in-person interviews to obtain information on settlement experiences and service needs, sources of help, service use and perceived barriers. The questionnaire included both closed-ended questions and open-ended questions. Volunteer Community Advisory Group members in all cities provided valuable support. To ensure cultural and linguistic comfort for respondents, trained female and male Sudanese interviewers conducted the interviews in English and in five Sudanese languages: Arabic, Arabi Juba, Dinka, Nuer and Bari. Recruiting of participants and interviewing adhered to ethics protocols approved by the Research Ethics Board of the Centre for Addiction and Mental Health.

The research team approached known Sudanese associations in the seven cities and also visited the sites to identify major areas of concern and to encourage wide community participation. We combined stratified purposeful (illustrating characteristic of subgroups of interest) and snowball (identifying participants from people who know others who are good examples) sampling to achieve a representative study sample (Patton, 1990), as random sampling was not possible. The survey sample represented approximately 10 per cent of Sudanese arriving between 2000 and 2003 and living in the seven cities. Within each city, the sample was further divided by Northern and Southern Sudanese adults as well as balanced by sex, age and length of time in Canada. Once data collection and entry was complete, cross-tabular analysis was performed to explore possible relationships between factors investigated in the study using SPSS (statistical and data management software). Descriptive statistics and frequencies were obtained, and selected open-ended questions were sorted, coded and analyzed.

STUDY SAMPLE DEMOGRAPHICS

On average, study respondents had lived 2.1 years in Canada. They were predominantly refugees, comprising 84 per cent of the total sample population. Most of these (62 per cent) were government-assisted refugees, 70 per cent of whom had come directly to Canada from refugee camps where living conditions were extremely harsh. One third of the total sample had been displaced within Sudan and, of this group, almost half had been displaced more than once. The remaining category of refugees were landed-in-Canada refugees (i.e., successful refugee claimants) or privately sponsored refugees. Only 16 per cent of the total study sample were family class, that is, people sponsored by or dependent on relatives or independent immigrants. Of the total study sample, 57 per cent were male and 43 per cent were female. About half of the sample were married with children.

FINDINGS

What follows are some settlement and integration challenges that the study participants identified as important for Sudanese newcomers in southern Ontario. One of the
most challenging areas of adaptation for Sudanese immigrants and refugees is in the
family sphere, often the source of essential social support for settlement and mental
health. Participants noted the importance of changing family forms, obligations and
meanings attached to marital roles and expectations within the family (that appear in
the context of various other psychological stresses), as well as loss of social supports.

Post-Migration Pressures and Stresses

The significance of the extended family as an important social unit for Sudanese cannot
be overstated. Pressures due to family obligations and separation affect settlement and
mental well-being in practical and psychological ways. For example, the need to send
money home to support family members is a significant strain for many Sudanese
newcomers, and inability or failure to do so was reported to cause distress. Of the total
survey sample, 79 per cent were trying to bring close family members to Canada. Of
these, 46 per cent were trying to bring parents, 15 per cent were trying to bring children
and 18 per cent were trying to bring a spouse. More than half of the respondents were
also trying to bring another family member, such as a sibling. (A "brother" or "sister"
may actually be a cousin, since most Sudanese languages do not linguistically distinguish between siblings and cousins.) The primary reason reported for difficulty in
family reunification was "low income." The consequences of this situation for respondents included "increasing sense of loneliness," ongoing "worries about their safety,"
"high phone bills" and "having to send a lot of money home"—a situation not exclusive
to Sudanese newcomers.

Mental Health Challenges

Responses to self-reported general health questions indicated that Sudanese
newcomers were coping, although under mental stress. Most respondents felt
"reasonably happy, all things considered." However, a majority also reported that
they "have lost much sleep over worry" and that they "felt under strain." As well, 43
per cent reported that they have "been upset or disturbed by bad memories" while 43
per cent also reported "feeling unhappy and depressed," suggesting a need for
further assessment by health professionals. Subsequent open-ended probes about
health status elicited many comments about mental distress, including loneliness,
frustration, worry and stress. In this regard, both male and female respondents
noted similar mental health concerns.

Women in our study also reported being stressed by the demands of their multiple
roles inside and outside the home. This finding is supported by the previously
mentioned qualitative study of Sudanese refugee women's mental health in Hamilton.
In the words of one woman: "I work outside and I work inside. . . . Since I have been in
Canada, I am not tired, but exhausted" (Bhaloo, 2005, p. 31). The potential for marital

conflict and family breakdown in such situations is of great concern in the community, as previously discussed.

The cultural onus of placing primary parenting on women—especially in the absence of the customary support of the extended family network—is also a potential source of stress as it occurs in a very different socio-cultural context with different norms and expectations regarding child care and child-rearing. In addition to having to learn new ways of parenting in a cultural context that they may not always understand, they also have a tangible fear of losing their children to the Children's Aid Society. Attesting to the different roles of Sudanese women and men in child rearing, 51 per cent of women in our study reported feeling "conflicted" about raising their children in Canada—compared to only 37 per cent of men. Only 22 per cent of women reported that they were happy to be raising their children in Canada, compared to 50 per cent of men. In this context, the gendered cultural tasking of mothers with primary parenting—in the general absence of customary extended family support, and in a new and unfamiliar socio-cultural environment—becomes a potential source of stress likely to affect Sudanese women's mental health.

Changing Gender Relations

Respondents living with spouses who revealed that their marital relationships had changed since arrival in Canada attributed the change to "having more worries and stress." The majority identified as contributing factors changing gender roles and expectations (especially gender role reversals as women become significant or principal sources of family income), greater financial pressures, increased workload (as women work both inside and outside the home), and changes due to the absence of the extended family. Respondents who reported a change in their conjugal relations also reported a greater number of psychological symptoms than those who did not.

Coping with the possibility of divorce and family disintegration was identified as a problem that also affects family members in Sudan. Marriage not only binds spouses, but also their families in a *de facto* contractual relationship: dowry or bridal wealth customs carry obligations, responsibilities and penalties, as do customary rights and obligations toward children. The dowry or bride price, paid to the woman's family to compensate them for losing her (in cash or other forms of wealth in the north and in cattle in much of the south), is practised widely in Sudan. It generally transfers to the husband all rights to his wife's sexuality, her labour and her future children. If the marriage breaks up, the bride price or dowry must usually be returned. Dowry repayment makes it difficult for women to seek divorce as the extended family in Sudan must then repay the bride price to the husband's family. Often racked with guilt and worried over the well-being of immediate and extended family members left behind in Sudan, Sudanese immigrant and refugee women whose marriages are at risk often face a dilemma that has obvious implications for their mental well-being.

More positively, however, 64 per cent of the study participants reported that in Canada they "talk more often" to their spouse and 54 per cent that they received "more respect from their spouse." Women tended to report these changes in their relationships in higher proportions than men, suggesting the heightened salience of these family changes for women.

Unmet Emotional and Social Support Needs, and Resilience

Although family members are often primary sources of emotional support, the proportion of responses indicating *unmet* emotional needs were highest among family class respondents, who are predominantly female: 44 per cent of these indicated a need for "someone to confide in and share feelings"; 44 per cent also reported they needed "someone to relax with and keep me company." These may indicate that Sudanese women experience social adjustment difficulties characterized by loneliness and social isolation.

Many Sudanese spouses who customarily depend on wider social networks struggle to communicate and build personal and emotionally intimate relationships with one another. One Sudanese man explains this predicament:

> So here [in Canada] then, the first problem is that you are the only two adults [in the household]. You are supposed to talk to one another and . . . you don't know how to talk to one another. The relationship begins right from the beginning . . . my wife used to have people she could talk to [back home] . . . I'm not there to talk to her, and she can't really talk to me. (Simich et al., 2004, p. 29)

Study respondents suggested that both Sudanese women and men need to be more flexible and supportive of each other. As one man said, Sudanese men have to assume more responsibilities in household chores, but then Sudanese women also need to accept that "if the woman is the one earning the money, she doesn't have to hold that against the man, that [he is] useless" (Simich et al., 2004, p. 30). A woman echoed the principle that the onus is on both Sudanese men and women to modify culturally defined roles in this radically altered socio-cultural environment.

> The problem I see is the family, they are holding on to their culture [customary gender roles] . . . It doesn't work that way here. So at this point, they need encouragement from both sides. (Simich et al., 2004, p. 30)

When asked what helps them to cope with difficulties, most respondents reported "support from friends" or "support from larger Sudanese community," and, to a lesser extent, "support from family." Such support networks signify a potentially strong community resource, although they may function differently for men and women. Approximately 35 per cent of respondents cited religious beliefs as a source of support, but very few cited support from settlement and social service providers. Nearly half reported that "hope for a better life in Canada" helped them cope with difficulties. Women were somewhat more likely to say that "hope for a better life for my children in Canada" helped them to cope (39 per cent) than were men (24 per cent).

Elusive Economic Integration

Like many newcomers to Canada, Sudanese are faced with barriers to economic integration (Badets & Howatson-Leo, 2000; Kazemipur & Halli, 2000). *Economic integration*, defined as employment commensurate with educational qualifications and work experience, remains elusive for most Sudanese newcomers. Only 39 per cent of the study sample was employed at the time of the study, though many had not been in Canada long (an average of 2.1 years). Government-assisted refugees, who formed the majority of our sample, are given modest financial assistance in their first 12 months in Canada, but the support payments are low, debts for travel loans are high and jobs are hard to find.

Many Sudanese experience mental distress associated with economic hardship during these critical early years in Canada (Simich, Hamilton & Baya, 2006). At the same time, they must navigate in an entirely new society, seek employment, achieve language proficiency and send money to family members still living in Sudan. Almost half of our study participants were currently looking for work. Women (especially those from Southern Sudan) had substantially lower education than men, and were consequently more disadvantaged in employment: only 22 per cent of female respondents were employed compared to 53 per cent of males. While the majority (70 per cent) of employed men held full-time jobs, only about half of employed women did. Even where they had the same or similar educational qualifications, women seemed to have more difficulty finding jobs than men—although proportionately more men reported seeking employment services. A higher proportion of men reported being "treated unfairly" than did women, perhaps because more men were employed and were thus likely to be more exposed to workplace discrimination. Both men and women regard the ubiquitous employment prerequisite of "Canadian experience" (they variously referred to this as "a small devil" or "a vicious cycle") and the non-recognition of pre-migration education, professional training and work experience as exclusionary and discriminatory and, ultimately, inherently racist (Bhaloo, 2005; Simich et al., 2004).

Initial Settlement Challenges

Women were more affected by certain challenges during the first year of resettlement than men. For example, 60 per cent of women, but only 40 per cent of men, reported inability to get around independently as a problem. Issues of language and communication mirror this imbalance. The highest proportions of those reporting difficulty communicating were women (58 per cent).

When asked about recent adverse life events, which are associated with mental distress, significantly more women (37 per cent) reported difficulties due to language than men (24 per cent). Respondents reported having the most difficulty communicating with doctors and other medical professionals—suggesting the importance of both cultural interpretation and cultural competence as distinct strategies. Furthermore, 78 per cent of respondents overall indicated that they needed health care information.

The cost of housing was a significant problem for 81 per cent of respondents. Most live near other Sudanese, a choice that 79 per cent reported as important, with women reporting this in higher proportions than did men. The primary reasons given included emotional support, social interaction and assistance. Half of female respondents reported not having used basic settlement services, compared to only one-fifth of male respondents. These female respondents did not use settlement services due to a combination of perceived cultural insensitivity on the part of service providers, lack of awareness of available settlement services and other barriers such as language and lack of access to transportation. The proportion of those with no knowledge of how to seek help was higher among women. (See Chapter 7 on services for immigrant women.)

DISCUSSION

Gender role changes due to resettlement present both advantages and disadvantages. Changing gender roles and conjugal relationships provide opportunities for Sudanese women and men to renegotiate their identities and obligations in a more equitable and beneficial way. The gendered construction of customary family responsibilities generally assumes that women are the principal custodians of family well-being. It is not surprising then that while many Sudanese women are willing to take on any job, however menial, to ensure the survival of their families, many Sudanese men are unwilling to perform jobs below their professional or educational level. Contributing to family income is status-enhancing (Bernard, 1987), and through employment Sudanese women who may not have had formal work opportunities back home have the chance to develop a stronger sense of autonomy. These changes can be threatening to men because they challenge accustomed familial patterns of power wherein women are expected to submit to male authority. Thus, as more Sudanese women become breadwinners, family power configurations change and the need to make adjustments in the couple relationship becomes important to maintaining marital and family harmony.

Still other challenges persist for women. Since English language proficiency is a prerequisite for employment, Sudanese women lacking English language proficiency tend to be relegated to low-level jobs with long hours and no security. With mothers acting as the primary parent in the absence of extended family support—and with lack of accessible and affordable child care—it is difficult for them to access and use English language training or upgrading programs, skills-training programs and adult education programs. However, without acquiring new skills from such training, they cannot find rewarding waged work but only low-paying, low-status, part-time, unskilled or semi-skilled employment with no job security or benefits. The financial stresses of low family incomes are further aggravated by obligations to send money to help extended family members left behind in Sudan or elsewhere. Inability to do so adds to the mental anguish. Lack of language skills further keeps newcomer Sudanese women isolated from the wider society. If they experience abuse and violence, they may not be aware of spousal assault legislation and the support services available to deal with abuse. (Chapter 15 focuses on intimate partner violence.)

Unmet family expectations can also generate frustration and stress for men. Their inability to care and provide for their families and fulfill their culturally defined responsibilities becomes an ongoing source of shame and emotional difficulty for men, resulting in strained family relationships and mental distress (Simich et al., 2006). Institutional and everyday racism such as barriers to employment further undermine precarious family relationships (Kafele & Khenti, 1999). This volatile mix creates potential for conflict and requires creative ways of thinking and acting to negotiate new relations between spouses. In Sudan, domestic conflicts tend to be mediated and resolved with the help of elder relatives when or before conflicts erupt into violence. We note that Sudanese women and men express misgivings about how marital disputes are handled in Canada once reported to authorities, because they feel little room is left for negotiation and reconciliation.

In Canada, the situation of married Sudanese women parenting alone also raises challenges. Lack of employment commensurate with qualifications leads some Sudanese husbands to seek work in other parts of Canada, the United States and the Middle East, thus living away from their families for extended periods. Their wives assume sole responsibility for their families and often face loneliness, isolation and new responsibilities without the accustomed support of extended family. Because sponsorship can be so lengthy, many women also struggle alone with the challenges of resettlement as single parents for years while waiting for their husband. However, these situations also present opportunities for women to gain independence, self-reliance and new knowledge and skills.

Neither privileged by their sex or race, they additionally face simultaneous discriminations based on their class position (lower socio-economic status and education), and other statuses such as "immigrants" and "refugees." The results of our study suggest that the interaction of these multiple identities do not bode well for Sudanese women's mental wellness.

The language limitations of Sudanese women affect their health and mental well-being. Women in our study reported that language difficulties make it hard to access and receive adequate health care because some clinics did not have trained cultural interpreters to help them to communicate their symptoms or health issues. This problem assumes even more importance given that language is pivotal in western mental health therapy. Thus, inability to easily and accurately articulate issues of their physical and mental well-being is likely to negatively affect Sudanese women's overall health. The same problem of language difficulties is likely to replicate itself when dealing with other mainstream institutions—and may not only result in tension, fear and anxiety, but may also have a detrimental effect on help-seeking. (Chapter 6 addresses issues around cultural interpretation and the implications of language barriers to immigrant women obtaining services.)

Because of structural discrimination embedded in assumptions about their intellectual abilities and competence (as captured in the demands for "Canadian experience" and the lack of recognition of pre-migration credentials), Sudanese immigrants experience difficulty gaining professional jobs. Discriminatory employment structures and practices that interact with gender barriers make it more difficult for Sudanese women respondents with similar qualifications as their male counterparts to find jobs. Our study also indicates that working conditions for employed Sudanese women may be worse than for employed Sudanese men (Simich et al., 2004). In looking at the barriers Sudanese women face in accessing employment, it is evident that their race, culture, gender and class intersect in ways that are likely to be harmful to their mental well-being—especially given the central role that employment plays in maintaining and promoting mental well-being.

Practice Guidelines

Our discussion of the resettlement experiences and mental well-being of Sudanese immigrant and refugee women draws primarily, but not exclusively, from the first major study of newcomer Sudanese immigrants and refugees in Ontario (Simich et al., 2004). It also includes information based on our prior work within this community. As community members and service providers, we draw as well on our own observations and knowledge of Sudanese immigrant and refugee women.

While the findings of our study may not appear new, they confirm that the existing mental health care system consistently fails to provide appropriate services for and effective outreach to recent newcomer women. We suggest the following as practice guidelines.

WORKING WITHIN A HISTORICAL, SOCIAL, ECONOMIC AND CULTURAL FRAMEWORK

- Openness to and familiarity with a client's socio-cultural norms can help to provide reassurance and a supportive environment for discussing problems.
- Service providers must consider Sudanese women's expectations, possible language difficulties and lack of familiarity with white Canadian society and norms, all of which can generate discomfort and stress. Cultural interpretation may be necessary.
- Although awareness alone cannot address fundamental issues of systemic discrimination and power differences that may exist in client-provider relationships, cultural awareness is a fundamental element of culturally competent psychotherapy (Lo & Fung, 2003).

UNDERSTANDING THE POSITION OF SUDANESE WOMEN IN CANADIAN SOCIETY

- Health care providers need to be aware of how the intersecting identities and status of Sudanese women as racialized newcomers may affect their mental well-being.

They also need to recognize how their own social position, with its associated power relations, plays out in therapeutic relationships, as well as possible sources of biases, stereotyping and labelling.

OVERCOMING BARRIERS TO HELP-SEEKING

- The very idea of active help-seeking from health care institutions and formal social service organizations may be unfamiliar to many Sudanese and other newcomer women. Thus, active outreach to immigrant women's groups to provide health promotion is needed to create open communication and help-seeking pathways.
- Fear of stigma due to breaches of confidentiality is a barrier to help-seeking and service use among many newcomer women, especially for mental health or family matters that are considered private. Therefore, health service providers need to be aware of the centrality of ensuring confidentiality as a pathway to facilitating help-seeking for Sudanese women.
- To this end, privacy and/or confidentiality protocols must be explained both in individual care contexts but also in partnership with community organizations on a group level to enable individual women to feel reassured about confidentiality enough to seek services when needed.

WORKING WITH DIVERSE BELIEFS REGARDING MENTAL HEALTH

- Mental health professionals must be receptive to diverse beliefs about mental well-being and cultural definitions of health and illness. This is especially important given the multiplicity of cultures and languages among Sudanese. The diversity within the community and the resulting diverse needs of women must be recognized.
- To develop culturally appropriate services, health providers must also be aware of how such different belief systems and practices may influence positive and negative health practices (Airhihenbuwa, 1992; Scrimshaw, 2001).
- Working with women to incorporate helpful indigenous beliefs and practices in their care is important. Perhaps a cultural consultation model would be used to supplement existing services by seeking advice from relevant community and religious service providers, cultural psychiatrists, Sudanese peer-support workers and other culturally competent care providers (Airhihenbuwa, 1992; Global Forum for Health Research, 2004; Kirmayer et al., 2003).
- Exploring a client's "explanatory model" or understanding of a problem (Kleinman, 1980)—that is, the causes, precipitating factors, effects, severity, desired outcomes, fears and perceptions about treatment—can help the care provider and client to arrive at mutually agreeable and effective solutions.

INCORPORATING DIVERSE PAST EXPERIENCES THAT AFFECT WOMEN'S MENTAL HEALTH

- Health service providers may have to deal with the psychological effects of sexual and other forms of violence, dislocation and the loss of loved ones in addition to resettlement stresses in Canada. However, while traumatic experiences are common among refugee women, they do not necessarily lead to posttraumatic stress disorder.

- Women from Northern Sudan may have specific health issues related to the experience of female genital cutting that can affect their gynecological, obstetrical and mental health (Global Forum on Health Research, 2004; Royal Australian College of Obstetricians and Gynaecologists, 1997; Toubia, 1995; World Health Organization, 1995). Because health practitioners have limited awareness of female genital cutting and its negative mental health consequences, the needs of women who have experienced it are not generally being met.

APPROACHING SERVICE PROVISION USING HEALTH PROMOTION AND EMPOWERMENT STRATEGIES

- Bearing in mind how mental distress is experienced and communicated, the primary goals of mental health promotion should be prevention, fostering self-help and coping skills, and providing high-quality, accurate and accessible information on mental health (National Electronic Library for Mental Health, 2003; World Health Organization, 2001). Thus, culturally informed health promotion strategies should be a main thrust when providing services to Sudanese immigrant and refugee women.

- Mental health promotion activities may be more acceptable when they are not directly related to mental disorders but are instead perceived to address social determinants of mental health that collectively affect the community.

- Health professionals could build on strengths that already exist in the Sudanese community by forming supportive alliances with women's informal social networks or ethnocultural associations that can act as kin groups providing mutual aid, emotional support, economic assistance and social interaction. For example, peer support programs, and social and self-help groups may provide individual Sudanese women with a degree of empathy and understanding that professionals alone are unlikely to provide.

- Mental health education programs must aim to demystify mental illness, address the stigma attached to it and inform community members of available mental health services to enable help-seeking and increase community capacity to support people with mental illness.

- Since problems of transportation, child care and low income may limit women's access to services, health promotion programs need to be community based and close to where Sudanese women live.

- To be relevant and accessible, mental health promotion programs and activities must be linked with refugee reception houses, settlement services, Settlement Workers in Schools (SWIS) programs and community health centres. This approach is consistent with principles of effective community outreach.

Conclusion

This chapter revealed a multiplicity of needs that cuts across disciplinary and sectoral boundaries. We suggest, therefore, that a multidisciplinary and/or multi-sectoral approach is necessary to improve Sudanese immigrant and refugee women's mental well-being. Such an approach requires the collaborative involvement of the settlement, social services and mental health sectors. Culturally appropriate community outreach and collaboration will be a key factor in achieving these and other research and practice objectives such as identifying specific mental health needs and health promotion objectives.

To gain a deeper understanding of the lives of Sudanese immigrant and refugee women, it is important to understand how their multiple identities are socially constructed and how these identities intersect to shape and influence their lives. The many ways that Sudanese women are discriminated against create social inequalities that inevitably affect their mental health and overall well-being. The fact that they must cope with poverty; low socio-economic standing; restricted access to employment, education and training; and lack of access to needed services are ultimately linked to a politics of discrimination that includes some and excludes others.

We need to remember, however, that despite the difficulties and marginalization they have encountered in the post-migration context, Sudanese women are agents making choices with critical perspectives on the circumstances and contexts of their lives. They are resourceful and resilient, frequently exhibiting a philosophy of hope and optimism, even in situations where the challenges seem enormous and possibly overwhelming.

We thank Citizenship and Immigration Canada, Ontario, for research funding and all Sudanese community members who assisted with and participated in this study. Research team members in Toronto were Dr. Laura Simich, Dr. Hayley Hamilton, Dr. Haile Fenta (University of Toronto), Khamisa Baya, Huda Bukhari, Sarah Bukhari, Huda Abuzeid (Anisa'a Association of Sudanese Women in Research and Development) and David Lugeron and Iman Ahmed (research assistants).

References

Abusharaf, R.M. (1997). Sudanese migration to the new world: Socio-economic characteristics. *International Migration, 35* (4), 513–536.

Abusharaf, R.M. (2002). *Wanderings: Sudanese Migrants and Exiles in North America.* Ithaca, NY: Cornell University Press.

Ahmed, I.M., Bremer, J.J., Magzoub, M. & Nouri, A. (1999). Characteristics of visitors to traditional healers in central Sudan. *Eastern Mediterranean Health Journal, 5* (1), 79–85.

Airhihenbuwa, C.O. (1992). Health promotion and disease prevention strategies for African Americans: A conceptual model. In R.L. Braithwaite & S.E. Taylor (Eds.), *Health Issues in the Black Community.* San Francisco, CA: Jossey-Bass.

Al-Krenawi, A. & Graham, J. (1999). Gender and biomedical/traditional mental health utilization among the Bedouin-Arabs of the Negev. *Culture, Medicine and Psychiatry, 23* (2), 219–243.

Angel, R. & Williams, K. (2000). Cultural models of health and illness. In I. Cuellar and F.A. Paniagua (Eds.), *Handbook of Multicultural Mental Health* (pp. 25–44). San Diego, CA: Academic Press.

Badets, J. & Howatson-Leo, L. (2000). Recent immigrants in the workforce. *Canadian Social Trends, 3* (52), 15–21. (Statistics Canada Catalogue No. 11-008-XPE).

Beiser, M. (2003). Why should researchers care about culture? *Canadian Journal of Psychiatry, 48* (3), 154–160.

Beiser, M. (2005). The health of immigrants and refugees in Canada. *Canadian Journal of Public Health, 96* (Suppl. 2), S30–44.

Bernard, J. (1987). *The Female World from a Global Perspective.* Bloomington: Indiana University Press.

Bhaloo, S. (2005). *Refugee Women from Sudan and Their Mental Health: Project Report.* Hamilton, ON: Funded by the Community Care Research Centre and the Arts Research Board at McMaster University.

Boddy, J. (1988). Spirits and selves in Northern Sudan: The cultural therapeutics of possession and trance. *American Ethnologist, 15* (1), 4–27.

Boddy, J. (1995). Managing tradition: "Superstition" and the making of national identity among Sudanese women refugees. In W. James (Ed.), *The Pursuit of Certainty: Religious and Cultural Formulations* (pp. 15–44). London: Routledge.

Brown, T., Sellers, S., Brown, K. & Jackson, J. (1999). Race, ethnicity and culture in the sociology of mental health. In C. Aneshensel & J. Phelan (Eds.), *Handbook of the Sociology of Mental Health* (pp. 167–182). New York: Kluwer Academic/Plenum Publishers.

Chen, Y., Subramanian, S.F., Acevedo-Garcia, D. & Kawachi, I. (2005). Women's status and depressive symptoms: A multilevel analysis. *Social Science & Medicine, 60* (1), 49–60.

Citizenship and Immigration Canada. (2005, Spring). *The Monitor.* Ottawa: Author. Available: www.cic.gc.ca/english/resources/statistics/monitor/issue09/05-overview.asp. Accessed January 15, 2008.

Denton, M., Prus, S. & Walters, V. (2004). Gender differences in health: A Canadian study of the psychosocial, structural and behavioural determinants of health. *Social Science & Medicine, 58* (12), 2585–2600.

Edward, J.K. (2004). *Understanding Socio-cultural Change: Transformations and Future Imagining among Southern Sudanese Women Refugees.* Unpublished doctoral dissertation, Ontario Institute for Studies in Education/University of Toronto.

Ensink, K. & Robertson, B.A. (1999). Patient and family experiences of psychiatric services and African indigenous healers. *Transcultural Psychiatry, 36* (1), 23–43.

Frode, J. (1998). *Theories of Sickness and Misfortune among the Hadandowa Beja: Narratives as Points of Entry into Beja Cultural Knowledge.* London: Kegan Paul International.

Galabuzi, G.E. (2004). Social exclusion. In D. Raphael (Ed.), *Social Determinants of Health: Canadian Perspectives* (pp. 235–252). Toronto: Canadian Scholars' Press.

Global Forum for Health Research. (2004). *Mental and Neurological Health and the Millennium Development Goals.* Geneva: Author.

Good, M.J., James, C., Good, B.J. & Becker, A. (2002). The culture of medicine and racial, ethnic and class disparities in healthcare. In B.D. Smedley, A.Y. Stith & A.R. Nelson (Eds.), *Unequal Treatment: Confronting Racial and Ethnic Disparities in Health Care* (pp. 594–625). Washington, DC: National Academies Press.

Goodman, J. (2004). Coping with trauma and hardship among unaccompanied refugee youths from Sudan. *Qualitative Health Research, 14* (9), 1177–1196.

Gureje, O. & Alem, A. (2000). Mental health policy development in Africa. *Bulletin of the World Health Organization, 78* (4), 475–482.

Guruge, S. & Khanlou, N. (2004). Intersectionalities of influence: Researching the health of immigrant and refugee women. *Canadian Journal of Nursing Research, 36* (3), 32–47.

Hale, S. (1997). *Gender Politics in Sudan: Islamism, Socialism and the State.* Boulder, CO: Westview.

Hoeing, W. (2004). *Self-Image and the Well Being of Refugees in Rhino Camp, Uganda: New Issues in Refugee Research* (Working Paper No. 103). Geneva: United Nations High Commissioner on Refugees, Evaluation and Policy Analysis Unit.

Hutchinson, S. & Jok, M.J. (2002). Gendered violence and the militarization of ethnicity: A case study from South Sudan. In R. Werbner (Ed.), *Postcolonial Subjectivities in Africa* (pp. 84–109). London: Zed Books.

Janzen, J.M. & Green, E.C. (2003). Continuity, change, and challenge in African medicine. In H. Selin (Ed.), *Medicine across Cultures: History and Practice of Medicine in Non-Western Cultures* (pp. 1–26). Dordrecht, The Netherlands: Kluwer Academic Publishers.

Jeppsson, O. & Hjern, A. (2005). Traumatic stress in context: A study of unaccompanied minors from Southern Sudan. In D. Ingleby (Ed.), *Forced Migration and Mental Health: Rethinking the Care of Refugees and Displaced Persons* (pp. 67–80). New York: Springer.

Jok, J.M. (1998). *Militarization, Gender and Reproductive Health in South Sudan.* Lewiston, NY: Edwin Mellen.

Kafele, P.K. & Khenti, A. (1999). *The Healing Journey, Phase III Report: Men of Colour and Mental Health.* Toronto: Sponsored by Across Boundaries in Partnership with the Trillium Foundation.

Karasz, A. (2005). Cultural differences in conceptual models of depression. *Social Science & Medicine, 60* (7), 1625–1635.

Karunakara, U.K., Neuner, F., Schauer, M., Singh, K., Hill, K., Elbert T. et al. (2004). Traumatic events and symptoms of post-traumatic stress disorder amongst Sudanese nationals, refugees and Ugandans in the West Nile. *African Health Sciences, 4* (2), 83–93.

Kayango-Male, D. & Onyango, P. (1984). *The Sociology of the African Family.* London: Longman Group.

Kazemipur A. & Halli S. (2000). Immigrants and "new poverty": The case of Canada. *International Migration Review, 35,* 1129–1156.

Kirmayer, L. (1989). Cultural variations in the response to psychiatric disorders and emotional distress. *Social Science & Medicine, 29* (3), 327–339.

Kirmayer, L., Groleau, D., Guzder, J., Blake, C. & Jarvis, E. (2003). Cultural consultation: A model of mental health service for multicultural societies. *Canadian Journal of Psychiatry, 48* (3), 145–153.

Kleinman, A. (1980). *Patients and Healers in the Context of Culture: An Exploration of the Borderland between Anthropology, Medicine, and Psychiatry.* Berkeley: University of California Press.

Lo, H-T. & Fung, K. (2003). Culturally competent psychotherapy. *Canadian Journal of Psychiatry, 48* (3), 161–170.

Lock, M. & Scheper-Hughes, N. (1996). A critical interpretive approach in medical anthropology rituals and routines of discipline and dissent. In C. Sargent & T. Johnson (Eds.), *Medical Anthropology: Contemporary Theory and Method* (pp. 41–70). Westport, CT: Praeger.

Loewy, M., Williams, D. & Keleta, A. (2002). Group counselling with traumatized East African refugee women in the United States: Using the *Kaffa* ceremony intervention. *Journal of Specialists in Group Work, 27* (2), 173–191.

Minkler, M. & Wallerstein, N. (2004). Introduction to community-based participatory research. In M. Minkler & N. Wallerstein (Eds.), *Community-Based Participatory Research for Health.* San Francisco, CA: Jossey-Bass.

Muecke, M. (1992). New paradigms for refugee health problems. *Social Science & Medicine, 34* (4), 515–523.

Murthy, R.S. (1998). Rural psychiatry in developing countries. *Psychiatric Services, 49* (7), 967–969.

NeLMH (National electronic Library for Mental Health) & *Mentality.* (2003). *Mental Health Promotion: Making It Happen.* Available: www.nelmh.org/page_view.asp?c=22&did=2354&fc= 004002: Accessed January 5, 2008.

Nogid, O. (2003). *Situational Analysis of IDPs in Sudan: A Field Account.* Trondheim, Norway: Norwegian University of Science and Technology, IDP Research Network. Available: www.idp.ntnu.no/ Register/UpLoadFiles/Paper%20Osama%20Abu%20Zied%20Nogid.pdf. Accessed January 5, 2008.

Patton, M.Q. (1990). *Qualitative Evaluation and Research Methods* (2nd. ed.). Newbury Park, CA: Sage Publications.

Pelzer, K. (1999). Trauma and mental health problems of Sudanese refugees in Uganda. *Central African Journal of Medicine, 45* (5), 110–114.

Rousseau, C., Bekki-Berrada, A. & Moreau, S. (2001). Trauma and extended separation from family among Latin American and African refugees in Montreal. *Psychiatry, 64* (1), 40–59.

Royal Australian College of Obstetricians and Gynaecologists. (1997). *Female Genital Mutilation: Information for Australian Health Professionals.* Melbourne: Author.

Scrimshaw, S.C. (2001). Culture, behavior and health. In M.H. Merson, R.E. Black & A.J. Mills (Eds.), *International Public Health: Diseases, Programs, Systems and Policies* (pp. 53–78). Gaithersburg, MD: Aspen Publishers.

Simich, L., Hamilton, H. & Baya, B.K. (2006). Mental distress, economic hardship and expectations of life in Canada among Sudanese newcomers. *Transcultural Psychiatry, 43* (3), 419–445.

Simich, L., Hamilton, H., Baya, B.K., Neuwirth, G. & Loh, B. (2004). *The Study of Sudanese Settlement in Ontario: Final Report.* Submitted to Citizenship and Immigration Canada, Ontario Settlement Directorate. Available: http://atwork.settlement.org/downloads/atwork/Study_of_ Sudanese_Settlement_in_Ontario.pdf. Accessed January 15, 2008.

Siqwana-Ndulo, N. (1998). Rural African family structure in the Eastern Cape Province, South Africa. *Journal of Comparative Family Studies, 29* (2), 407–418.

Sue, S. (2006). Cultural competency: From philosophy to research and practice. *Journal of Community Psychology, 34* (2), 237–245.

Thurston, W.E. & Vissandjée, B. (2005). An ecological model for understanding culture as a determinant of women's health. *Critical Public Health, 15* (3), 229–242.

Toubia, N. (1988). Women and health in Sudan. In N. Toubia (Ed.), *Women of the Arab World: The Coming Challenge* (pp. 98–109). London: Zed Books.

Toubia, N. (1995). *Female Genital Mutilation: A Call for Global Action.* New York: Rainbo.

Williams, D. & Williams-Morris, R. (2000). Racism and mental health: The African-American experience. *Ethnicity and Health, 5* (3–4), 243–268.

Wing, A.K. (Ed.). (1997). *Critical Race Feminism: A Reader.* New York: New York University Press.

World Health Organization. (1995). *Female Genital Mutilation: Report of a WHO Technical Group.* Geneva: Author.

World Health Organization. (2001). *The World Health Report 2001: Mental Health—New Understanding, New Hope.* Geneva: Author.

Young, A. (1982). The anthropologies of illness and sickness. *Annual Review of Anthropology, 11,* 257–285.

Chapter 10

Separation and Reunification Challenges Faced by Caribbean Women and Their Children

AGATHA CAMPBELL AND ZORINA FLAMAN

Caribbean people[1] may immigrate to Canada as part of a nuclear or extended family or may leave family members behind. Due to economic factors and the high percentage of female-headed households in the Caribbean, more Caribbean women than men migrate. This chapter focuses on issues that Caribbean women may face as a result of being separated from and later reunited with their children.

As early as the 1940s, Caribbean people began immigrating to other English-speaking countries such as the United States and England. Following changes in the Canadian immigration laws in 1967, the number of Caribbean people immigrating to Canada has increased. Most Caribbean immigrants to Canada have settled in Ontario, particularly Toronto, and in Quebec, mainly in Montreal (Anderson & Grant, 1987; Rambally, 1995). The main reasons for migration are to seek educational and job opportunities and, ultimately, economic advancement.

Caribbean people who immigrate to Canada work in a range of fields, including nursing, teaching and domestic labour (Baptiste et al., 1997; Sharpe, 1997). Many professionals who came alone and had jobs awaiting them were able to establish themselves quickly and sponsor their families. However, many single mothers immigrated as

---

1. The term "Caribbean" refers to the primarily English-speaking countries of Barbados, Belize, British Virgin Islands, Cayman Islands, Dominica, Grenada, Guyana, Jamaica, Monsserrat, St. Christopher-Nevis (St. Kitts), St. Lucia, St. Vincent and the Grenadines, Trinidad and Tobago, and the Turks and Caicos Islands. The older term "West Indies" can be used interchangeably with "Caribbean." While the majority of people in the Caribbean are black, the population consists of diverse racial, ethnic and language groups.

domestic workers or labourers, often leaving their children behind with relatives and/or friends (Crawford, 2004; Lashley, 2000). They often experienced delays in sending for or returning to their children due to economic hardships and immigration policies and other structural barriers (Flynn & Henwood, 2000; St. Joseph's Convent [sjc] Young Leaders, 1999).

The impact of the separation is felt both by the mother and by the children left behind. Separation and reunion difficulties may be minimal or non-existent if the duration of separation is short. However, if the period of separation is lengthy, as in the case of those experiencing economic hardships, the challenges are many. Due to gender norms, Caribbean women tend to bear most of the childcare responsibilities. Therefore, children left behind tend to focus on their mother's absence during the migration process. Limited research indicates that girls are more affected by their mother's absence than boys are (Jones et al., 2004; sjc Young Leaders, 1999), and that girls experience and cope with this separation differently than boys do. However, due to the lack of sufficient research on how gender differences factor into children's response to the separation from their mother, we apply the concepts to children in general.

In this chapter, we:

- discuss the challenges faced by Caribbean immigrant women and children through separation and reunification, and highlight some reasons for these challenges
- consider the impact these challenges have on the mental and emotional health of both the mother and the children
- review past interventions used to support the family
- consider attachment theory as an approach to addressing the issues facing mothers and children in the separation and reunification process
- present practical strategies for working with Caribbean women and their children
- suggest areas for further research to help Caribbean women and children deal with the challenges of separation and reunification.

Separation Issues

CHALLENGES FACING THE MOTHERS

Only a small percentage of Caribbean families conform to the nuclear family structure. Gender, culture and class are all factors that influence the family's formation. Caribbean family structures vary, with women-headed households making up a significant number. Consequently, caring for the child often shifts to someone else when the biological mother migrates (Senior, 1991).

It is understandable that separation contributes to increased stress both for the mother and for the child left in the Caribbean (Smith, 1996). After coming to Canada, the mother often maintains some semblance of parenting by frequently calling, visiting and sending money, food and clothing (Glasgow & Gouse-Sheese, 1995; Lashley, 2000). In some cases, however, children do not have an opportunity to maintain ongoing communication with their mother for several months or to receive regular financial support. This limited contact and/or support can result in children's feelings of abandonment, resentment and bitterness toward the mother (Evans & Davies, 1997; Jones et al., 2004; Mohammed, 1998).

The mother may have inconsistent contact with the child for various reasons, including economic, immigration and environmental hardships. For instance, she may have difficulty adapting to a different climate, and finding housing and a well-paying job. She may also lack or be alienated from support systems (Christiansen et al., 1984; Lashley, 2000). Some women arrive as domestic workers or labourers or find themselves streamed into low-status and low-paying jobs (Crawford, 2004) requiring lengthy work hours in multiple jobs. As a result, it is more challenging for Caribbean women to accumulate adequate financial resources to facilitate reunification with their children in a short period of time. In addition, women may begin new families, which may further extend the period for reuniting with their children. These hardships contribute to feelings of increased emotional turmoil and instability for mothers and their children.

Although the goal of reunion remains a driving force for the mother, the realities of living in Canada present a different picture. Most of the research indicates that the longer the separation, the more difficult the reunion will be emotionally and psychologically for mothers and children (Crawford, 2004; Glasgow & Gouse-Sheese, 1995).

CHALLENGES FACING THE CHILDREN

Children in the Caribbean may undergo a number of adjustments in their lives while the mother seeks a better life for them. Separation from their mother can be traumatic and stressful for children, particularly for adolescents. Teachers in the Caribbean have noted effects in the school environment (Rambally, 2002). One primary school teacher in the Caribbean who has been teaching for more than 30 years noted that children are unhappy and sad as they wait tirelessly to join their mothers. Known as "barrel children," because their mothers regularly send them clothes, gifts and other necessities in barrels, these children often do not develop a "normal" pattern of coping with their grief at the loss of their mothers (L. Gomez-Coppin, personal communication, December 20, 2004; Crawford, 2004).

Research indicates that most fathers are not guardians of the household when the mother migrates. In fact, the child is generally left in the care of a grandmother, an aunt or another female relative. Girls who are left behind may be placed in the position of caregiver for their younger siblings. The whereabouts of the biological father may be unknown, and even when the child is left with the father, his involvement is limited (Jones et al., 2004; sjc Young Leaders, 1999). However, children may still idealize and mourn their fathers.

While often children grieve their mother's departure, particularly if the children had a secure attachment with her, children may become attached to their new caregiver, leading to a renewed sense of stability and comfort. These unofficial adoptions may not always be stable for the children, and in such cases children may spend their childhood and/or part of adolescence in a number of households (Russell-Brown et al., 1997; Senior, 1991). If the caregiver is emotionally neglectful or physically, sexually and/or emotionally abusive, the children will have little confidence that they will be responded to when in need (Mennen & O'Keefe, 2004). This leaves them vulnerable in times of stress, and at a higher risk of developing mental and physical health problems (Atkinson & Goldberg, 2004). In addition, if reunification takes much longer than expected, the children may get frustrated and angry, and may become involved in criminal activities.

Reunification Issues

The literature indicates that Caribbean women and their children are reunited in Canada anywhere from one to six years after separation; however, it can take as long as 15 years in some cases (Anderson & Grant, 1987; Glasgow & Gouse-Sheese, 1995). The age of the child at the time of the mother's departure is generally between one and six years. Therefore the child can be reunited with the mother as a child or an adolescent. Glasgow and Gouse-Sheese's (1995) study on Caribbean adolescents reuniting with their parents in Canada indicated that the ages of their sample at reunification ranged from 14 to 21 years, with the participants having lived apart from their parent(s) for four to 15 years.

Stressful reunification experiences may lead the mothers and their children to seek counselling from (or to become the focus of attention by) social agencies. However, many other parents may avoid seeking help from and/or referrals to social services. Research reveals that families in the Caribbean do not readily accept help from mental health professionals (Baptiste et al., 1997; Gopaul-McNicol, 1993; Razack, 2003). They generally seek help from their church and extended family, believing that problems should be kept and solved within the family. Most Caribbean people also believe that there is a stigma attached to seeking counselling, and that only "crazy" people need mental health counselling. Consequently, they may only access external help as a last resort (Baptiste et al., 1997).

CHALLENGES FACING THE MOTHER AND CHILDREN

Mothers and their children may face various challenges when reunited in Canada. The mother may see reunification as an ultimate act of love because she has made many sacrifices to bring her child to Canada. Christiansen et al. (1984) reported that parents usually go to great lengths to prepare for the arrival of their child (e.g., creating a welcoming space for the child in the home). However, in some cases, mothers are psychologically unprepared for the reunion, having lived separate lives for an extended period and being unfamiliar with the child's experiences during the separation. Personal stories we have heard from the families who went through the reunification process indicate that the mother may have idealistic or unrealistic expectations of the reunification with her child. For example, a mother who left a six-year-old in the Caribbean and is later introduced to her 16-year-old in Canada may expect to relive the relationship that she had from the past. However, relating to this 16-year-old may seem like adopting a new person into her life.

Data show the problems in adjustment for the child seem to reach crisis proportions within three years after arrival in Canada (Christiansen et al., 1984). Some younger children and youth may challenge parents' authoritative child-rearing practices, including the use of physical punishment as a form of discipline. The use of physical discipline by mothers may result in the involvement of child protection agencies.

Most children do not believe that reunification with their mother demonstrates an ultimate act of love (Glasgow & Gouse-Sheese, 1995; Lashley, 2000). Many studies indicate that this reunion produces tension, especially for youths who may have had a lengthy period of separation (Anderson & Grant, 1987; Rambally, 1995). If the separation was unplanned, or the child was not involved in the decision-making process, the child may not have dealt with the separation experience. In some instances, attachment to the biological mother may never have occurred because the mother left the child at a young age. In other cases, children react strongly to separation, believing that they were disliked or rejected by their mother.

Some children may have experienced further separation and multiple losses as they were shifted from one caregiver to another prior to and after their mother's migration. This may be due to abuse and neglect, or to the hospitalization or death of a caregiver. As a result, the child's ability to establish trusting relationships with adults may have been compromised (Glasgow & Gouse-Sheese, 1995; Jones et al., 2004; Wilkes, 1992).

For those children who did have sustained relationships with caregivers in the Caribbean, it may be quite difficult to leave these significant relationships. Insufficient time to say goodbye to those who were significant to the child while the mother was away may leave the child or adolescent with a prolonged sense of loss (Glasgow & Gouse-Sheese, 1995; Jones et al., 2004). In Canada, the mother may be looking ahead and may discourage the child from reaching out to or discussing caregivers in the Caribbean whom she or he has recently left. Such disconnections may lead to an incomplete grieving process for the child, and possibly subsequent behavioural issues.

Other challenges may occur if the child is brought into a new family, with step-siblings and a step-parent. The child's responses and reactions may create emotional upheaval and turmoil for the mother who may not have anticipated these added challenges. In addition, members of the new family may have unrealistic expectations of each other. The extended family and social support systems that the child had in the Caribbean are generally not available in Canada, adding to the child's feelings of separation, loss, stress and anxiety. Girls who were left behind may have been placed in the position of caregiver for their younger siblings and may be expected to carry on with these responsibilities when they are reunited with their mothers, particularly if their mother has begun a new family. These responsibilities increase the girls' feelings of resentment and anger, and her sense of feeling ignored, unwanted and alone (Flynn & Henwood, 2000; Jones et al., 2004).

If the period of separation was very long, frustration and anger may have played a role in a child becoming involved in the criminal justice system in the Caribbean—a problem that may continue here, with involvement in Canada's criminal justice system as well (Wilkes, 1992).

Practice Implications

PAST STRATEGIES

The presenting problems of the reunion of the Caribbean mother and her child appear to be similar in Canada, the United States and England. The literature reveals that most studies on therapeutic intervention to deal with mental health issues were carried out 10 to 15 years ago. Moreover, very few clinical studies have been conducted specifically addressing the difficulties and stressors experienced by Caribbean mothers related to separation from and reunification with their children. Limited data were available on the impact of severing ties within Caribbean families and the strategies that women use in coping with stress in the new cultural environment (Arnold, 1997). Many researchers and social service workers in Canada, the Caribbean and the United States have called for research supporting alternative interventions to help these families in transition (Jones et al., 2004).

The more recent literature in Canada on issues of reunification of Caribbean mothers and children reveal that intervention focused on the problems faced by youths in the school system (Anderson & Grant, 1987; Glasgow & Gouse-Sheese, 1995; Rambally 1995). Other studies focused on family counselling, with particular emphasis on separation and depression resulting first from the loss of the biological mother and then from the loss of a surrogate mother when the child emigrated, and on problems associated with the reunion process (Christiansen et al., 1984; Glasgow & Gouse-Sheese, 1995). The intervention methods have been crisis and family counselling, and group work that concentrated on the youths. Some authors (Christiansen et al., 1984; Glasgow & Gouse-Sheese, 1995; Rambally, 1995) felt that group work offered the young people an opportunity to be heard by supportive adults and helped them find meaning in their past experiences and current conflicts.

Research has shown that there is increased interest in the concept of attachment as relevant to explaining the function and dysfunction in children, families and society (Atkinson & Goldberg, 2004; Levy & Orlans, 1998). Some research was completed in the Caribbean on the issues of separation and loss as a consequence of parental migration from the perspective of children themselves. In their 2004 study, Jones et al. found that children separated from parents because of migration were more than twice as likely as other children to have emotional problems. The other study by sjc Young Leaders (1999) polled 419 children whose mothers had migrated from four Caribbean islands, and spoke with some of the mothers who had migrated to the United States. This study suggests that the effects of separation are especially negative for the children, whose dominant feelings were of abandonment, rejection and loss. In addition, the data reveal that "girls, more than boys, tend to speak out actively on the issue of the loss of the mother" (p. 50).

Jones et al. (2004) indicate that there is a need for urgent and focused policy reformulation as well as structured support systems for children and their caregivers who are separated through migration. It is conceivable that children from the Caribbean will continue to experience negative psychological effects if they do not receive appropriate intervention in the Caribbean and/or when they reunite with their mother in Canada. We agree with Jones et al. (2004) that intervention programs are urgently needed to assess the correlation between consistent parenting and the psychological well-being of children. Mental health professionals and social workers who work with Caribbean children and families on issues of migration acknowledge that the issues of separation and loss are very relevant to migration.

NEW STRATEGIES

Attachment Theory

Mental health professionals might consider attachment theory and attachment interventions to explore how Caribbean women respond to and cope with the separation from and reunion with their children. An analysis of this intervention may provide mental health professionals with further strategies to help Caribbean mothers, children and families to better prepare for separation and reunification challenges. The knowledge and use of attachment theory and its implications can be useful when working with this population, whether it is in the Caribbean, Canada, England or the United States (Arnold, 2003; Jones et al., 2004).

Attachment theory deals with the important bond between parents and children, generally with the mother as the main caregiver. The quality of that attachment, particularly in the early years, has implications for the quality of parent-child interactions, the child's mental and emotional health, and parenting in future generations. It is therefore essential to explore all avenues to address and reduce the emotional costs that migration can have for children and parents. Healthy attachment to parents can reduce children's vulnerability to being abused or exposed to criminal activity, and can help them seek more appropriate ways to meet their emotional needs.

Attachment theory provides a framework that is suited to working with this population. The issues of separation and reunification deal with the implications as well as the applications of attachment. In addition, the goals of attachment-based treatment are to interrupt the symptomatic cycle in family relationships and increase the parent's acceptance of the child and the child's confidence in the parent's availability (Atkinson & Goldberg, 2004).

Bowlby (1982, 1997, 1998) initially outlined the concepts of attachment theory, and recently many others have expanded on this theory and its implications for treatment and intervention, particularly in relation to psychopathology, child abuse and neglect, and child welfare (Atkinson & Goldberg, 2004; Howe, 2005; Mennen & O'Keefe, 2004). According to Bowlby (1997), attachment theory considers the way humans form strong affectional and emotional bonds to particular people, especially mothers, who, in most cases, are the primary caregivers. Bowlby states that within one year, most infants develop a strong attachment to a person who provides "mothering" but who may not necessarily be the biological mother. Attachment is considered different from bonding. *Bonding* is the biological, genetic and emotional connection between a mother and her baby during pregnancy and at birth. *Attachment* is learned after birth through interactions between the person who provides mothering and the child during the first three years of life (Levy & Orlans, 1998). Research shows that attachment is a lifespan concept, with children maintaining attachment to their parents throughout childhood and perhaps into adulthood (Ainsworth et al., 1978). The young child relies on the attachment figure and seeks physical proximity especially when the child is sad, ill or frightened. While the need for physical proximity lessens for older children, they expect the attachment figure to be available for communication, and to be accessible and responsive when they seek help (Kerns et al., 1996).

According to Scroufe (1983), the quality of attachment is the cornerstone that moulds children's behaviour in interacting with others throughout their lifespan. If a child enjoys a secure attachment, she or he is emotionally stable in relationships, and develops leadership and social skills as well as positive interaction with others. The pattern of attachment a child shows toward the mother figure is, to a high degree, the consequence of the pattern of mothering received (Bowlby, 1982). Worldwide, research indicates that 65 per cent of infants are securely attached to their mother, 25 per cent avoidantly attached and 10 per cent resistantly attached (Van Ijzendoorn, 1992). Children with secure attachments embrace life opportunities, form better relationships with their peers, have effective leadership and social skills, and are more confident (Levy & Orlans, 1998; Scroufe et al., 2005). The benefits of secure attachment continue beyond the early formative years. Children and teenagers with secure attachment histories excel in social and emotional skills and at each stage of development. In addition, parenting behaviours are transmitted from one generation to another. Hence, securely attached children grow into parents who are responsive and sensitive to their own children (Egeland & Erickson, 1999). Insecure attachment (i.e., avoidant and resistant attachment) manifests in attachment behaviours that result in children who are anxious, more dependent and manipulative, and who take pleasure in others' distress (Levy & Orlans, 1998).

Parents' attachment patterns have also been documented. In their study about the stability and transmission of adult attachment across three generations, Benoit and Parker (1994) noted that one of the breakthroughs in attachment research was the development of empirical means for "measuring" working models of attachment in infants. Developed by George et al. (1985), the test known as the Adult Attachment Interview (AAI) assesses adults' internal working model for attachment relationships. These *internal working models* "refer to the kind of memories, experiences, outcomes, feelings and knowledge about what tends to happen in relationships, particularly with attachment figures at times of need" (Howe, 2005, p. 28). The AAI can stimulate subjects to retrieve and evaluate attachment-related autobiographical memories and has increasingly been used to predict the quality of parent-child interactions and infant-parent attachments.

The AAI may help to determine the quality of the attachment relationship between the Caribbean mother and children who were reunited, and help to devise appropriate intervention to deal with reunion challenges. As previously stated, many Caribbean children will have several caregivers. Bowlby (1982) stressed that it is incorrect to suppose that young children diffuse their attachment over many figures without forming a strong attachment to anyone, and consequently would not miss any particular person when that person is away. Based on a substantial body of evidence on attachment theory and practice, Bowlby (1982) concluded that the loss of a child's mother (or mother figure) is by far the most significant loss in spite of other variables that may determine a child's distress. We hope that the use of attachment theory and interventions provide a framework that will not only address the important emotional aspects of child-parent relationships, but will also shed light on the broader child-rearing practices of parents in the Caribbean in relation to economic and social conditions.

Recognizing Each Family's Unique Situation

Mental health professionals who deal with Caribbean families need to recognize that each family has unique issues and circumstances. To determine the extent and quality of attachment between the Caribbean mother and child, mental health professionals can ask each person questions separately. The following list of questions is not exhaustive, but can serve as a guide when assessing an individual family situation.

For the mother, questions include inquiring about her background and decision to immigrate to Canada, and asking about both the positive and negative challenges of living in Canada. For the child, questions include inquiring about living in the Caribbean without her or his mother, about the caregivers in the Caribbean and about experiences once in Canada.

Examples of questions for the mother:
• Did you have family in Canada before you arrived?
• What did it feel like for you to move to a new country?
• In general, how do you think your child felt about your going to Canada without her or him?
• What was the age of your child when you left?
• Who cared for your child in the Caribbean while you were in Canada?
• Were there other children where your child lived? How were they related to you?

- How did you keep in touch with your child (e.g., by letters and pictures, by phone, in person)?
- How often did you contact your child?
- How often did your child contact you?
- How well do you feel your child was cared for in the Caribbean?
- How did it feel to leave your child?
- How does it feel to have daily contact with your child again?
- How are you and your child coping with living together?
- After your child arrived in Canada, did she or he contact family and friends in the Caribbean? If so, how often and how did the communication go? If not, why not?
- What do you think are the main challenges (positive and/or negative) for families moving from the Caribbean to Canada?
- Which, if any, services or supports offered to you in Canada were helpful during this time?
- What services or supports that were not offered would you have liked?

Examples of questions for the child (depending on the child's age):
- What has it been like for you to move from the Caribbean to Canada?
- Who took care of you in the Caribbean? How long did this person or these people take care of you?
- Did you live with other children? If yes, how were you related to them?
- Did you keep in touch with your mother? If yes, how did you keep in touch? How often did you contact her?
- Did your mother keep in touch with you? If yes, how did she keep in touch? How often did she contact you?
- How did you feel when your mother moved to Canada?
- How does it feel to live with your mother again?
- After you came to Canada, did you get in touch with your family and friends in the Caribbean? If so, how often? If not, why not?
- What helps you feel comfortable here in Canada?

Responses to the previous questions can help mental health professionals provide appropriate support, guidance, counselling and referrals to Caribbean mothers and their children. In asking the mother and child questions to determine appropriate intervention, it is necessary to understand the parent-child problems associated with reunification in a broader perspective to include the Caribbean family's history, support networks, economic and social conditions, migration patterns, adaptation and survival mechanisms, coping skills and child-rearing patterns (Rambally, 1995). In addition, it is important to obtain information about successful reunions, in which mothers and their children coped well with the challenges of reuniting and did not need referrals to social services. Knowing what works can be helpful information to other families, to mental health professionals and to social agencies.

Dealing with Attachment Concerns

The following factors may facilitate the best attachment outcomes:

- mother and child were securely attached in the Caribbean
- an ongoing attachment pattern was maintained while the mother and child were separated
- the child had a secure attachment caregiver while in the Caribbean (e.g., the grandmother).

Better attachment outcomes may result in fewer referrals for counselling, psychotherapy and group therapy to child protection and other social agencies because the mother and child are better able to cope with challenges. However, if there is an insecure attachment between the mother and child, it will be more difficult for them to deal with problems effectively; the following strategies to deal with attachment concerns may help.

Thomas (2000) documented several strategies to use with children who have been diagnosed with *attachment disorder*, a break in the bond with parents that causes trauma. However, some of these strategies may also be appropriate for mental health professionals who provide services to Caribbean women and children experiencing separation and reunification issues in Canada. These strategies include the following:

USE ATTACHMENT THERAPY

This form of therapy dispels enough of the internalized bitterness and anger and leaves an opening for warmth, affection and love. The goal of attachment therapy is for the child to see the adults in the world not as the ones who left them or hurt them, but as those who are capable of helping and being trusted (Thomas, 2000). This provides the opportunity for the Caribbean woman to inform the child of her love and affection. As indicated in the studies by Jones et al. (2004) and SJC Young Leaders (1999), young girls, in particular, are quite affected by their mother's emigration. They greatly miss their mother's guidance, advice and expressions of love, especially at a young age. These children might display psychological and emotional trauma affecting their self-esteem, peer relationships and sense of identity. Young boys tend to display their emotional difficulties through aggressive behaviour.

CONSIDER UNIQUE ATTACHMENT PRACTICES

Although the attachment relationship is universal, the manner in which attachment behaviours are displayed varies among different cultures (Mawani, 2001; Mennen & O'Keefe, 2004). Therefore mental health care professionals need to be open-minded and aware of the various child-rearing styles and attitudes of Caribbean families when working with this community. It is also important to recognize the cultural differences among Caribbean families who may experience attachment difficulties.

UNDERSTAND THE CHILD

The mother has to recognize that her child has probably experienced abandonment and loss, and may feel unloved, lost and in pain. According to Thomas (2000), the more years that are lost to separation, the more likely the child is to develop unhealthy coping mechanisms in handling close relationships with others, including the mother. Therefore, if separation has been prolonged, the mother needs to understand these coping strategies. Jones et al. (2004) reported that children from their Caribbean study were more vulnerable in terms of exposure to both risks of abuse and criminal activities but also in seeking appropriate ways to meet their emotional needs. These children were significantly more likely to report depressive symptoms than those who were not separated from their parents—a situation that increases risks of alcohol and other drug use as well as, later, mental illness.

Attachment-based interventions can help the mother understand how the broken attachment bond affected her child. These interventions can enhance maternal sensitivity, provide social support and promote change in the mother's inner working models of attachment—the experience and knowledge of relationships, especially with attachment figures in a time of need (Atkinson & Goldberg, 2004; Howe, 2005).

KNOW HOW CHILDREN DEVELOP AND HOW SEPARATION AFFECTS THEM

The mother needs to be knowledgeable about the child's development and about the impact of separation on her or him. Depending on their age and the length of separation, some children may be angry, distant or rejecting, pushing away the mother who tries to reconnect with them. Other children may constantly need attention. These behaviours may cause stress between mother and child because of their unfamiliarity with each other and unresolved feelings about their separation. Professional help is recommended to help mother and child recognize and deal with the impact of their separation experiences.

GATHER A SUPPORT TEAM

It is essential that both the mother and child gather a circle of support that includes people who can help: grandparents, friends, a therapist, a teacher, a social worker, a church community and anyone else interested in the child's welfare. The child might benefit from the involvement of the extended family members who have cared for and cared about the child. Individuals who have knowledge of Caribbean families, for example, ethno-specific Caribbean agencies, can be helpful. The people in this support circle need to be non-judgmental. They also need to be aware of how other issues such sexism, racism, socio economic, socio cultural and political issues affect the family formation and parental reasons for migration and separation from their child.

FACE THE PROBLEM

The mother needs to acknowledge and accept that the child's behaviour may reflect an attachment disruption that is a result of the separation. In addition, the mother has to acknowledge the child's life in the Caribbean while they were separated. It is important that the mother attempt to see the child's past experiences through the child's eyes. Separation from her or his mother can be traumatic and stressful for a child, particularly for an adolescent. The child in the Caribbean may have suffered physical, sexual and emotional abuse. It is essential that the mother acknowledge with honesty and openness any additional emotional and physical issues facing the child.

TAKE TIME OFF

If at all possible, the mother needs to take time off work when the child first arrives. According to Thomas (2000), prioritizing and committing to the child's needs demonstrates the mother's commitment to the child's emotional survival. Taking time off from work, if feasible, can allow the extra time necessary for reuniting, healing and bonding. The child should not be moved from caregiver to caregiver, especially during the first three years of healing from previous attachment trauma. The mother may be inclined to continue the practice of "child shifting," which may lead to further ruptures in the attachment process. If it is not financially possible for the mother to take time off, she at least needs to be available to deal with issues that may occur (e.g., at school).

Research Implications

There is a paucity of research on how Caribbean parents and children cope with separation and reunion in Canada. A few recent studies from the Caribbean and Canada have addressed the significant impact of migration on children and parents, with particular emphasis on girls and women (Flynn & Henwood, 2000; Jones et al., 2004; SJC Young Leaders, 1999). These studies and limited previous research recognize the significant need to address the psychological and emotional impact of separation and reunification among Caribbean women and children. We believe that attachment theory and its implications and applications are relevant to the assessment and treatment of such families. We recommend that further research be conducted in Canada and the Caribbean to gain more evidence-based data to help Caribbean women and children understand and cope with the challenges of separation and reunification. Suggestions for specific topics follow:

IMMIGRATION PROCESS

Further research can advise on the immigration processes in both the Caribbean and Canada, and hopefully reduce the length and challenges of the separation and reunification process. Research should focus on length of the immigration process that prolongs the separation of parents and children.

PARENTING PROCESS

Research is needed to examine attachment theory in connection with the parenting practices in the Caribbean, and how separation and reunification are affected by these practices.

SOCIAL, ECONOMIC, HEALTH AND CULTURAL FACTORS

As indicated previously, other factors affect the reunification process and these must be considered along with attachment theory. Socio-economic status, education, life stressors, family circumstances, health, family and social supports, and culture will affect the impact of attachment on the mother and the child. Research should focus on how these factors affect the outcome of the reunification process.

INFLUENCE/NON-INFLUENCE OF FATHERS

The composition of the household before and after migration to Canada, and the influence of the father will be factors in the outcome of reunification. Research indicates that most fathers are not guardians of the household when the mother migrates. Therefore, the influence or non-influence of fathers must be considered in researching separation and reunification issues with mothers and children.

SUCCESSFUL REUNIONS

It is important to research reunions that are successful to isolate variables that contribute to or hinder the success or failure of reunions.

LINK BETWEEN ATTACHMENT THEORY AND COPING MECHANISMS

Both the available research and the many needs reported by service providers and families (E. Bonner, personal communication, November 6, 2000; R. Hackett, personal communication, October 31, 2000; Mohammed, 1998) link attachment theory with coping mechanisms of Caribbean mothers and their children during separation and reunification. More quantitative and/or qualitative research is urgently needed in this area to determine whether attachment interventions are indeed applicable to this immigrant community in Canada. We recommend that the research be conducted both in Canada and the Caribbean.

Conclusion

We hope that the use of current research, and investment in further research, on attachment strategies will offer new and effective methods of intervention. The results of the research would benefit not only Caribbean immigrant women; rather, they could be applied to most immigrant women who leave their children in their homeland and are later reunited with them.

References

Ainsworth, M.D.S., Blehar, M.C., Waters, E. & Wall, S. (1978). *Patterns of Attachment: A Psychological Study of the Strange Situation*. Hillsdale, NJ: Lawrence Erkbaum Associates.

Anderson, W.W. & Grant, R.W. (1987). *The New Newcomers: Patterns of Adjustment of West Indian Immigrant Children in Metropolitan Toronto Schools*. Toronto: Canadian Scholars' Press.

Arnold E. (1997). Issues of reunification of migrant West Indian children in the United Kingdom. In J.L. Roopnarine & J. Brown (Eds.), *Caribbean Families: Diversity among Ethnic Groups* (pp. 243–258). Greenwich, CT: Ablex Publishing Corporation.

Arnold E. (2003). Inter-cultural counseling in a social services setting. In A. Dupont-Joshua (Ed.), *Working Inter-culturally in Counselling Settings* (pp. 195–209). New York: Brunner-Routledge.

Atkinson, L. & Goldberg, S. (2004). *Attachment Issues in Psychopathology and Intervention*. Mahwah, NJ: Lawrence Erlbaum Associates.

Baptiste, D.A., Jr., Hardy, K.V. & Lewis, L. (1997). Clinical practice with Caribbean immigrant families in the United States: The intersection of emigration, immigration, culture, and race. In J.L. Roopnarine & J. Brown (Eds.), *Caribbean Families: Diversity among Ethnic Groups* (pp. 275–303). Greenwich, CT: Ablex Publishing Corporation.

Benoit, D. & Parker, K.C.H. (1994). Stability and transmission of attachment across three generations. *Child Development, 65* (5), 1444–1456.

Bowlby, J. (1982). *Attachment and Loss: Volume I. Attachment* (2nd ed.) London: The Hogarth Press Ltd.

Bowlby, J. (1997). *Attachment and Loss: Vol. III. Loss: Sadness and Depression*. London: Pimlico.

Bowlby, J. (1998). *A Secure Base: Parent-Child Attachment and Healthy Human Development*. New York: Basic Books.

Christiansen, J.M., Thornley, A., Robinson, J.A. & Herberg, E.N. (1984). *West Indians in Toronto: Implications for Helping Professionals*. Toronto: Family Service Association of Metropolitan Toronto.

Crawford, C. (2004). African-Caribbean women, diaspora and transnationality. *Canadian Woman Studies/les cahiers de la femme, 23* (2), 97–103.

Egeland, B. & Erickson, M.F. (1999). Findings from the parent-child project and implications for early intervention. *Zero to Three*, Nov/Dec, 3–10.

Evans, H. & Davies, R. (1997). Overview of issues in childhood socialization in the Caribbean. In J.L. Roopnarine & J. Brown (Eds.), *Caribbean Families: Diversity among Ethnic Groups* (pp. 1–24). Greenwich, CT: Ablex Publishing Corporation.

Flynn, K. & Henwood, C. (2000). Nothing to write home about: Caribbean Canadian daughters, mothers and migration. *Journal of the Association for Research on Mothering, 22* (2), 118–129.

George, C., Kaplan, N. & Main, M. (1985). *Adult Attachment Interview* (3rd. ed.). Department of Psychology, University of California, Berkeley.

Glasgow, G.F. & Gouse-Sheese, J. (1995). Themes of rejection and abandonment in group work with Caribbean adolescents. *Social Work with Groups, 17* (4), 3–27.

Gopaul-McNicol, S. (1993). *Working with West Indian Families*. London: The Guilford Press.

Howe, D. (2005). *Child Abuse and Neglect: Attachment, Development and Intervention*. Hampshire: Palgrave MacMillan.

Jones, A., Sharpe, J. & Sogren, M. (2004). Children's experiences of separation from parents as a consequence of migration. *The Caribbean Journal of Social Work, 3*, 89–109.

Kerns, K.A., Klepac, L. & Cole, A. (1996). Peer relationships and preadolescents' perceptions of security in the child-mother relationship. *Developmental Review, 33* (3), 457–466.

Lashley, M. (2000). The unrecognized social stressors of migration and reunification in Caribbean families. *Journal of Transcultural Psychiatry, 37* (2), 203–217.

Levy, T.M. & Orlans, M. (1998). *Attachment, Trauma, and Healing: Understanding and Treating Attachment Disorder in Children and Families*. Washington, DC: Child Welfare League of America.

Mawani, F.N. (2001). Sharing attachment practices across cultures: Learning from immigrants and refugees. *Infant Mental Health Promotion Project, 32*, 38–42.

Mennen, F.E. & O'Keefe, M. (2004). Informed decisions in child welfare: The use of attachment theory. *Child and Youth Services Review, 27*, 577–593.

Mohammed, S. (1998). Migration and the family in the Caribbean. *Caribbean Quarterly, 44* (3 & 4), 1–14.

Rambally, R.T. (1995). The overrepresentation of black youth in the Quebec social service system: Issues and perspectives. *Canadian Social Work Review, 12* (1), 85–97.

Rambally, R.T. (2002). *Practice Imperfect: Reflections on a Career in Social Work*. Ste-Anne-de-Bellevue, QC: Shoreline Press.

Razack, N. (2003). Social work with Canadians of Caribbean background: Postcolonial and critical race insights into practice. In A. Al-Krenawi & J.R. Graham (Eds.), *Multicultural Social Work in Canada: Working with Diverse Ethno-racial Communities* (pp. 338–364). Don Mills, ON: Oxford University Press.

Russell-Brown, P.A., Norville, B. & Griffith, C. (1997). Child shifting: A survival strategy for teenage mothers. In J.L. Roopnarine & J. Brown (Eds.), *Caribbean Families: Diversity among Ethnic Groups* (pp. 223–242). Greenwich, CT: Ablex Publishing Corporation.

Scroufe, L.A. (1983). Infant-caregiver attachment and patterns of adaptation in preschool: The roots of maladaptation and competence. In M. Perlmutter (Ed.), *Minnesota Symposium in Child Psychology: Vol. 16* (pp. 41–83). Hillsdale, NJ: Lawrence Erlbaum Associates.

Scroufe, L.A., Egeland, B., Carlson, E. & Collins, W.A. (2005). The development of the person: The Minnesota Study of Risk and Adaptation from Birth to Adulthood. New York: Guilford Press.

Senior, O. (1991). *Working Miracles: Women's Lives in the English-Speaking Caribbean.* Indianapolis, IN: Indiana University Press.

Sharpe, J. (1997). Mental health issues and family socialization in the Caribbean. In J.L. Roopnarine & J. Brown (Eds.), *Caribbean Families: Diversity among Ethnic Groups* (pp. 259–273). Greenwich, CT: Ablex Publishing Corporation.

Smith, R.T. (1996). *Matrifocal.* New York: Routledge.

St. Joseph's Convent Young Leaders. (1999). *Mothers Don't Come in Barrels.* Port-of-Spain, Trinidad and Tobago: Author.

Thomas, N.L. (2000). Parenting children with attachment disorders. In T.M. Levy (Ed.), *Handbook of Attachment Interventions* (pp. 67–109). San Diego, CA: Academic Press.

Van Ijzendoorn, M.H. (1992). Review: Intergenerational transmission of parenting: A review of studies in nonclinical populations. *Developmental Review, 12,* 76–99.

Wilkes, J.R. (1992). Children in limbo: Working for the best outcome when children are taken into care. *Canada's Mental Health, 40* (2), 2–5.

Chapter 11

Counselling Lesbian and Bisexual Immigrant Women of Colour

FARZANA DOCTOR AND SILVANA BAZET

Lesbian and bisexual women of colour face multiple challenges in their lives. Systemic and interpersonal racism, sexism and heterosexism affect their self-esteem, relationships and quality of life. They have complex identities and develop unique mechanisms to survive and sustain themselves.

This chapter explores the complexities of counselling lesbian and bisexual immigrant women of colour in the context of the tremendous impact that racism and heterosexism have on their well-being. Most of the information in this chapter is practice-based and stems from our direct experience counselling lesbian and bisexual women of colour, many of whom are immigrants and refugees. Case examples presented in this chapter also derive from our clinical experience, and have been fictionalized for confidentiality purposes. The purpose of this chapter is to heighten awareness of the complexities in counselling these clients in a variety of counselling, social service and health settings. Although it is understood that multiple social locations such as gender, class, religion, age, body size and ability intersect in the lives of immigrant and refugee lesbian and bisexual women of colour, due to space limitations, this chapter mainly addresses the impact of racism and heterosexism.

The terms "lesbian," "bisexual" and "queer" are used in this chapter. The term "lesbian" refers to women whose primary emotional, sexual and romantic attractions are to women. Bisexual women have attractions to more than one gender.[1] The term

---

1. Traditionally, bisexual women have been understood to be attracted to women and men. However, current criticisms of binary notions of gender state that there are more than two genders (i.e., transgender people). Some people may prefer to use the terms "queer" or "pansexual" to refer to their sexual orientation.

"queer" reclaims a previously derogatory term for lesbian, bisexual, gay and non-heterosexual transgender and transsexual people. The term "queer," like "dyke," tends to be used only by those people within the lesbian, gay, bisexual, transgender and transsexual (LGBTT) communities. Clients may use different words to identify themselves including some that we do not use here, such as "gay woman" or "woman-loving woman." For more information about these terms, see Barbara et al. (2004). Many of these terms, while used around the globe, are rooted in western ideas of sexuality and some clients may use other words that are more culturally congruent to them.[2]

Gay, lesbian and bisexual people immigrate to Canada for many reasons. Some may be motivated to do so in order to both live in a country where there are greater perceived[3] and legal rights and freedoms for them and to avoid family or community pressures to marry (Sullivan & Jackson, 1999). Although exact numbers are not available, Canada is seeing a greater number of people claiming refugee status based on persecution for sexual orientation or gender identity (Hughes, 2002; Jimenez, 2004). Other motivations can include political persecution not related to their sexual orientation, the quest for a better socio-economic status or the desire to pursue a relationship with a Canadian citizen (Holt, 2004).

Theoretical Framework

This chapter uses an anti-oppression framework and is grounded in the authors' private psychotherapy practices and their long-time involvement in community and activist work. This framework is informed by the knowledge and understanding that counselling does not occur in a social vacuum and that societal power structures affect both counselling practice and clients' lives (Pollack, 2004). It is the service provider's role to acknowledge and address oppression when working with clients (Chen-Hayes, 2003). Service providers need to be aware of how sexism, racism, heterosexism and other oppressions have an impact on both themselves and their clients and how this informs and affects the counselling process.

In this chapter, the term "clients" is used interchangeably with "lesbian and bisexual women of colour." We do not make a distinction between women who are in therapeutic settings and women outside of such settings. This is done intentionally as part of our anti-oppression approach to counselling, where power differentials between therapist and clients are deconstructed.

---

2. An example of this is the New York–based lesbian Latina group called Las Buenas Amigas, The Good Friends. For more information about this group, see www.lasbuenasamigas.org.

3. There is a widespread perception among service providers that Canada is enlightened and free for LGBTT people, while previously colonized nations are "backward" and oppressive in this regard. This false polarization does not reflect the complex realities of living as an LGBTT person in either the colonizing or colonized nations.

Literature Review

There is a clear paucity of research and academic writing about counselling issues for lesbian and bisexual immigrant and refugee women of colour. Much of what does exist focuses on sexual orientation or race, but not both. Much of our knowledge about sexual orientation has come from research focused on the lives of American white gay men (Graziano, 2004; Parks et al., 2004; Savin-Williams, 1996). In studies including lesbians as "subjects" of research, lesbians of colour and those who are immigrants are rarely mentioned (Moreno, 2002). Bisexuals are often poorly represented in studies and their issues tend to be "lumped in" with lesbian and gay issues in general. Literature on immigrant and refugee women of colour rarely acknowledges the existence of lesbians and bisexual women. In fact, there is a scarcity of research dealing with immigrant and refugee women's sexuality in general (Espín, 1999).

The available literature indicates some common themes related to the "triple jeopardy" status that queer women of colour face; they experience oppression based on race, gender and sexual orientation from mainstream society, queer and ethno-specific communities (Washington, 2001; Poon & Ho, 2002; Rosario et al., 2004; Green & Boyd-Franklin, 1996). The impact of this "triple jeopardy" status includes identity conflicts, confusion or anxiety (Moreno, 2002); greater vulnerability to sexually transmitted diseases (Poon & Ho, 2002); increased risk for mental health problems (Zea et al., 1999); less access to preventative health care services; and higher prevalence of alcohol and tobacco use (Mays et al., 2002).

The literature also suggests that multiple marginalization can be a source of strength in that it helps lesbians of colour manage more flexibly (than white lesbians) stressors associated with oppression. This may be because lesbians of colour learn to function within minority and majority cultures from an early age, and sometimes with family or community guidance (Liu & Chan, 1996; Parks et al., 2004).

Complex and Interrelated Identities

Lesbian and bisexual women of colour have complex and interrelated identities. They share many of the issues and concerns of other immigrant and refugee women and children of immigrants. Due to space limitations, refer to Chapter 7 for a discussion of some of the common issues. Given that first-, second- and third-generation Canadians of colour are often viewed by mainstream culture as immigrants even when they are born in Canada, the issues below may relate to them as well. Included below are examples of ways in which race and sexual orientation intersect in the lives of lesbian and bisexual women of colour.

AGE AT IMMIGRATION

The age at which a client immigrated is useful information because age of immigration affects identity. For example, a client who immigrates at a younger age and enters the Canadian school system as a child (compared to someone who immigrated as an adolescent or adult) will have a different sense of belonging, identity and community. Adolescents or adults who have grown up in their country of origin may have a clearer sense of their country of origin's culture and history, and of their own identity (Razack, 2003). They may also have a stronger sense of the LGBTT communities in their country of origin, and the status of queer people there. Some clients experience migration and coming out concurrently. Espín (1996) describes each process as "the crossing of geographical borders and identity borders," a process that involves significant losses and transitions as well as gains. Attending to both experiences will be important in therapy. A client may express this by talking about losses related to her country of origin or her heterosexual privilege. She may also express the joys related to new freedoms and experiences in Canada and in LGBTT communities.

LEGAL STATUS IN CANADA

A client's legal status in Canada can also add complexity. For example, if the client does not have permanent residency or citizenship, the system can reinforce her feeling of alienation or what clients describe as "being in limbo." This is particularly dangerous for lesbian and bisexual women as they are often forced to remain in the closet about their sexual orientation due to fears that disclosing such information could affect their chances of remaining in Canada.

COMING OUT EXPERIENCES

Therapists should ask about coming out experiences in the country of origin. Was she part of lesbian or bisexual communities in her country of origin? How are those communities similar or different from where she lives now? What has it been like to adapt to these differences? What is her sense of belonging in LGBTT communities here?

MIGRATION EXPERIENCES

A client's experience of migration, changes in socio-economic status and reasons for leaving her country of origin are important. A person's experience of migration will be different based on her own financial resources or those of her family; whether she suffered persecution or torture, and for what reasons (sexual orientation may be one of them); whether she grew up in many countries before coming to Canada; or whether she lived part of her life in refugee camps. Clients who experienced persecution may be coping with symptoms of posttraumatic stress (Lacroix, 2003).

Lesbian and bisexual women's experiences of persecution based on sexual orientation may manifest differently from men's. According to one immigration lawyer in Toronto who specializes in refugee claims based on sexual orientation, women tend to report control, threats and violence from inside their homes while men report more violence from strangers outside their homes (E. Khaki, personal interview, January 13, 2005). This may be related to differences in gender roles and norms in that women may be less likely to be "out" in the streets compared to men.

SYSTEMIC RACISM IN CANADA

Service providers should research (through reading, searching the Internet, speaking with colleagues) what people in a client's community have faced in Canada. Systemic racism suffered by the client's community over generations can affect acculturation. For instance, the Japanese internment; the Chinese Head Tax; the *Indian Act*; and racial profiling of Black, Arab and Latin American communities have all had a tremendous impact on those communities (Chinese Canadian National Council, 2005; Ontario Human Rights Commission, 2003). These governmental actions have shaped the ways in which communities of colour perceive themselves and their right to belong. One Black bisexual woman stated that she did not want to be out at work because "there is enough against me as it is."

LANGUAGE

Language plays an important role in how clients view their identity. It may be useful to find out whether a client learned her parents' first language. Pressures by parents and society to assimilate, as well as internalized racism and rebellion toward parents who expect their children to speak their mother tongue, can result in the loss of language. The consequences of this loss include an inability to communicate with segments of the same ethno-racial community and/or extended family that may not be proficient in English or French. A client who has not learned the parents' first language can experience feelings of alienation from her own community, a feeling she may already experience as a sexual minority.

Bilingual children sometimes act in the role of translator for immigrant parents, performing the roles of adults in stressful situations such as visits to hospitals or government offices. This can alter parent-child dynamics in profound ways (Espín, 1999). For instance, a client may be overly responsible as a child and "grow up too fast." Some children have to deal with societal, institutional and/or interpersonal racism by themselves if parents are unable to advocate for them. In the case of a lesbian or bisexual youth, she may also be experiencing homophobic bullying on her own without the support of parents who can help her.

If English or French is a second language, clients may experience difficulties expressing their feelings in their second language while in therapy. On the other hand, the second language can be used as a tool to avoid shame associated with being lesbian or bisexual. For example, a client may feel freer to speak about her sexuality, her body and sexual practices in her second language than in her mother tongue because the English or French words may not carry the same negative cultural connotations as the first language (Espín, 1999). For example, a client who was taunted in the schoolyard with the word "tortillera" may have difficulty using this Spanish word but might proudly use the English equivalent "dyke" to describe herself. This is particularly true for clients who immigrated to Canada as adults. This may not be true for those who grew up in Canada since they have been heterosexually socialized in English or French as well. This does not mean that cultures that speak languages other than English or French are more lesbophobic or biphobic. Rather, the issue is that many cultures embed and teach heterosexism through language.

BICULTURAL ISSUES

A bicultural person is one who participates in and is able to navigate both the new and original cultures (LaFramboise et al., 1993). The degree of biculturalism experienced by a woman will be determined by the age of immigration and the length of time she has been in Canada. Clients may bring questions to therapy such as how to belong to both cultures, the validity and equality of both cultures and the ways in which people from each perceive them. They may feel conflicted about which culture is less or more likely to respect their sexual orientation identity and, given that, to which they must be most aligned or loyal. For example, one Latin American client stated during a counselling session, "Latinos are all macho homophobes," revealing her internalization of a common negative stereotype about her community. Clients may also face tensions between collectivist and individualist orientations of cultures. For example, a bicultural client from a collectivist-oriented family culture may feel both liberated and selfish for coming out; she may feel freedom for being able to express herself fully while worrying about the possible negative community reaction and subsequent impact on her family.

MIXED RACE ISSUES

As with bicultural women, mixed race women often have questions related to belonging to more than one ethno-racial community and the validity and equality of each community in relation to the other. How they are treated and perceived by each community is also an issue of concern (Razack, 2003). Discussion about privilege and discrimination connected to having light or dark skin and an exploration of family dynamics and what parents have conveyed about this may be important.[4]

Women who have lighter skin and who are regarded by others as white, or who attempt to "pass" as white, can experience difficulties in integrating their identity. This is because the white identity is more highly valued in a white-dominated society, making it more difficult for the client to fully integrate all aspects of her racial identity. Also, clients may be rejected or mistrusted by people of colour who unfairly assume that their lighter skin makes them less conscious of and resistant to racism.

RELIGION

Clients for whom religion is important may need to explore the issue of whether they can be both a religious or spiritual person and be queer. For service providers who do not feel competent addressing issues of religion or spirituality, it may be important to refer the client to a queer-positive provider or organization that will address these issues. Examples of such organizations are Salaam Queer Muslim Community (www.salaamcanada.com) and the Metropolitan Community Church of Toronto (mcctoronto.com). For those who need and want to reject their religion, the task may be to do so in a way that preserves their sense of moral integrity. Deconstructing false moral tenets may be a part of the therapy process and clients may need to explore alternative or progressive interpretations of their religious texts and be linked with queer-positive faith-based groups in order to reject the notion that it is evil or sinful to be lesbian or bisexual. The degree of internalization of false moral tenets can have a tremendous impact on the well-being of clients.

This list of complex identities is not exhaustive. There are many other factors that contribute to the complexity of identity development such as education, adoption, class, gender identity, ability and age.

Coming Out

This term "coming out" is used to describe the process of accepting one's sexual orientation, and it is often assumed to be stage-based, linear and progressive. Rarely does coming out occur in this manner. It is a non-linear process that can have simultaneous avenues of understanding and acceptance as well as obstacles. All decisions regarding coming out

---

4. Because complexions can vary among biological siblings, the issue of light-skin privilege may play out even in families where children are born to two parents of colour. For example, a child with lighter skin may be favoured, while a child with darker skin may be the "ugly one." Perceptions about how families view different complexions may be later complicated by a mixed race woman's sexuality, and the family's response to her coming out. One bisexual client spoke about her coming out experience: "My mother told me I could still get a man, because I am not too dark." Her mother felt that the client's relatively lighter skin colour would allow her to attract a man from their ethno-cultural community, even if others found out about her sexual orientation.

must be made by the client. This includes if, when and to whom to come out. The client may have valid reasons for choosing not to do so. Parks et al. (2004) found differences in coming out milestones between lesbians of colour and white lesbians. Compared to white women, women of colour questioned their sexual orientation at a younger age, took more time to decide they were lesbian but more quickly disclosed their identity to others—a result that contradicts studies that suggest that ethnocultural factors such as religion, the importance of family, traditional gender roles and homophobia delay or arrest the coming out process for queer people of colour (Savin-Williams, 1996).

When health practitioners work with lesbian and bisexual women of colour, it is important to take into consideration the following questions:

- Is the client coming out now?
- If the client is out, for how long has she been out and to whom?
- Where did she come out? Was it in a rural or urban area? Was the client's family the only family of colour around?
- Did she come out before or after coming to Canada? If she came out before, was she a part of lesbian or bisexual communities in her country of origin? If not, what assumptions do she or her family make about how the migration experience has affected her sexual orientation?
- Does the client believe that she will be hurt or rejected by her family and community if she is out to them?
- How old was the client when she came out and in which era? For example, a client who came out in the 1980s will have a different sense of herself compared to a woman coming out now in a context where more resources are available to queer women of colour.
- Does the client have dependants (children, parents or extended family) abroad? This can include non-biological family as well, such as people who grew up together. How do these relationships impact on her degree of "outness"?
- Has the client had previous heterosexual relationships or marriages? If children are involved, are there issues of custody and/or visitation rights that may affect the client's desire or ability to be public about her sexual orientation?
- What is your client's legal status? Clients who do not have secure legal status in Canada may not feel free to be out.
- Is she aware of queer people, groups or associations from her ethno-racial community in Canada or in her country of origin? Has she ever participated in any of these?

Impact of Racism and Heterosexism on Clients

Oppression, specifically racism and heterosexism, affects lesbian and bisexual immigrant and refugee women of colour. Below are some examples of common experiences that clients face.

PRESSURES TO ASSIMILATE

Queer immigrant women of colour experience significant pressures from LGBTT, ethno-specific and white communities to assimilate. Assimilation is a process that requires a person to reject the marginalized culture while wholeheartedly adopting the mainstream one. This pressure also affects and is reproduced in mainstream LGBTT communities. An alternative response to the dominance of the mainstream culture is integration, a process whereby a person participates in both communities, retaining a strong sense of ethno-racial identity while thriving in the mainstream culture. With integration, a person can also challenge and resist mainstream culture (Al-Krenawi & Graham, 2003). Below are some specific examples of pressures lesbians and bisexual women of colour can face when accessing the health and social service systems:

A client seeking help from an agency that supports LGBTT people was told that to be a lesbian she had to give up her identity as a woman of colour and separate from her ethno-racial/cultural heritage because she would never be accepted as lesbian by her ethno-racial community.

A client seeking help from her doctor was sent to a community centre that serves her ethno-racial community. The counsellor there thought that introducing her to a "reformed lesbian" (a lesbian who now claims to be heterosexual) would be helpful.

These examples also illustrate the common myth that being queer is a "white thing," that a person cannot be both queer and a person of colour.

STEREOTYPING OF COMMUNITIES OF COLOUR AS MORE BI-/HOMOPHOBIC THAN WHITE COMMUNITIES

One manifestation of oppression is stereotyping. Racist stereotypes deem cultures and races to be monolithic and homogenous rather than diverse and heterogeneous. A common stereotype about minority ethno-racial communities is that they are less willing to address their heterosexism, homophobia, lesbophobia and biphobia. An example of this stereotype can be seen in Canada's debates about same-sex marriage. The media has often focused on how "traditional" immigrant groups will react negatively to the change in legislation, as though this is one large voting block with one agenda. Although it is true that some people in communities of colour oppose changing the definition of marriage to include same-gender marriages, others support the change (Loghi, 2005; Wong-Tam, 2004). The impact of this stereotyping on clients is that the racism within the message, and the belief that their communities are more homophobic than white communities, becomes internalized. The perception that communities of colour are more bi-/homophobic is rooted in a racist belief that communities of colour are more "backward" and "ignorant." Washington (2001, p. 119) challenges this negative perception:

> [R]ecent studies suggest that lesbians and gay men of colour may experience higher degrees of acceptance within their families and communities of colour than do their white counterparts . . . such acceptance is often limited and typically means . . . communities do not for the most part disown or expel their lesbian and gay members.

This can be a confusing issue given the pervasiveness of the misperception and the fact that many people from ethno-racial communities may reinforce the belief that their communities are less supportive of queer rights. Service providers can help clients to deconstruct racist stereotyping by pointing out that their communities and cultures are not monolithic and homogenous and by helping the client to seek queer-positive allies within their communities. In doing so, service providers can help a client to address internalized racism and heterosexism.

This is not to deny that ethno-racial minority communities hold and act on homophobic beliefs (as other communities do). Lesbian, bisexual women and other women who don't conform to traditional gender roles challenge their community's values and norms. However, as Espín (1996, p. 101) states,

> Paradoxically, these values also provide the pathway to reconciliation . . . when the love of children and the value of family ties are strong, nothing, including homosexuality, will permanently split the family. Ultimately, when the family system is bound by love and respect, a way is found to embrace the homosexual member.

Sometimes, a family's tolerance of a lesbian or bisexual daughter is contingent on her remaining silent about her sexual orientation beyond the family (Green & Boyd-Franklin, 1996). In examining a community of colour's homophobia, it is important to recognize the context of racism. Many immigrant communities of colour carry a legacy of colonialism; and homophobia is part of that legacy (Seabrook, 2004). Colonization has also played a role in repressing indigenous beliefs and practices vis-a-vis queer sexualities, the result being that cultural acceptance and celebration of non-heterosexual and gender non-conforming people has been lost or suppressed in many societies. Most people are not even aware that their ethno-racial communities may have once had a rich history of queer pride and inclusion. In fact, most societies have long precolonial histories of the existence and celebration of queer people (Feinberg, 1996).

Some lesbian and bisexual women of colour lose their ethno-racial community and family connections when choosing to be open about their sexual orientation.

Losing connection to one's ethno-racial community in a racist society can take away the only shelter from racism a client may have, a place where they feel validated and are taught how to deal with the pain it causes (Greene & Boyd-Franklin, 1996). They may also lose the only place where they can see themselves reflected as people of colour until they can connect with other LGBTT people of colour. While most white queer people also suffer if they lose their families and communities, those who are from dominant ethnic groups (i.e., of Caucasian European ancestry) do not lose their sense of ethno-racial identity because it is reflected everywhere.

INTERNALIZED OPPRESSION

Racist, sexist and heterosexist messages are pervasive and become internalized. This internalization affects client well-being (Chen-Hayes, 2003). As stated by Hardiman and Jackson (1997, p. 21),

> People who have been socialized in an oppressive environment and who accept the dominant's group ideology about their group have learned to accept a definition of themselves that is hurtful and limiting. They think, feel and act in ways that demonstrate the devaluation of their group and of themselves as members of that group.

Therapists should gently challenge internalized oppression while validating clients' fears and hurtful past experiences. A common comment clients make is: "The lesbian of colour community is so messed up." Address the comment by asking some of the following questions: Is that true in all situations? What makes you feel that way? Are there any examples that suggest something different? How does the thought that the community may be "messed up" make you feel about yourself?

The work of dismantling internalized oppression with clients during the counselling process is slow, often painful, but necessary and ongoing. As a client recently put it: "I have been working on this for so long. Shouldn't I be done by now? Shouldn't I be able to come out to people without thinking?" It is also important to note that clients who are politicized—and can talk freely about racism, sexism, heterosexism and the other oppressions they experience—have not necessarily worked on the emotional impact that discrimination has had on them.

Sometimes service providers shy away from confronting expressions of internalized oppression, but to do so can be seen as accepting of and colluding with racism, sexism and heterosexism. Service providers can avoid this by learning to "hear" the ways that internalized oppression can subtly manifest itself.

RACISM IN SAME-GENDER INTERRACIAL RELATIONSHIPS

Lesbian, gay and bisexual people who have interracial relationships are discussed in the literature, in terms of racism that people of colour face from white partners and lovers (Graziano, 2004; Ayres, 1999) and the need for therapists to address differences related to privilege and oppression in interracial relationships (Addison & Brown, 2003).

LGBTT people are often inexperienced at discussing racism, and partners of colour in interracial relationships may find themselves tacitly agreeing to not talk about race and privilege (Addison & Brown, 2003). Interracial same-gender couples may draw more public attention than couples who share the same ethno-racial identity and may experience more homophobia. It may be the first time that a white partner has to contend with the realities of racism and she may feel guilty about her privilege and attempt to overcompensate in ways that are not helpful (Greene & Boyd-Franklin, 1996). For example, a white partner might unilaterally decide to avoid an event to protect her partner from anticipated racism rather than discussing the issue with her partner.

While not limited to same-gender relationships, racism can take a variety of forms, including exoticization of the person of colour, refusals to acknowledge racism from oneself or others, and using accents or language difficulties to undermine a partner's self-esteem. One form of racism in interracial relationships that may be unique to same-gender partners is the demand from a white lover that her partner distance herself from, or cut ties with, her family or community, alleging that they are homophobic. Examples the authors have heard are "Your family is not good for you," or "You either come out to them or I leave you." When this type of comment comes from a white lover who does not understand how the ethno-specific community operates or its importance to her partner, the remark is typically informed by racism. This sort of comment often increases a woman of colour's isolation, rather than giving her support. Although homophobia from her family may be real, and she may in fact need to cut ties, it is a decision that must be made by the woman of colour and not her white partner.

When listening to clients' narratives about their relationships, it is important for service providers to "tune in" to examples of racism. Clients may have learned to minimize or deny the racism they experience. Exploring relationship dynamics and asking clients how they felt about comments and behaviours by partners will be important.

Clients' Strategies for Dealing with Racism and Heterosexism

Lesbian and bisexual women of colour find ways to cope, survive and thrive in a context of heterosexism and racism. Below are some strategies the authors have found to be commonly used by clients. Some of these strategies may be used concurrently and don't necessarily reflect linear stages of growth. For example, a client may strategize with her family about how to deal with heterosexism, while taking a stand against her friends or colleagues' heterosexist or racist comments and assumptions.

Compartmentalization
A client leaves parts of herself at home depending on which community event or family gathering she is attending. She is not out or is only partially out. For example, she may attend a community of colour event but ensure that no one finds out she is lesbian or bisexual. Or, she may spend time only with white LGBTT people. While with them, she

may want to be seen as "just the same" and actively distance herself from communities of colour by ignoring racist comments. She might participate in racist jokes or avoid places where LGBTT people of colour might gather.

Strategizing

A client begins to strategize how to bring more of herself into the picture. For example, she is out to family and/or community, but does not bring her lover to a family wedding. She may go out with white LGBTT friends and make mention of her different ethno-racial status (e.g., tell them about a social, political or support group from her own ethno-racial community), while expressing loyalty to her friends (e.g., by saying that she would rather spend time with them than attend the meeting with the group from her ethno-racial community).

Negotiating

A client uses a more direct approach and makes compromises in order to meet others' needs. For example, she is out to her family and/or community, and brings her lover as a date to the family wedding. However, she may not tell people that her date is her lover and compromises by not displaying public affection. With a white lover, she may choose to go to the meeting mentioned in "Strategizing" but ensure that her relationship is not jeopardized by saying, "I am going out tonight, but we can spend all day tomorrow together."

Taking a Stand

A client is out to her family and/or community and refuses to compromise, demanding to be accepted as queer and a person of colour. For example, while at social gatherings, she may correct heterosexist assumptions by telling people that she is lesbian when they ask about her husband or she may confront racist comments. She may attend the ethno-specific meeting mentioned in the previous two strategies and expect her friends and partner to support her. She then deals with subsequent consequences, for example, homophobic reactions from family and/or community or racist reactions from friends or a partner who may feel excluded from the meeting.

Creating Communities with Other Queers of Colour

A client seeks friends and allies who will share a common understanding regarding racism and lesbo-/biphobia. She may continue to take a stand with family and/or community while also creating a community where she feels "at home" and can receive support. This could take the form of a group or social circle for queer people of colour.

THERAPIST'S ROLE IN CONFRONTING RACISM AND HETEROSEXISM

It is the therapist's role to actively confront his or her own and the client's racism and heterosexism in therapy. Here are some tips for doing so:

- Do your own work regarding oppression. Anti-oppression work is ongoing for everyone, no matter what their social location. Often, there is a misconception that if one attends some diversity training or does some reading, then the work is over. Being an ally to lesbian and bisexual women of colour requires ongoing training, learning, self-reflection and supervision.

- Understand your own social location and the privilege you hold. Therapists who haven't examined and understood their own privilege and oppression cannot comfortably support and challenge a client in her process of doing the same. Hardiman and Jackson (1997, p. 21) refer to this as internalized domination:

    Internalized domination refers to the behaviours, thoughts, and feelings of agents, who through their socialization as members of the dominant group, learn to think and act in ways that express internalized notions of entitlement and privilege.

- Understand power in the counselling dyad. Therapists have power over clients, and understanding differences in social location and how this may affect the therapy is crucial. Address this directly in the counselling dyad. It is up to the therapist to raise these issues. As clearly stated by Bell (1997, p. 13),

    Dominants also have an important role to play in challenging oppression and creating alternatives. . . . Dominants too need to identify the role they play in maintaining the system and the price they pay for privileged status in an unequal hierarchy.

- Don't collude with societal racism, sexism and heterosexism. Examples of collusion can include ignoring and not confronting internalized oppression in your client, or doubting a client's reports of racism or heterosexism.

- Validate the client's experience of racism, sexism and lesbo-/biphobia. When a client is silent about being oppressed or begins to doubt her own experiences, she may be blaming herself.

- Gently challenge internalized oppression while validating fears. Ask direct questions about race and sexual orientation (Barbara et al., 2004). It can be difficult for clients to raise taboo issues, especially with a therapist who does not share their social location. It is much better for the therapist to ask direct questions such as "How do you identify your sexual orientation?" or "Is your girlfriend a white woman or woman of colour?" The therapist should practice these questions in advance so that they are delivered in a non-judgmental and comfortable manner. Clients can sense the slightest signs of a therapist's discomfort with these subjects.

- It is inappropriate to ask a client to teach others (her partner, friends, the therapist) about racism and heterosexism. She may at times choose to be involved in a "teaching moment" with others, but it is not her job. There is a difference between asking a client for information about *her life* and asking her to educate you about her community.

- Be intentionally inclusive by ensuring that your client is aware that you are welcoming of queer people of colour. Do your walls and waiting areas show that you understand the issues of lesbian and bisexual women of colour? What artwork, posters, publications show this? Be mindful that some artwork does not positively portray people of colour but rather appropriates their cultures.

- Do specific research for resources and information that will help you understand and support your clients. Become more aware of the client's communities, but use the information cautiously. Much of the "cultural literacy" information available overgeneralizes and oversimplifies cultures.

- Get appropriate supervision. Does your supervisor understand racism and heterosexism? Is your supervisor doing his or her own work around oppression so that he or she can challenge you? Also, supervision needs to be a safe place to talk about one's own racism, sexism, heterosexism, lesbophobia and biphobia. Seek a supervisor who will challenge you instead of reassuring you that you are not racist, lesbophobic or biphobic. Supervisors must be willing and able to explore with you the complexities and layers of counselling a queer person of colour, and how societal and interpersonal racism and lesbo-/biphobia play a role in the counselling dyad.

Conclusion

This chapter addressed the struggles that lesbian and bisexual women of colour experience: their complex identities, the impact of societal oppression on identity development and relationships, and the strategies developed to cope with this oppression. Given these struggles, lesbian and bisexual women of colour are often in constant negotiation to sustain wholeness. What makes this journey difficult is not necessarily the demands from each community but society's power inequities and the prejudices and discrimination that sustain those inequities. Psychotherapy takes place within this context and it is a psychotherapist's role to be aware of societal oppression and her or his own social locations in order to avoid colluding with racist and heterosexist social structures that affect clients' well-being.

References

Addison, S.M. & Brown, M.M. (2003). Working with couples on ethnicity and sexual identity: The "parts" interview. In J. Whitman & C. Boyd (Eds.), *The Therapist's Notebook for Lesbian, Gay and Bisexual Clients* (pp. 110–114). New York: Haworth Clinical Practice Press.

Al-Krenawi, A. & Graham, J.R. (2003). Introduction. In A. Al-Krenawi & J.R. Graham (Eds.), *Working with Diverse Ethno-racial Communities* (pp. 1–20). Toronto: Oxford University Press.

Ayres, T. (1999). China doll, the experience of being a gay Chinese Australian. *Journal of Homosexuality, 36* (3/4), 87–97.

Barbara, A., Chaim, G. & Doctor, F. (2004). *Asking the Right Questions 2: Talking about Sexual Orientation and Gender Identity in Mental Health and Addiction Settings.* Toronto: Centre for

Addiction and Mental Health.

Bell, L.A. (1997). Theoretical foundations for social justice. In M. Adams, L.A. Bell & P. Griffin (Eds.), *Teaching for Diversity and Social Justice* (pp. 3–15). New York: Routledge.

Chen-Hayes, S. (2003). Challenging multiple oppressions with GLBT clients. In J.S. Whitman & C.J. Boyd (Eds.), *The Therapist's Notebook for Lesbian, Gay and Bisexual Clients: Homework, Handouts, and Activities for Use in Psychotherapy* (pp. 174–177). New York: Haworth Press.

Chinese Canadian National Council. (2005). *The Chinese Head Tax and Exclusion Act.* Available: www.ccnc.ca/redress/history.html. Accessed January 5, 2008.

Espín, O.M. (1999). *Women Crossing Boundaries: A Psychology of Immigration and Transformations of Sexuality.* New York: Routledge.

Espín, O.M. (1996). Leaving the nation and joining the tribe: Lesbian immigrants crossing geographical and identity borders. *Women & Therapy, 19* (4), 99–108.

Feinberg, L. (1996). *Transgender Warriors: Making History from Joan of Arc to Dennis Rodman.* Boston: Beacon Press.

Graziano, K.J. (2004). Oppression and resiliency in a post-apartheid South Africa: Unheard voices of Black gay men and lesbians. *Cultural Diversity and Ethnic Minority Psychology, 10* (3), 302–316.

Green, B. & Boyd-Franklin, N. (1996). African American lesbians: Issues in couples therapy. In J. Laird & R. Green (Eds.), *Lesbians and Gays in Couples and Families* (pp. 251–271). San Francisco: Jossey-Bass.

Hardiman, R. & Jackson B.W. (1997). Conceptual foundations for social justice courses. In M. Adams, L.A. Bell & P. Griffin (Eds.), *Teaching for Diversity and Social Justice* (pp. 16–29). New York: Routledge.

Holt, M. (2004). "Marriage-like" or married? Lesbian and gay marriage, partnership and migration. *Feminism & Psychology, 14* (1), 30–35.

Hughes, D. (2003). Correlates of African American and Latino parents' messages to children about ethnicity and race: A comparative study of racial socialization. *American Journal of Community Psychology, 31* (1/2), 15–33.

Jimenez, M. (2004, May 20). Gay Jordanian now "gloriously free" in Canada: Sent to Canada to "straighten out," he founded support group for Muslims. *Globe & Mail.* Available: www.sodomylaws.org/world/canada/canews021.htm. Accessed January 5, 2008.

Lacroix, M. (2003). Culturally appropriate knowledge and skills required for effective multicultural practice with individuals, families and small groups. In A. Al-Krenawi & J.R. Graham (Eds.), *Working with Diverse Ethno-racial Communities* (pp. 23–46). Toronto: Oxford University Press.

LaFramboise, T., Coleman, H.L.K. & Gerton, J. (1993). Psychological impact of biculturalism: Evidence and theory. *Psychological Bulletin, 114* (3), 395–412.

Liu, P. & Chan, C.S. (1996). Lesbian, gay, and bisexual Asian Americans and their families. In J. Laird & R. Green (Eds.), *Lesbians and Gays in Couples and Families* (pp. 137–152). San Francisco: Jossey-Bass.

Loghi, B. (2005, February 8). Tories blast Harper for same-sex warning. *Globe and Mail*, p. A5.

Mays, V.M., Yancey, A.K., Cochran, S.D., Weber, M. & Fielding, J.E. (2002). Heterogeneity of health disparities among African American, Hispanic, and Asian American women: Unrecognized influences of sexual orientation. *American Journal of Public Health, 92* (4), 632–639.

Moreno, C. (2002). *Invisible Lesbians: Latina Immigrant Lesbian Coming Out Experiences.* Unpublished doctoral dissertation, Maimonides University, Miami, Florida.

Ontario Human Rights Commission. (2003). *Paying the Price: The Human Cost of Racial Profiling— Inquiry Report*. Available: www.ohrc.on.ca/english/consultations/racial-profiling-report.pdf. Accessed January 5, 2008.

Parks, C.A., Hughes, T.L. & Matthews, A.K. (2004). Race/ethnicity and sexual orientation: Intersecting identities. *Cultural Diversity and Ethnic Minority Psychology, 10* (3), 241–254.

Pollack, S. (2004). Anti-oppressive social work practice with women in prison: Discursive reconstructions and alternative practices. *British Journal of Social Work, 34* (5), 693–707.

Poon, M.K. & Ho, P.T. (2002). A qualitative analysis of cultural and social vulnerabilities to HIV infection among gay, lesbian and bisexual Asian youth. *Journal of Gay and Lesbian Social Services, 14* (3), 43–78.

Razack, N. (2003). Canadians of Caribbean background: Postcolonial and critical race perspectives for practice. In A. Al-Krenawi & J.R. Graham (Eds.), *Multicultural Social Work in Canada: Working with Diverse Ethno-racial Communities* (pp. 338–364). Toronto: Oxford University Press.

Rosario, M., Schrimshaw, E.W. & Hunter, J. (2004). Ethnic/racial differences in the coming-out process of lesbian, gay, and bisexual youths: A comparison of sexual identity development over time. *Cultural Diversity and Ethnic Minority Psychology, 10* (3), 215–228.

Savin-Williams, R.C. (1996). Self-labeling and disclosure among gay, lesbian and bisexual youths. In J. Laird & R. Green (Eds.), *Lesbians and Gays in Couples and Families* (pp. 153–183). San Francisco: Jossey-Bass.

Seabrook, J. (2004, July 3). It's not natural: The developing world's homophobia is a legacy of colonial rule. *The Guardian Weekly*.

Sullivan, G. & Jackson, P.A. (1999). Introduction: Ethnic minorities and the lesbian and gay community. *Journal of Homosexuality, 36* (3/4), 1–28.

Washington, P. (2001). Who drinks from the fountain of freedom? Homophobia in communities of colour. *Journal of Gay and Lesbian Social Services, 13* (1/2), 117–131.

Wong-Tam, K. (2004, February 18). Are queers projecting homophobia onto people of colour? *Xtra!*

Zea, M.C., Reisen, C.A. & Poppen, P.I. (1999). Psychological well-being among Latino lesbians and gay men. *Cultural Diversity and Ethnic Minority Psychology, 5* (4), 371–379.

Chapter 12

Practice Implications for Working with Refugee Women

JAIRO ORTIZ

This chapter addresses ethical, moral and clinical dilemmas that mental health professionals face when working with women going through the immigration process. The chapter focuses on the care of women who, for the most part, are Spanish speaking and come from Central and South America. I discuss the experience of refugee women negotiating the health care and immigration systems, the impact of this experience on their mental health and the significant influence that the therapeutic alliance has on successful therapeutic outcomes.

Many of my observations are drawn from my experiences as a clinical social worker at the community mental health clinic of a Toronto hospital. My work is also informed by my own migration experience: I came to Canada from Colombia in 1979 and, like many of my clients, have struggled to navigate the system here as an immigrant.

At the clinic where I work, our services are offered in the several languages spoken by our staff, including Spanish, Portuguese, Chinese and Italian. We provide services to immigrants and refugees from many communities, including Latin America, Africa, the Middle East and China. Clients vary in terms of where they are in the immigration process, either as permanent residents or in the process of achieving "status."

Our program uses the *collaborative care model*. Every client is assigned a clinician—who is a trained therapist with a background either in social work, psychology education or occupational therapy and who performs the initial psychosocial assessment—and a psychiatrist, who works with the clinician to complete the psychiatric assessment and develops the treatment in consultation with the clinician. We often refer clients to other clinics and services either in the hospital or in other centres, depending on the complexity of the issues they present (e.g., sleep disturbances, diabetes, neurological problems, addictions). We sometimes also collaborate with other agencies, such as community centres, settlement services and shelters, to form a "circle of care." This model allows us to offer a holistic approach that goes beyond the medical model to helping clients deal with their concerns.

The women seeking refugee status who come to our clinic are often affected by the same psychiatric illnesses seen in the general population. This chapter highlights the social issues such as poverty, isolation and distrust that are common in this group of women and that are significant stressors that can affect treatment. Of special concern are women fleeing domestic violence, sexual abuse and discrimination based on sexual orientation in their home countries, as well as women sponsoring a same-sex partner who is also a refugee claimant. Case studies toward the end of the chapter highlight four women's experiences of migration and of accessing services at different levels in the health care system, as well as the consequences of going "underground" with no legal status, no health coverage and no ability to work.

My review of the literature on refugee women was collected by the U.S. Department of Health and Human Services through what was formerly their Center on Women, Violence and Trauma (now the National Center for Trauma-Informed Care). This literature review indicates that while migration per se does not result in higher rates of mental disorders, both immigration and forced migration can affect the well-being and subsequent integration of immigrants into the host society. Women who do attend our community mental health clinic generally come with health issues that arise from their experience as refugees travelling through, in some cases, a number of countries to reach Canada.

Forced migrants often share a traumatic past, including exposure to war-related violence, sexual assault, torture, incarceration and genocide. (Please see Chapter 14 for more information about working with trauma.) It is not uncommon for many women and couples to have to flee their country without the resources to pay for their children's journey, or the journey may be too dangerous for their children. Their hope is to reunite with the children as soon as possible. Many women are forced to flee their home countries due to gender violence, which in many cases takes the form of sexual assault and other forms of sexual violence perpetrated by government authorities, military personnel and/or insurgents. They may also leave due to domestic or community violence that their governments tolerate or encourage. During flight, they are often re-victimized by pirates, border guards, army personnel, resistance members, male refugees and others. Unfortunately, violence against women and children may not abate upon reaching the supposed safety of an asylum country.

Clinical Encounters

While a claim for refugee protection is being considered, claimants in Canada are, in theory, entitled to health services (through the Interim Federal Health Program rather than through provincial health insurance) as well as to public assistance, employment and education (for themselves and their children). In reality, however, these services are not easy to access (Mosher et al., 2004). Women who are not fluent in English have a harder time finding a doctor. Women who are refused status and choose to live underground or illegally have either very limited access or no access to these services. In our clinic, many women who seek services due to mental health problems have been referred by community-based organizations or immigration lawyers. Many women are referred by family physicians after reporting symptoms such as pain, lack of energy and general malaise, which have been explored and found to be unrelated to a particular physiological condition. If women come to our clinic before they have seen a physician, we help them find physicians so that physiological causes can be ruled out. However, before referring a woman to a family physician, we need to explore the woman's perception of the services that would be provided. Many women fear that an immigration-related medical examination (necessary to secure work permits) will reveal less visible conditions (e.g., epilepsy, blood disorders), sexually transmitted diseases, past pregnancies, abortions, sexual assault and other health concerns. Since such findings would likely be viewed negatively in their community and culture, women often try to avoid or delay this part of the immigration process, which curtails their ability to gain legal work.

Theoretical Stance and Treatment Models

Michael J. Lambert and Benjamin M. Ogles indicate that several factors play a role in effective therapeutic intervention. The therapeutic relationship contributes 30 per cent to successful therapeutic outcomes; factors external to the therapeutic relationship contribute another 40 per cent; hope and/or expectancy contribute 15 per cent; and the therapeutic method contributes 15 per cent (Lambert & Ogles, 2004). Lambert and Ogles' work has been confirmed by Scott Miller, Barry Duncan and Mark Hubble in their seminal work, *Escape from Babel: Toward a Unifying Language for Psychotherapy Practice* (1997). In this book, the authors state that to assess the effectiveness of therapy, the focus needs to shift from the process to the outcome. In other words, rather than focusing on such factors as the type of therapy and length of sessions, the therapist should focus on results: on whether the client's symptoms decrease. Their data came from a meta-analysis of factors that contribute to the effectiveness of therapy. These findings indicate that the therapeutic alliance significantly influences the outcome of the intervention. Because of the complexity of issues clients face, the therapeutic alliance becomes even more central to their treatment, and the type of clinical interventions we use become less relevant. Given that our clinic's root philosophy is capacity building—the process of creating an environment that helps clients strengthen their knowledge, abilities and skills—our approach to a woman's problems requires the integration of factors beyond the clinical diagnosis and treatment available.

Because we have not found a model that is suited to all of our clients, we tailor treatment according to the particular circumstances of the client. The following are some of the models we use:

- solution-focused therapy
- psychodynamic psychotherapy
- cognitive-behavioural therapy
- mindfulness meditation.

SOLUTION-FOCUSED THERAPY

"Solution-focused brief therapy has been described as part of a 'mega trend' in psychotherapy in which the focus of treatment has shifted away from the explanations, problems and pathology, and toward solutions, competence and capabilities" (O'Hanlon & Weiner-Davis, 1989, p. 6).

This approach allows the client to develop concrete goals broken down into small, objective steps, and it enables her to use different sets of skills to make changes in her life. The basic premise is that the client is the expert on her life, and the therapist is no longer the "traditional expert" but a catalyst for change. The emphasis is on acknowledging and building on strengths rather than on "fixing deficiencies."[1]

Women clients consistently report that solution-focused therapy's approach makes them feel respected, empowered and motivated to use their own resources—many of which they were not aware they had. They appreciate the implicit respect for the client as an expert on herself, the focus on the client's strengths, the non-judgmental approach of the interviewer and the dynamic nature of the therapy, in which the therapist follows the direction of the client. We have found the work of Heather Fiske (1998) particularly useful in trying to prevent suicide, a risk factor that is quite prevalent in the women who attend our clinic, especially among clients with symptoms of depression and trauma.[2]

---

1. For a detailed description of the 12 basic principles of solution-focused therapy, see Walter and Peller's work *Becoming Solution Focused in Brief Therapy* (1992). Also, Peter De Jong and Insoo Kim Berg (2002), in their book *Interviewing for Solutions*, provide a comprehensive guide on how to set the different stages in the process to help clients develop solutions to their problems.

2. Fiske has developed a protocol of intervention for the client as well as the family in the document *Living with a Suicidal Person: What Families Can Do* (www.communitylifelines.ca/WhatFamiliesCanDo.pdf), which we have translated in different languages for our clients.

PSYCHODYNAMIC PSYCHOTHERAPY

Common to all psychoanalytic theory is the assumption that we, as psychological beings, have unique genetic constitutions, developmental histories, and internal or imaginative responses to external events. Many of these internal responses become part of unconscious thought patterns, which, along with conscious thought, influence a person and his or her symptoms. In cases of mental health problems, a client's developmental history may be inhibited, fixated or arrested, leading the person to act inappropriately in an effort to manage his or her emotions (Doidge & Freebury, 1998).

Personal change through psychodynamic psychotherapy occurs in three key ways. First, the therapist and client develop a therapeutic alliance; second, the therapist and client seek understanding of the client, and the patterns of maladaptive defence mechanisms (how emotions and thoughts are managed); third, the client applies the insights gained in treatment to the challenges she faces (Luborsky, 1993).

COGNITIVE-BEHAVIOURAL THERAPY

Cognitive-behavioural therapy (CBT) is considered by many experts to be the number one way to treat depression and anxiety, which are common among the women we work with. CBT focuses on helping clients become aware of how certain negative automatic thoughts, attitudes, expectations and beliefs contribute to feelings of sadness and anxiety. Clients learn how these thinking patterns and belief systems, which may have been developed in the past to deal with difficult or painful experiences, can be identified and changed to bring about lasting emotional and behavioural changes (Beck, 1995). They learn to have more control over their moods by having more control over the way they think.

Judith Beck argues that since CBT assumes that clients have the language skills necessary to follow written instructions and write journal entries, CBT needs to be adapted to those who have no formal education and to those who are not fluent in English (Beck, 1995). For example, a CBT workbook entitled *Mind over Mood: Change How You Feel by Changing the Way You Think* (Greenberger & Padesky, 1995) has been translated into Spanish. However, some of our clients—many of whom have only basic academic skills, such as a primary education—may find this workbook still too academic. In these cases, instead of using journals, reports or other written exercises, we apply CBT principles through discussions with clients: in other words, orally.

While some of CBT's principles coincide with the solution-focused approach, CBT's emphasis on the problem and its formal structure (the exercises exploring how thoughts are related to emotions) makes its basic assumptions different from those of solution-focused therapy.

MINDFULNESS MEDITATION

Mindfulness meditation is based on Jon Kabat-Zinn's work at the Stress Reduction Clinic of the University of Massachusetts Medical Center, which he published in his book *Full Catastrophe Living* (1990). This approach helps to reduce anxiety and, sometimes, chronic pain. It includes group meditation, mindfulness stress reduction, yoga and relaxation.[4]

Mindful breathing and sitting (meditation) helps to relax and focus the mind. Mindfulness meditation has been shown to help people manage stressful situations by increasing their awareness and by helping them to be more receptive to their current situation and internal states (Kabat-Zinn, 1990). This method encourages them to embrace with minimal resistance their current life situation and internal states.

With mindfulness meditation, people can learn to be less judgmental, which brings about a more relaxed state. They can learn to be aware of anger and other emotional states with compassion. This enables them to eventually let go of these states or, at least, not intensify them.

The yoga component of mindfulness meditation encourages slow, gentle stretching and strengthening exercises done with awareness of one's breathing and of the sensations that arise. Yoga can be particularly helpful for getting clients in touch with their bodies; they learn to identify changes in their body when emotional pain is reduced and to see connections between the mind, body and spirit. Yoga helps to improve their health and vitality.

Factors Affecting Access to Treatment

Many clients had not been identified as needing mental health services either in their countries of origin or initially in Canada, for several reasons:
- stigma and lack of services
- poverty
- lack of information
- risk of deportation
- distrust
- social isolation.

STIGMA AND LACK OF SERVICES

Stigma—negative attitudes (prejudice) and negative behaviour (discrimination) toward people with mental health problems—may have prevented people from seeking

4. See Kabat-Zinn's (2005) *Coming to Our Senses: Healing Ourselves and the World through Mindfulness* for more information on this topic.

help (Centre for Addiction and Mental Health, 2007).[5] Mental health services that may have been lacking in their home countries may still not be easily accessible in Canada. For example, long distances to urban centres may make it difficult for people in rural communities to access services. Even in larger centres, it can be difficult to get into programs with limited capacity. Because of this, one of the first steps in care is to orient clients to the services we provide.

(For more information about services for immigrant and refugee women, see Chapter 7.)

The therapist also needs to provide psychoeducation to dispel the stigma surrounding the use of mental health services. The comment, "But I don't know why I'm here. I am not crazy" is common: clients we see are often reluctant to seek psychiatric care, believing that it is reserved for crazy people or people of weak character. As well, they are frequently afraid of taking psychotropic medication, viewing it as for "sick people" only. They may describe physical symptoms such as headaches and fatigue rather than depression because they see physical problems as more acceptable. By discussing the stigma around mental health problems, clients will be more likely to open up about their difficulties and develop trust in the therapist.

In the initial assessment, in addition to the clinical issues, the therapist needs to address social issues that could be significant stressors for the client, and that may influence the treatment plan. Addressing social issues related to poverty, social isolation, distrust, previous formal education and sexual orientation requires knowledge and skills on the part of the clinician. Though this chapter is not an exhaustive analysis of such issues, the following discussion may help to clarify what we have observed in our clinic.

POVERTY

Most of the women who attend our clinic report similar socio-economic concerns. Their accounts of poverty corroborate the findings of studies of women who are on welfare (Mosher et al., 2004). For those refugee claimants who are able to obtain social assistance, the amount is grossly inadequate. Women spend most of the allowance on rent, which leaves almost nothing for other expenses such as food, clothing, transportation, medicine and telephone services. The struggle to meet basic needs demands all of their attention and energy, and failure to meet these needs increases their sense of hopelessness, alienation and despair. Although economic hardship is an issue for many

---

5. Stigma involves stereotypes, labels, myths and judgments, such as thinking that people with mental health problems are abnormal, that they caused their own problems or that they could easily resolve their problems if they really wanted to. As people often fear and avoid what they don't understand, people with mental health problems are often excluded from regular aspects of life, such as social activities, friendships and other relationships—sometimes even from their own families. People with mental health problems can internalize the prejudice and discrimination they face and may come to believe the negative messages they receive from others, which often lowers their self-esteem and causes guilt and shame. It is not surprising that stigma may have even contributed to people keeping their mental health problems a secret, which means that these concerns are less likely to decrease or go away.

new immigrants, the plight of women who attempt to live underground is particularly daunting. Neither the women nor the children can work legally, attend school or have access to health services. For those women who have children requesting additional goods and entertainment, not having enough money to provide these affects their self-esteem and causes them to question their ability to parent.

The effects of poverty on health are clear. There is a strong link between poverty and inadequate diet, which is linked to compromises in overall health. The limited social assistance clients receive affects their ability to attend clinic appointments, further undermining their access to health services. Therefore, the clinic allocates funds to provide bus fare to whoever needs it. Another significant issue we deal with is clients' inability to get the medications they need—either because they receive little or no social assistance, or the prescribed drug is not on the province's subsidized medications list. In these cases, clients depend on the samples doctors get from pharmaceutical companies—clearly nor a reliable source for getting needed medication.

Additional Cost Burdens

Completing the documentation to settle as a landed immigrant in Canada requires additional expenses that are not covered by welfare, such as work permits, studying authorizations and landing fees. Mosher et al. (2004) found that in many cases, when women manage to save enough to cover the expenses, they raise suspicion, and they are investigated for fraud. For women at our clinic, this is a significant source of stress, anxiety and despair.

Lack of Recognition of Foreign Qualifications

Many immigrants are affected by the lack of recognition of foreign-acquired qualifications. Some immigrant and most refugee women are unable to work in occupations for which they were qualified in their home countries. As a result, they are kept in minimum-wage jobs. This factor has two major consequences. First, it forces the women to live on an income below the poverty level. Second, it has a negative effect on the person's sense of identity, pride and self-esteem. Both of these factors can negatively affect their mental health.

LACK OF INFORMATION

Many women come to our clinic without an understanding of the Canadian social system and the government resources available to the public. A significant amount of time and energy is dedicated to help clients learn about their rights and how to negotiate the social system to access resources. Even though this is a traditional role for the settlement worker, rather than the clinician, it becomes an integral part of our care and support to the client. Often, they need basic information—such as how to access food banks, where to buy affordable clothing or where to learn English.

Many clients have received inadequate advice about the use of government services.

In general, all refugees fear that seeking government services, social assistance, health care, shelters, police, support services or other help could have a negative impact on how their application will be considered by immigration, regardless of what stage the application is at. For example, the clinician often needs to develop a strong therapeutic alliance before a woman will request help with a basic issue such as birth control. A woman may be reluctant to discuss birth control for several reasons. Her partner may have asked her not to talk about it, perhaps because of misconceptions provided by others already living in Canada (e.g., that by using birth control she will be less scared of getting pregnant, and thus be more promiscuous); because of his own conservative beliefs about using birth control; or because of his desire to maintain control over her reproductive system. Or she may fear that any perception of a reliance on health care services would be a mark against them and their family's refugee application. This avoidance of support services compounds their disadvantaged situation (in health and other areas). This is especially problematic for women who live in abusive situations because they refuse to access services for themselves and their children, believing that it will negatively affect their refugee application. Convincing clients that access to health care and social services will not negatively affect their application for refugee status takes a significant amount of counselling. Clinicians need to be aware that this fear of jeopardizing their refugee applications is heightened in women who have full responsibility for children.

Clinicians need to provide women with information to enable them to use the services available, such as clinics and community centres. The level of comfort the woman has in approaching services in her own community will depend on her fear of gossip or reprisals (due to her partner's potential connection with the counsellors) or of loss of social status within her community (because it is taboo to discuss issues outside the immediate family that are considered culturally to be private and which may lead to perceived shame for the family).

English Language Ability

Learning about clients' social situation (e.g., housing, finances and transportation), which we normally look at during an assessment, is often complicated by their inability to speak English. If clients lack the social support of relatives or friends, and are isolated, the therapist needs to be much more active in calling social welfare offices or agencies that have the mandate to serve those without refugee or landed immigrant status.

We can reduce the fear and sense of helplessness common in the women by communicating with them in their own language. It is important to provide information about a range of services to which they are entitled and to connect them with other agencies that offer settlement services. However, we also need to educate them about how the social welfare system can further victimize them with rules and regulations (e.g., requiring them to report additional income; and give information about who they live with, the presence of a partner, maximum allowable rent limit), as this can be an abuse of power and force women into further alienation. The immigration status of women and their unfamiliarity with English, with Canadian laws and with social services can increase their marginalization.

Mosher et al. (2004) describe how the lack of proficiency in English makes it very difficult to access information, services and supports. They also point out how in cases of domestic abuse, which is a common problem for clients who come to the clinic, male partners manipulate communication to prevent support services from acting on behalf of the women. Such isolation clearly compromises the woman's safety. (For more information about intimate partner violence, see Chapter 15.)

While clients at the clinic are able to communicate in their mother tongue, this is not the norm for refugee claimants interacting with the legal system. It is highly unlikely that clients will be able to speak to lawyers and government officials and to testify at the hearing without an interpreter.

This raises several issues: The women feel a loss of voice—this is particularly so for women forced to tell their story through their male partners and then have the story retold by the interpreter. (Chapter 6 discusses issues around cultural interpretation.) The women experience fear and shame about disclosing personal stories if the interpreter is male and/or a member of their community. Women who seek refugee status fear that their story (e.g., sexual abuse) will become fodder for gossip within the community. A contributing factor to feelings of shame, fear and guilt is the prevalent cultural idea that if a woman is raped, she is somehow to be blamed for it. In our experience, female claimants often refuse to tell the whole story to the lawyer who is representing her in the immigration hearing, in which the Personal Information Form, which states the reasons for the refugee application to the immigration court, is reviewed. This may in part be because the interpreter (whether male or female) is a member of the woman's cultural community, and might have links to authorities or groups back in her home country, thereby placing her in danger. This situation can be extremely frustrating for the client. Instead of telling her story, she will often appear despondent when talking through the interpreter.

RISK OF DEPORTATION

Mosher et al. (2004) found that many abusive men try to intimidate their wives or partners by threatening to cancel their sponsorship, thereby putting the women at risk of deportation. As mentioned, this factor often prevents women from reporting abuse. People seeking refugee status whose claims are denied also face impending deportation should their claim be denied. The long wait to have the immigration hearing— some waits last years—is a significant obstacle to treatment because women continue to experience the possibility of returning to the place where the abuse occurred and may be being abused by their husbands while waiting for the process to unfold. The wait can be particularly traumatic for women already experiencing posttraumatic stress disorder due to abuse.

DISTRUST

The clinician needs to be skilled in how to create a solid therapeutic alliance with the client and overcome her distrust. An effective way to achieve this is through solution-focused therapy—by encouraging a person to acknowledge her own strengths, by respecting her as an expert on herself and by being non-judgmental. Some women may have come from countries where disclosing personal information to someone in authority is dangerous. A therapist's non-judgmental, patient attitude is extremely important in allowing the women to reveal their story as their trust builds. Practitioners need to develop a strong awareness of cues (e.g., decreased anxiety, safety in disclosing private information and continued reassurance that they are listened to) that indicate that women are ready to talk about their concerns. It is important that therapists do not judge the truthfulness of clients' stories. To be non-judgmental, clinicians need to deal with their own assumptions about the reasons why these women seek help, and to be alert to our own dynamics of counter-transference—the emotional reaction that we experience when confronted with issues that are salient in our own experience, and that influence the way we relate to clients. Such an approach can minimize the potential to re-traumatize women by forcing them to give an account of what happened before they are ready or by receiving their story with a judgmental attitude.

The clinician also needs to deliver services with a clear, patient-centred care philosophy. This entails being mindful of women's journey and the many challenges they have faced. Since this might be the first time some women here have received mental health care, the clinician needs to explain in detail about the rules regarding the confidentiality of information shared during the assessment and therapy, given that some women might perceive our role to be that of state agents. In many cases, women need to be reassured early in the process that only in exceptional circumstances would we have to disclose their status to anyone.

A particularly sensitive area is the case of women who are involved with child protection services and who become mandated clients. During the initial intervention, when the issues of confidentiality and the duty to report are discussed, we need to tell the client what our professional and civic responsibilities are. While it is important to present information about confidentiality to every client, in the case of mandated clients, we need to establish how our role differs from that of child protection workers, and how the clinical work can be instrumental in helping the client to overcome the problems that precipitated their involvement with child protection services. Sometimes it is necessary to call joint meetings with the child protection workers, the client and other pertinent players to clarify roles and expectations.

SOCIAL ISOLATION

Social isolation, lack of trust in authority figures, failed relationships, separation from relatives and friends in their country of origin, and strained relations with family members are common realities in immigrant and refugee women's lives. The process of integration in a new social environment can be extremely difficult. For Latin Americans, this can be particularly true: because many Latin American countries have been at war with each other and Canada has welcomed people from opposing sides, there is no integrated community here with shared political values. Therefore, some people can be very guarded with others. Clinicians need to explore, at the onset, if any situation or traumatic experience in their country of origin may be an obstacle to the treatment; for instance, if the client has beliefs about the identity of the clinician (e.g., of his or her nationality or political affiliation). This opportunity can be used to clarify perceptions and identify potential conflicts of interest.

Women who do attend our clinic often have a history of trauma, particularly those women who have survived war or war-like conditions. They experienced torture and kidnapping, and witnessed the killings of loved ones, comrades or bystanders. Some clients from Central America started their journey in their towns, and arrived in Canada after months of travel, which may have included planes, ships, boats, vehicles and walking. Some paid agents (people who, usually for a substantial fee, smuggle individuals into the United States or Canada). The people who were supposed to be helping them during these journeys may have further traumatized them.

Clients with symptoms of posttraumatic stress disorder (including generalized anxiety, social phobia, lack of trust, flashbacks, shame and a tendency to use avoidance as a defence mechanism), may not have sought care or accessed mental health clinics or programs even though they have been living in Canada for many years. This is also very much influenced by systemic racism and various structural barriers.

Women from countries where many refugees originate have less opportunity to pursue education and employment and less opportunity to participate in social and recreational activities than their male counterparts. This continues in Canada because of social expectations that do not allow women to integrate into the community. Women refugees are expected to stay at home and care for family (not just for children but often for elders and other extended family members as well) and their fear of using social resources limits their interaction with broader society. As such, clients often feel caught between their old life and new life and this exacerbates poor mental health. Women feel trapped by the expectation that they will stay at home in the role of caregiver despite their desire to pursue education and work—opportunities they may never have had in their country of origin. Women may feel re-victimized in Canada. Clients may appear angry or frustrated at themselves, their families and the system for keeping them trapped in the oppressive lifestyle they had in their country of origin.

Many women feel extreme guilt and shame for abandoning their children when fleeing the hardship that they and other family members faced in their country of origin. They often have no one to talk to about the impact of the separation and this is not something they typically discuss with their lawyers. Women refugees continually mourn the "loss" of their children left behind, particularly if there is little chance the child will be able to join the family. (The female children are the ones disproportionately left behind because the traditional roles assigned to girls dictate that they become productive workers both at home and outside the home at an early age. They become vulnerable to abuse when parents—especially the mother—are not there to protect them.) This is particularly distressing, not to mention guilt-inducing, for the mother who is aware that the child was selected to be left behind because of her gender. (For a discussion of separation and reunification of mothers and children, see Chapter 10.)

Our work cannot be accomplished without the development of and consistent access to support networks, such as community centres, schools, churches, support groups, clinics and doctors' offices.

Sexual Orientation

Many women who apply for refugee status as a result of persecution based on sexual orientation have lost the support of family and friends in their country of origin when they have either disclosed that they are lesbians or have been identified by others to be lesbians. Especially in Latin America, homophobia is rampant and even encouraged at different levels, including the legal, religious and social systems. This discrimination equally affects females and males. Their experience is further complicated when they try to integrate with social networks from Latin America that have already been established in Canada, where they find similar negative attitudes to the ones experienced at home, though often expressed more subtly and with less dire implications. These women frequently have ambivalent feelings about their orientation, having been conditioned by the moral and religious principles they grew up with, and the feeling that they have "shamed" their family. Their sense of social alienation and shame are commonly contributing factors to any depression and unresolved anger that originated in violence, discrimination or other unjust treatment they experienced. (Chapter 11 focuses on counselling lesbian and bisexual immigrant women of colour.)

Some women have confided in their therapist that they experienced trauma and assaults in their own country. Many women have recounted that police or secret service officers have perpetrated these assaults to, in the officers' own words, "teach them to become real women." Therefore, they have not been able to register complaints for fear of retaliation, or of their complaint being dismissed, bringing additional shame to the victim.

Because women often don't report assault, they don't have documentation to support their stories. This complicates their refugee claims; clinicians' and psychiatrists' professional opinions become critical to explaining the present symptoms as corroborating evidence. In addition, family physicians play an important role in documenting physical evidence of trauma.

Part of the clinician's role is to gather and share the information necessary to refer the client to available support groups and resources, to facilitate those connections and to provide support.

Psychological Issues

A review of the files opened at the clinic reveal that clients' most common complaints were depression and trauma-related symptoms, some of them complicated with psychosis—a state of mind in which thinking, reasoning and mood are significantly disrupted.

We commonly see three levels of psychological trauma in the clients we see. The two most immediate and pressing levels are the trauma of the migration itself (which is a journey usually fraught with exploitation, and a departure that generally involves a difficult separation from children) and the trauma involved in the long process of applying for refugee status and settling in Canada (which can be disappointingly mired in even more instability). The third level of trauma relates to the reasons the women had to leave their country of origin: reasons such as sexual abuse, the malnourishment and exploitation of their children, political unrest and in some cases civil war, and general instability and lack of opportunity. Almost all of the clients have experienced sexual abuse. The perpetrators may have been spouses, or the sexual attacks may have been perpetrated as part of interrogation and torture by political, military or police authorities. Recurring flashbacks, hypervigilance, anxiety and insomnia are common symptoms.

When child abuse is present, a woman usually benefits from multiple treatment modalities over a long period to address the complexity and intensity of her symptoms. Treatment modalities may include trauma therapy, art therapy, cognitive-behavioural therapy, individual psychotherapies, couple therapy, group therapy, medication, relaxation as well as connection with community services that provide opportunities to develop skills and integrate into Canadian society.

Along with trauma, depression is usually present. (For more about the social determinants of depression, see Chapter 4.) If we understand depression as a response to significant loss, the high incidence of depression in this population is not surprising. As noted in the case studies that follow, clients have lost their country and culture, and have often left family (sometimes their own children) behind. They may have lost their careers, professional status and respect. If they are raising children, they now have to do so without the help of extended family. Clinically, we have been faced with not only the incidence of depression but also its severity. Suicidal thinking or intent is common, as is psychosis.

Case Studies

The following case studies illustrate some of the issues raised in this chapter, and discuss the clinical interventions that have been tried in our clinic. The clients whose stories are described had symptoms of posttraumatic stress disorder.

CASE 1

Ms. D is from South America. She left her home country with her two daughters because she was being abused by her husband and had problems documenting the abuse. The Immigration Review Board had refused Ms. D's claim two years before she came to the clinic presenting with severe depression. She had been living underground, working illegally when she could, and moving regularly when she feared the immigration authorities would find her. Her two daughters, one now a teenager, had been attending school regularly and were well adapted to the social environment and culture of Canada. Immigration authorities had found them and, following a pre-removal risk assessment hearing, the client and her children were told to leave the country immediately. We were quite moved by the trials this family had been through having to keep their secret, unable to go to an emergency department when ill, and living as fugitives and in poverty. Even though the clinic's policy is to serve everybody regardless of medical insurance coverage, Ms. D refused to be admitted as an inpatient to the hospital that our clinic is part of. However, in this case, we were able to provide her with enough medication to be treated at home for her suicidal thoughts, and the acute psychosis generated by the removal order. Ms. D had access to us by phone, and her teenage daughter became a constant support to her.

This is one case in which the crisis intervention principles were stretched beyond customary safeguards, due to the alienation this family was enduring. Acting as an advocate, the clinician was able to gain access to the authorities directly. The case was stayed, and an appeal on humanitarian grounds was granted.

CASE 2

Ms. F is a 26-year-old woman who came to us with symptoms of depression and post-traumatic stress disorder. Ms. F indicated that she had left her country to escape persecution from army and drug dealers who had moved into the area where she and her husband had a small pig farm. Both sides were requesting their involvement, creating a situation that forced them to leave for Canada. Ms. F told us that when they first arrived, she and her husband slept on Toronto city buses because they didn't know how to access housing. She had a five-year-old daughter from a previous marriage who was living with Ms. F's mother, who became the girl's primary caregiver. They could not bring the daughter to Canada. Ms. F's immigration process took about four years, and only recently has she been accepted as a convention refugee.

While her main concern was her guilt about abandoning her daughter, her husband disclosed that they were having significant marital problems because Ms. F refused to have intimate contact with him. During the assessment, Ms. F confided that she was having significant difficulty engaging in sexual activities because she had flashbacks of the rape she endured by army members, who tried to force her to divulge information about the drug trade in the area and threatened to rape her daughter as well if she did not divulge the information. At the time, she had not disclosed the assault to her husband, for fear of his reaction and shame. She was also unsure whether her pregnancy had been the result of the rape. After her arrival in Canada, she had a miscarriage.

Her guilt at not having been able to prevent the rape and the flashbacks of the incident were overwhelming. A contributing factor to her feelings was the prevalent idea in her culture of origin that, if a woman is raped, she is somehow to be blamed for it. Ms. F was treated with an antidepressant and was supported through the process of disclosing to her husband within the safe environment of therapy. While shocked, he was eventually supportive, and over time she was able to overcome the trauma. However, depression persisted due to the separation from her daughter.

The government of Canada finally allowed her, her husband and their son, who was born a year later, to stay in Canada. She is arranging to bring her daughter to Canada. She is now employed, and her husband supported the family during her last pregnancy. Her anxiety and depression are in remission. Her prognosis is good, and she no longer requires our services.

CASE 3

Ms. M is a 57-year-old woman who was referred to our clinic by the psychiatric department of a Toronto-area hospital, where she was admitted after collapsing at work. Because of her lack of proficiency in English and the lack of translation services at the hospital, she was unable to disclose much of her history at this hospital.

During the initial interview at our clinic, she disclosed that she had been working two full-time jobs to support her children who had been left behind in her home country and who were now grown up. She had had to flee her country after she publicly confronted the politician who killed her son in a hit-and-run.

At this point in our treatment, her main presenting problem was the unresolved grief of the loss of her son and the separation from her family. She was actively suicidal, and even had an envelope with personal documents related to her ordeals. She wanted the clinician to forward it to her family if she killed herself. The clinician was able to contract with Ms. M not to take her life, and encouraged her to confront her past by looking at the documents during the session, while she dealt with the feelings elicited by the exercise. In addition to the presenting problem, Ms. M indicated that she had experienced physical and sexual abuse by a relative at an early age. At the core of her problems was the unresolved issue of her abandonment as a child and feelings of rejection, which she now projects on her grown children. (In other words, she attributes to them behaviours and attitudes that come from her own interpretation, not necessarily, from objective observation—that is, she feels rejected by her children, even when they are not being rejecting.) This only perpetuates her suffering. Because of the physical separation from her children, she continues to feel that she has failed as a mother. Her relationships with her children are strained because she insists on treating them as if they had remained at the age she left them, and not as the adults they have become.

Treatment gave Ms. M permission to care for herself, a skill that she had never learned. She participated in individual therapy and took antidepressant medications, which we have periodically had to change as they lost their effectiveness. She has attended several group therapy cycles that focused on addressing anxiety and depression. She has also received acupuncture treatment to deal with her symptoms of fibromyalgia (e.g., fatigue and widespread pain in the body). She has been supported to obtain subsidized housing, disability support payments and English-as-a-second-language classes. She has also been encouraged to be active in her church.

Despite these supports in her life, she continues to experience the chronic effects of trauma, including an intractable depression. Her inability to accept her limitations and unfulfilled dreams prevent her from enjoying her accomplishments.

CASE 4

Ms. T is 32 years old. She graduated from a recognized university in her country and had an executive position in her field. She became romantically involved with a married woman, whose husband learned about the affair. Because he was influential in their city, he began a campaign of harassment at her work, and she was fired. She left the country after she was raped by two police officers, "who wanted to teach her to be a woman. . . ." Her father and brother were in the military, and she has been unable to come out to her family. She had to hide from them her reasons for coming to Canada.

During her care and treatment with us, Ms. T wanted to deal with the fact that—at a very early age—while her family lived in a military compound, one of the soldiers sexually abused her. Over the years, several others had further abused her. Her goal was to learn to be comfortable with herself, to accept her sexuality and to become proficient in English. She was referred to a work program, and she successfully completed her first placement in a job in her field. The use of relaxation techniques, such as the body scan (a mindfulness meditation technique in which a person brings attention to the whole body, one part at a time) has helped her control her anxiety, and to be mindful of her body's sensations.

These cases illustrate the need to have a comprehensive approach in developing a plan of intervention and treatment. Due to clients' multiple needs and the complexity of their situations, the responsibility of securing needed resources and of accessing other services often falls to the therapist, who has the language skills, the knowledge and the ability to negotiate the system. The following section clarifies some of these issues.

Care and Intervention

THE CLINICIAN'S ROLE

As a clinician with a background in social psychology and social work, my practice is informed by the individual issues and social context of the clients I see. My professional role is guided by the theoretical and practical developments of Ignacio Martin-Baro, a social psychologist who laid the groundwork for what is known today as liberation psychology. His *Writings for a Liberation Psychology* (1994) presents a comprehensive description of his work. Martin-Baro argues that the role of the psychologist working with refugees and those displaced by violence is to use all interventions to promote *conscientization* in the individual—that is, to teach clients to identify the sources of oppression in the world, and to forge a future they can have control of and become self-sufficient in. Martin-Baro's work is also based on the work of Paolo Freire (1971), who developed the concept of conscientization in *Pedagogy of the Oppressed*. This concept has been central to my body of knowledge and ideology.

To have a comprehensive approach to supporting clients, therapists need to become well versed and sensitive to issues that directly affect the way the legal process of immigration affects women in general, and especially those with psychiatric problems. The following are some of the most common issues.

LEGAL AND ETHICAL CONCERNS

As often occurs in many patriarchal communities, the male partner usually oversees the legal process. The legal aid certificate is usually under the husband's name, and most husbands attend the lawyer's meetings, hold and control the woman's documentation and act as the interpreter. In all these ways, the husband is the "gatekeeper" to the woman having her refugee claim heard and to accessing the services that flow from gaining immigration status. In some cases, the husband threatens, blackmails and intimidates the woman, thereby blocking her from pursuing her claim on her own, perpetuating her dependency and ongoing abuse, and maintaining the power imbalance. As a woman learns about the rights and services available to protect her in Canada, her husband tends to impose social isolation, sometimes even preventing the woman from attending therapeutic sessions. Sometimes this is done by giving her false information or by stressing the widespread stigma about people with mental health problems and the rumours that a person's emotional status can result in the refusal of sponsorship or refugee status.

Women who seek refugee status are often reluctant to speak publicly about sexual abuse and exploitation. The trauma caused by the experience can be so overwhelming that it can adversely affect the woman's ability to speak in public and to remember events and articulate them in a formal forum such as the refugee hearing; in turn, adjudicators may doubt the testimony because of her difficulty in presenting the data.

This is further complicated because, unfortunately, some officials either don't under-stand the specific culture of origin, or impose the Canadian accepted points of view regarding rights and protection agencies.

Clients understand that the success of their family's refugee application depends on their ability to explain that they have a well-founded fear of persecution. However, the overwhelming fear and shame of describing sexual abuse or other sensitive issues, particularly through a male interpreter—and the possibility of facing stigma in her community if her story is leaked through the interpreter—often results in women self-censoring. The distrust that leads them to avoid disclosure causes women to feel extreme anxiety and sometimes repression by the system.

The following situations illustrate how difficult some of the issues previously discussed can be.

Regardless of whether an assault happened in front of a partner or was a form of retaliation by members of the secret police or army in their country of origin, many women keep it a secret. As a result, a woman's relationship with her partner tends to become strained, especially when the partner lacks sensitivity about the experience or is unaware of the process.

Often, it has taken months of care, support and treatment before changes are noticeable. Once this stage is reached, and if the woman chooses to disclose the issue and deal with her partner, the therapist needs to provide couple counselling to support the woman in opening the dialogue, and provide the necessary follow-up. However, couple counselling is not always appropriate. In such cases, the focus is on helping the woman continue with the healing process.

A co-ordinated strategy between the therapist and the client's immigration lawyer is vital to facilitate the process of disclosure prior to the court hearing—especially if the woman's lawyer is unaware of the issues. (Sometimes it is the lawyer who first hears about the abuse and then refers the woman to our services.)

Women's credibility is often undermined when they don't have documentation from their home country. Women (more often than men) are not expected to provide or do not have the opportunity to request and obtain official documents such as educa-tion certificates and driver's licenses. Often documentation is created ad hoc, by fathers and husbands who are inaccurate in their record-keeping (e.g., inaccurate birth dates). Adjudicators become suspicious about women who give birth dates and wedding dates that conflict with the information on the forms completed by their father or spouse.

Legal factors increase stress and anxiety levels, which in turn negatively affect the well-being of the family. Therapists need to help clients develop strategies to control their anxiety and improve their concentration and self-confidence. Role-playing and organizing mock hearings are useful tools. In addition, should the therapist become aware of inconsistencies in the documentation or in the facts of the story—either due to confusion or lack of accuracy in the original translation of documents—it is impor-tant that sufficient information be presented to the pertinent officials. In some instances, clinicians have been called to the court hearing either as an expert witness or as emotional support for the client.

ADVOCACY

While advocating for a client should be an aspect of all therapies, it is especially important in working with women who are seeking refugee status and who are recent immigrants. They often deal with a social and health care system without speaking the language of access. They also deal with a complex legal system. The therapist cannot adopt a neutral role in these matters by simply describing the facts. When speaking with relevant authorities, we need to clearly articulate the client's prognosis, and what the repercussions could be for the client, should she be deported to the country from which she fled. We are often involved in phoning or writing reports for lawyers, immigration services and social services. Our work needs to be grounded with solid documentation. Our reports provide concise, pertinent information and our clinical impressions provide a voice for clients, based on the credibility of our work. In other words, we provide "an equal footing" with the system.

Ms. D, as discussed in Case 1, was about to be deported with her two daughters. It seemed that she had exhausted all legal avenues. She had a relationship with a male Canadian citizen who wished to marry her. They were seen together by the therapist who then wrote a letter supporting her application to stay on humanitarian grounds (based on reasons such as her children being in school in Canada) and to give her time to be sponsored by her spouse-to-be. The clinicians intervened by directly contacting the pertinent official and presenting a verbal recommendation. This resulted in a revision of the application for refugee status, which had been initially denied.

INTENSE NATURE OF THE MATERIAL

The sexual content of these women's abuse history and the intensity of their emotions can make it difficult for the women to tell their stories and for the therapist to hear them. A solid empathic stance on the part of the clinician is paramount. We need to be aware of the socio-political issues prevalent in the environments where the abuse happened. Therapists should critically analyze the official reports and denials of abuse from the implicated governments, and gather information from reliable sources to form an objective and informed understanding of the stories that our clients share during treatment.

This work challenges the therapist to continuously analyze his or her personal experience, attitudes, values and behaviours regarding abuse. The therapist needs to develop enough resilience and understanding of the dynamics of abuse so he or she can be a committed and objective participant when the client discloses the abuse and through the woman's healing process. As a male therapist, I cannot claim that I have all the answers and sufficient understanding. However, previous work in child welfare with children who have been abused as well as my current work have helped me to gain insight into the devastating and lasting effects that abuse and trauma have on individuals and their families.

I have access to peer supervision, as well as consultation with a psychiatrist, in order to debrief and find support to deal with some of the especially serious cases, which revive memories of my own experience growing up in Latin America. To avoid burn out, the therapist needs to become familiar and skilled in dealing with the effects of *vicarious traumatization*—every time we witness a client or group of clients deal with trauma, we have an emotional response that needs to be integrated in a constructive way. In other words, we need to take care of ourselves, so we can care for others.

Strategies for Mental Health Practitioners

The following are some strategies for working with refugee claimants:
- First and foremost, the language barriers clients face must be addressed. Mental health services and clinics should provide language services. As well, practitioners should encourage multilingual students to apply to universities and colleges to ensure a culturally representative group of trained health care professionals: systematic needs assessments of the different communities would support such requests.
- Therapists who are fluent in a client's language need to become accurate cultural translators to facilitate communication between clients and other professionals who are not proficient in the client's mother tongue. (See Chapter 6 on the community interpreter.)
- To break down barriers to services, practitioners need to be aware of the client's housing situation when deciding whether to adhere to the rules of catchment areas that govern our hospitals and community agencies and which establish who is eligible to receive the services. In general, the people we serve are often not settled at a fixed address. Access to telephone communication is difficult or non-existent and the search for affordable accommodation may take a long time.
- Clinicians should try to work as a team to provide culturally sensitive care. Cultures are dynamic, varied and multilayered. The goal of the collaborative care model is to provide comprehensive treatment. Care teams facilitate peer support and supervision, important aspects of service delivery.
- Clinicians must learn about the immigration system, structure and current policies, so clients can be given accurate information about how to navigate the immigration system. Attending conferences, rallies and forums, and talking to settlement experts and lawyers are some of the practical ways to learn about this area. Learning from the experiences of other clinicians is also useful.
- When clients are entangled in the legal system, therapists should co-ordinate with the clients and their lawyers about the disclosure of information and how this should be done in order to minimize the impact of such premature or unplanned disclosure on the client.
- Counsellors' documentation should include pertinent and concise information. Such information should be kept private and therapists should inform clients of

circumstances in which counsellors could be forced to submit their notes. Therapists should address clients' concerns about the confidentiality of their information.

• Therapists need to be empathetic, non-judgmental and able to focus on the solutions that the client identifies as being pertinent to her life.

Conclusion

Clinicians who work with women who have come to Canada seeking refugee status need to understand that the nature of the work is not only challenging from the clinical perspective but from a political perspective as well. A clinical perspective demands solid theoretical grounding to allow for a comprehensive and varied approach that draws from several intervention models to respond to the diverse needs of clients. The sociological variables involved in working with women who have fled repressive environments introduces a political dimension necessary to understand the history and structural forces that precipitated and maintained the unhealthy environment from which these women came.

We are dealing with a marginalized sector of our society. In addition to providing clinical intervention, we are obliged to promote, facilitate and support the integration at many different levels, beginning with the legal, medical, educational and welfare systems, designed to provide the necessary supports to live in our society.

We need to be committed to providing services and support beyond the ones traditionally assigned to the clinician, avoiding paternalistic forms of intervention that would foster further dependency. We, as clinicians, do not rescue people; rather, we need to facilitate growth, critical judgment and free decision making in our clients.

References

Beck, J. (1995). *Cognitive Therapy: Basics and Beyond.* New York: Guilford Press.

Centre for Addiction and Mental Health. (2003). *Challenges and Choices: Finding Mental Health Services in Ontario.* Toronto: Author.

Centre for Addiction and Mental Health. (2007). *Understanding the Impact of Prejudice and Discrimination on People with Mental Health and Substance Use Problems.* Toronto: Author. Available: www.camh.net/Care_Treatment/Resources_clients_families_friends/stigma_ brochure.pdf. Accessed January 4, 2008.

Center on Women, Violence and Trauma. (n.d.). *Women Co-occurring Disorders and Violence Study Addressing the Impact of Violence and Trauma on Women & Adolescent Girls.* United States Department of Health and Human Services: Substance Abuse and Mental Health Services Administration. Bethesda, MD.

De Jong, P. & Berg, I.S. (2002). *Interviewing for Solutions* (2nd ed.). Pacific Grove, CA: Wadsworth, Thomson Learning.

Doidge, N. & Freebury, R. (1998). General guidelines for the practice of psychotherapy. In P. Cameron, J. Ennis & J. Deadman (Eds.), *Standards and Guidelines for the Psychotherapies.* Toronto: University of Toronto Press.

Fiske, H. (1998). Applications of solution-focused brief therapy in suicide prevention. In D. De Leo, A. Schmidtke & R.F.W. Diekstra (Eds.), *Suicide Prevention* (pp. 185–197). Dordrecht, Netherlands: Kluwer Academic Publishers.

Freire, P. (1971). *Pedagogy of the Oppressed.* New York: Herder and Herder.

Greenberger, D. & Padesky, C. (1995). *Mind over Mood: Change How You Feel by Changing the Way You Think.* New York: Guilford Press.

Kabat-Zinn, J. (1990) *Full Catastrophe Living.* New York: Dell Publishing.

Kabat-Zinn, J. (2005). *Coming to Our Senses: Healing Ourselves and the World through Mindfulness.* New York: Hyperion.

Lambert, M.J. & Ogles, B.M. (2004). The efficacy and effectiveness of psychotherapy. In M.J. Lambert (Ed.), *Bergin & Garfield's Handbook of Psychotherapy and Behavior Change* (5th ed.; pp. 139–193). New York: Wiley.

Luborsky, L. (1993). How to maximize the curative factors in dynamic psychotherapy. In N. Miller, L. Luborsky, J.P. Barber & J.P. Dochery (Eds.), *Psychodynamic Treatment Research: A Handbook for Clinical Practice.* New York: Basic.

Martin-Baro, I. (1994). *Writings for a Liberation Psychology.* Cambridge, MA: Harvard University Press.

Miller, S.D., Duncan, B.L. & Hubble, M.A. (1997). *Escape from Babel: Toward a Unifying Language for Psychotherapy Practice.* New York: W.W. Norton & Company.

Mosher, J., Evans, P., Little, M., Morrow, E., Boulding, J. & VanderPlaats, N. (2004). *Walking on Eggshells: Abused Women's Experiences of Ontario's Welfare System—Final Report of Research Findings from the Woman and Abuse Welfare Research Project.* Available: http://dawn.thot.net/walking-on-eggshells.htm. Accessed January 4, 2008.

O'Hanlon, W.H. & Weiner-Davis, M. (1989). *In Search of Solutions: A New Direction in Psychotherapy.* New York: W.W. Norton & Company.

Walter, J. & Peller, J. (1992). *Becoming Solution Focused in Brief Therapy.* Levittown, PA: Brunner/Mazel.

Chapter 13

Addressing Older Women's Health

A Pressing Need

SEPALI GURUGE, PARVATHY KANTHASAMY AND EDWARD JASON SANTOS

While Canadian researchers have been increasingly focusing on the health of immigrant and refugee women, the mental health of older immigrant women has garnered little attention. Of Canada's foreign-born population, approximately 3.5 million are older immigrants, and approximately half of this group is women (Statistics Canada, 2007). Even though the literature does not substantiate whether or not older immigrant women are more likely to experience mental illnesses, we do know that they are more likely to be dependent on their children and to live in poverty. They are also less likely to have health care coverage and access to care than their native-born counterparts. They often engage in unpaid work in the form of child care; in taking care of other older or ill family members; and in cooking, cleaning and running errands for adult children who are employed in paid labour. Older women who have lost their extended family and friends owing to resettlement in a new country can also become socially and emotionally isolated, especially when they outlive their husbands. The concerns, needs and well-being of these older women deserve special attention.

We begin this chapter with a brief literature review on the key concerns of older immigrant women, paying particular attention to the diverse social, cultural and economic forces that influence their mental health and well-being. We use the example of older Sri Lankan Tamil women in Canada to highlight general issues and concerns faced by older women immigrants. Since the 1983 riots and the ensuing civil war in Sri Lanka, more than 500,000 Tamils have been internally displaced and more than one million Tamils have fled Sri Lanka seeking refuge elsewhere. From 1996 to 2001, the Sri Lankan Tamil community in Canada increased by 38 per cent (Hyndman, 2003), making it the largest Sri Lankan Tamil community outside of Sri Lanka. As is the pattern with most immigrants to Canada, the majority of Tamils have settled in major urban centres. According to community leaders, more than 250,000 Tamils are now living in the Greater Toronto Area.

In this chapter, references to the Tamil community are based primarily on our health and/or settlement work as well as a number of research studies that we have conducted in the Tamil community (including Guruge, 2007; Hyman et al., 2006; Kanthasamy, 2005; Morrison et al., 1999). We also draw on other study reports, such as the Tamil Mental Health Survey (TMHS) conducted by Beiser et al. (2006) involving 1,110 study participants; and Nathan (2006) and Shu (2005) studies that examined intimate partner violence (IPV) in the Tamil community in the Greater Toronto Area.

Like other immigrants in Canada, the life of Tamil seniors is considerably different post-migration than it is pre-migration due to a number of interconnected factors surrounding their life in a new country. For this reason, we apply a social determinants of health approach to address the impact of such factors as employment and income, living and working conditions, social support and isolation, and health practices and health service utilization on the health of all Canadians (Health Canada, 2002). While not all social determinants we discuss are specific to age or gender, most social determinants exert a greater negative influence on older women immigrants. According to Wyn and Solis (2001), "there are both social and medical markers that change as women age, such as child and family responsibilities, work commitments, economic security, and health status" (p. 148). (For a discussion of theoretical perspectives surrounding social determinants of health approaches, see Chapter 2.)

Finally, we make recommendations for health care professionals, settlement workers and policy-makers to address the barriers older immigrant women face, with the goal of improving care, support and services for them.

Background and Literature Review

We conducted a literature review on the mental health needs of older women using several databases, including Sociological Abstracts, Social Sciences Citation Index, Academic Search Premier, CINAHL and ProQuest. A combination of key words and text words were used, including mental health, mental illness, elder, older and senior.[1] The initial search using these key words captured approximately 1,300 articles published between 2000 and 2007. When refining the search to include the term "immigrant," the result included less than 10 per cent of the initial search result for most of the above-noted databases.

A review of the accessible publications from this search indicated certain limitations in the existing literature. Most articles mentioned "elderly," "older" and "senior

---

1. While there might be slight differences in the use of the terms "older," "senior" and "elderly," we use them interchangeably in this chapter.

immigrant" sporadically, while only a few articles focused on the topic. This was especially the case for Canadian articles: of the 10 Canadian articles retrieved, five focused on older immigrants' mental health. Of the 12 articles from the United States, 11 focused on older immigrants' mental health. Eight articles retrieved were based on the work conducted in international settings. Approximately 75 per cent of all articles retrieved focused on the concerns of older Chinese or Korean immigrants. Of these, the number of articles that focused on the mental health and illness concerns of older immigrant *women* was further limited. Despite these limitations, we were able to identify several recurring themes related to the mental health of older immigrants and their experiences in the post-migration context; these are presented next.

RELATIONSHIPS AND MULTIPLE BURDENS WITHIN THE FAMILY

Grewal et al. (2005) study findings showed that relationships with family are important to South Asian women and a major influencing factor on their health and health care decision-making. The 47 women participants (aged 25 to 80) in this qualitative study, conducted in the lower mainland of British Columbia, noted that women experienced unexpected role changes in the post-migration context. Many of the older women were sponsored by their children and were dependent on them for basic needs such as food, accommodation, clothing and medical care. As such, they perceived that they had lost their sense of autonomy. The participants also noted that older women were not "traditionally" required to carry out household chores; however, because they were dependent on their family members in Canada, the older women felt obligated to do household chores even when they had health problems.

During our work in the Sri Lankan Tamil community, we observed similar themes. Most older Tamil women come to Canada sponsored by their sons and daughters, while a small number also arrive sponsored by their husbands. Owing to the delays in family sponsorship and the reunification application process in Canada,[2] some adult children spend large amounts of money to bring their aging parents from Sri Lanka to Canada "illegally." These sponsorship obligations often create a sense of obligation for the older women to do household work, including cooking, providing child care and cleaning the house for the extended family. During her work with the Tamil community, one of the authors (P.K.) learned that some older women prepare food for several families, each with several children, who come to pick up food on their way to paid work. The stresses associated with these burdens are sometimes exacerbated for the women by being separated from their husbands. For example, an older woman might be living in Scarborough with her daughter to take care of her grandchildren, while the older woman's husband lives in Oakville to care for their son's children. In the TMHS report (Beiser et al., 2006), participants over 50 noted "the burden of housework" in the following manner: 14 per cent indicated that they were "babysitting most of the time"

---

2. At time of publication, the sponsorship of parents' applications took approximately four years.

and 39 per cent reported "cooking most of the time," compared to one per cent and 30 per cent respectively among their younger counterparts who reported having to do similar work (p. 11). These burdens, and the associated stresses that seniors in such situations face, are often not discussed within families, nor have they received much attention from researchers or service providers.

LANGUAGE AND COMMUNICATION BARRIERS

Another common theme in the literature on the mental health needs and concerns of older immigrants is the language barrier they often face upon moving to a new country. Aroian et al.'s qualitative study (2005) on the patterns of health care and social services use among elderly Chinese immigrants in Boston (n=27; women = 63.6%) identified language as one of the key reasons for their lower health care and social service utilization. Language barriers were also cited by Lai (2004) in a quantitative study on the prevalence of depressive symptoms among elderly Chinese immigrants in Canada (n=444; women = 53.8%). Lai noted that while public health education and preventive mental health services are available to the Canadian public, many of the services were inaccessible to elderly Chinese immigrants due to language barriers and "cultural incompatibility" between users and providers of health care services. A similar finding was noted by Sohng et al. (2002) on health-promoting behaviours among a group of elderly Korean immigrants (n=110; women=70.9%) in Washington state. The authors found that none of the study participants engaged in "community health programs, and health information via media was hardly available to them because of their lack of English fluency" (p. 298).

In our work with older Tamil women, we found that they had concerns around communicating with their own family members as well as those outside of the family. While in Sri Lanka, the elderly were respected and cared for; in Canada they are more likely to be perceived as a burden. Concerns regarding the seniors' relationships with their children and grandchildren were noted in Beiser et al.'s (2006) TMHS report: 12 per cent of those aged 50 and over reported that grandchildren hardly communicate with them, 14 per cent reported that "their children hardly communicated with them, and 12 per cent reported feeling lonely although they were living with children" (p.12). The relationships between the elderly and their adult children or grandchildren can be strained "because of the separation caused by their flight from Sri Lanka" (Kandasamy, 1995, p. 18), which is further exacerbated if the elderly comment negatively on the newly adopted behaviour of their children and/or grandchildren in Canada.

Tamil seniors who are from rural areas and/or war-torn areas of Sri Lanka or those who belong to lower socioeconomic backgrounds often do not speak English. As a result, they are wholly dependent on their family members for activities such as banking, sending mail, visiting relatives or places of worship, shopping and/or getting around the city, or visiting health care providers. In one of our recent studies (Guruge,

2007), the language barrier was noted as one of the key reasons for the difficulties Tamil women face in seeking care and support to deal with intimate partner violence.

ABUSE AND TRAUMA

Just as intimate partner violence is a key concern among every community and society, so too is elder abuse, defined as any intentional, unintentional or negligent act that causes harm or serious risk of harm to an older person. Abusive acts can be physical, sexual, psychological, emotional, financial or involve neglect and abandonment. While the abuse can occur in the home or in institutions, here we focus on the abuse that elderly women experience at home, in the hands of their family members.

While both older and younger victims are more likely to be abused by someone known to them, the likelihood is greatest for older people (Statistics Canada, 2005). More than 35 per cent of people who perpetrate violence against older people were their adult children and 31 per cent were their current or previous intimate partners. Numerous studies have focused on this topic (for example, see Anetzberger, 2005; Brandl, 2007; Gorbien, 2005; Summers & Hoffman, 2006). However little health research attention has been paid to the topic within immigrant communities in Canada.[3]

Like older women from other communities, older Tamil women describe experiencing various forms of violence including emotional, physical, sexual and financial abuse. These abusive acts are often committed by husbands, children, children-in-law and/or grandchildren or other family members. In a recent report by Hyman et al. (2006) on intimate partner violence, older Tamil women reported that they considered the following as abusive acts or behaviour: physical abuse, suspicion, beatings every day, insulting and criticizing wife's parents or family, "hurting the mind," and strong words or "calling animal names."

We also learned about other forms of abusive acts. For example, Tamil seniors are sometimes excluded from family gatherings or are asked to remain in the basement or in their bedrooms while children have visitors. They may also be left at home because there is no space in the car; so that they can babysit; because the presence of older adults or in-laws makes younger men uncomfortable to drink alcohol; or because they are perceived as dressing or behaving inappropriately or not speaking properly. Older women are more vulnerable when they become widows since the women's social status is often tied to that of their husbands. As widows, they are frequently not allowed to take a central role in various rites of passage such as at marriage or puberty ceremonies of their children and grandchildren (Guruge, 2007).

From our health and settlement work and research in the Tamil community (Guruge, 2007; Hyman et al., 2006; Kanthasamy, 2005; Morrison et al., 1999; Nathan, 2006; Shu, 2005), we have noticed the following barriers to disclosing abuse: lack of

---

3. We did not search Grey literature.

awareness of their rights; feeling shame and embarrassment; feeling that it would be disloyal and a betrayal; feeling they deserve the abuse; not wanting to be responsible for hurting the abusive family member; fearing reprisal or other consequences such as abandonment, being moved to an institution, breaking up the family or being alone; being concerned about confidentiality and the desire to protect their own and their family's standing in the community; believing that family problems should be kept within the family; limited social support and geographical isolation; and financial and language difficulties.

These barriers are similar to those reported in the literature for women from diverse ethnoracial backgrounds. The vulnerability of older Tamil women dealing with abuse was compounded by their experience during the civil war and related trauma, as well as by the loss of loved ones. In addition, not unlike most older women in many other communities, older Tamil women might empathize with their abusive family member if the abusive family member is their sponsor or caregiver for the burden and obligations that she or he has assumed in caring for them. Or they may fail to recognize the abuse for what it is. Usually their children and grandchildren's angry and/or abusive behaviours are perceived as occurring due to the stressful lives they lead in Canada (Guruge, 2007).

SOCIAL ISOLATION

The literature points to social isolation as a factor that negatively affects the mental health and well-being of the elderly. By contrast, social support creates a buffering effect against adverse life events and living conditions (Beiser, 1988; Beiser & Hou, 2001; Lai, 2004; WHO, 1998;) and curtails symptoms of acute and chronic mental stress (Cohen & Willis, 1985). For example, in a quantitative study in a Baltimore area (n=205; women = 63.4%) by Han and colleagues (2007) on the correlates of depression among a group of Korean American elderly, a higher appraisal of social support was predictive of lower depressive symptoms. Eleven per cent of the elderly Korean sample indicated having no social support. Based on the data from 1,537 elderly Chinese immigrants who participated in a cross-sectional multi-site survey in Canada on health and well-being, Lai (2004) also found that elder immigrants strongly needed social supports. According to Lai, social support within similar ethnic groups promoted ethnic identity, which seems to "indicate a positive impact on the amount of depressive symptoms experienced by the elderly Chinese immigrant" (p. 682).

Similarly, informal social support from families, friends and like-ethnocultural community networks is important to Tamils. In Sri Lanka, most live as joint extended families, and within these family situations, elders are usually the family heads, and are deferred to around key decisions on such issues as marriage, buying property and managing resources. Even though the older men hold more status and authority and women's status is often linked to that of their husbands, older women also hold much respect, status and associated authority within the extended family. Older Tamil women's identities, activities, roles and responsibilities as well as their emotional and physical well-being revolve around their immediate and extended families. By contrast, in Canada, they have limited access to and participation in familiar social networks when they resettle, a situation exacerbated by such factors as weather, transportation and finances.

Nostalgic feelings for their own home and for their life in Sri Lanka tend to affect older women more when they are homebound. As noted in a previous study (Morrison et al., 1999) in the Sri Lankan Tamil community in Toronto, doors and windows in Canada are often kept locked and regular contacts with neighbours limited; and the environment is "much more exclusionary and enhances the isolation and loneliness these women feel" (p. 155). In addition, the language barrier makes it difficult for older women to make new friends, especially those from communities other than their own.

WEATHER AND TRANSPORTATION CONCERNS

Weather can be a problem for anyone arriving in Canada from a predominantly warm country. For older immigrant women coming from these countries, this can be an even greater concern, reducing their opportunities to meet others and maintain informal social networks. Unable to afford appropriate winter clothing and footwear, and feeling scared of falling in the snow or on ice, many remain indoors during the colder months. The structure of homes and apartments can also be problematic; for example, narrow stairs can be difficult for the women to manage, especially if they are also carrying grandchildren and/or are wearing saris or long skirts. Travel can be particularly difficult for women who live in the suburbs and thus rely more on cars. Those who do not speak English comfortably may avoid travelling alone on public transit for fear of getting lost in a large city. This, in turn, limits them from regularly attending a place of worship or from visiting their children and grandchildren living in another part of the city more often.

Similar concerns were captured in the TMHS report by Beiser et al. (2006): 31 per cent of those over 50 reported that they depend on children to take them around while 49 per cent reported that they "do not like being dependent on children." For those over 60 years and older, these percentages increased to 46 per cent and 66 per cent, respectively (p.12). These changes are a major concern for older Tamil women who, in their homeland, were used to having frequent contact with other family members, friends and neighbours, and regularly attending local social, cultural and religious functions.

CONCEPTUALIZATION OF HEALTH

The literature also reveals how culture influences older immigrants' conceptualization of health and their decisions about health and health care needs. A qualitative study by Marwaha and Livingston (2002) noted how culturally based beliefs and assumptions influence conceptualizations of depression in the mental health service usage patterns among older Black African-Caribbean participants who are well-established long-term immigrants in London (n=19; women = 9). The study participants viewed the etiology of depression to be related to "some sort of spiritual nature" and thought that it would be inappropriate to seek medical help for this problem. Those who had been depressed believed that they felt this way because of being alienated from aspects of their culture. Based on qualitative semi-structured interviews with a purposeful sample of 10 older Thai immigrant women (and 10 older men) in the United States, Soonthornchaiya and Dancy (2006) reported that depression was defined as "feeling disappointment and pressure in the mind and included symptoms of isolation, pounding heart, and dissatisfaction" (p.681). Their perception of coping strategies included practising Buddhism and acceptance.

In a Canadian study, Lai (2004) noted cultural values, beliefs and expectations to play a positive role in enhancing Chinese immigrants' mental health. And Chappell's 2005 quantitative study of older Chinese immigrants in seven Canadian cities (n=2,272; women = 55.8%) revealed how "seniors are valued as wise and contributing members of society, who deserve and are to be provided with care and respect" (p. 70). Older immigrants could experience a better quality of life and valuation of their old age if such an attitude and status could be maintained in the post-migration context.

In our work in the Tamil community, we found that cultural values and beliefs influenced how Tamils conceptualized health and illness: generally, they believe that problems are caused by divine will or are a result of their activities in the previous life. Because of this, the elderly especially believe that they can do little to extricate themselves. Beliefs and attitudes were found to significantly influence the decision to seek help among the study participants in the recent TMHS report (Beiser et al., 2006). Their findings showed that the belief that health problems would go away by themselves influenced women more than men in the Tamil community. "Almost a third of the study sample identified rituals as a source of problem relief" (p. 35); however, the types of rituals or how they provide relief was not explored in this quantitative study.

ACCULTURATION AND ACCULTURATIVE STRESS

In the literature, acculturation and acculturative stress were also found to contribute to mental health problems among older immigrants. Han et al. (2007) noted that "immigrants are considered a high-risk group for mental health problems such as depression, a resulting phenomenon that is commonly explained by theories of acculturative stress" (p. 116). Similarly, Cuellar et al. (2004) found acculturation to play a role in feelings of stress and depression on the subjective well-being of elderly Mexican immigrants (n=353; women = 74.2%) in their quantitative study in Texas. The authors found that immigrants, in general, experienced more stress than those born in the United States, and that these effects were strongly moderated by income, gender, age and acculturation.

Given that the age at which people immigrate influences the rate of acculturation, it is also likely that older immigrants' attempts to maintain previously valued beliefs, attitudes and role expectations in the post-migration context are in conflict with those of their children and grandchildren who might acculturate at a faster rate, potentially creating further stress. There is no research on the particular impact of acculturation and differential rates of acculturation among family members.

FINANCIAL STRESSES

For older women, lack of or loss of finances and financial dependency create considerable stress, fear of poverty, loss of social status at home and in the community, and loss of self-esteem. Owing to the immigration rules, seniors are dependent on their sponsors for 10 years following their immigration to Canada. Even at age 65, many are not entitled to the social security fund due to their late arrival in Canada. They are unable to secure employment in the new setting due to language differences, lack of prior "Canadian experience," ageism and racism, and as a result, are often dependent on their children. These conditions present a considerable role reversal for the elderly, who often would have been the head of households in their home country. Even if they receive a pension, usually such income is given to or taken away by their children, and only a few older women have their own bank accounts. Some seniors feel uneasy about asking for money for their daily expenses, including for transportation to visit a health care professional or social or settlement worker. An older Tamil woman told one of the authors (P.K.) that her whole body trembles when she has to ask for a bus or train ticket. This financial dependency on children often limits older women's activities, which, in turn, keeps them further isolated. In the 2006 TMHS, Beiser et al. found that financial stresses negatively affected Tamils over 50. Even with limited finances, some women feel obligated to assist their children financially. Thirty-three per cent of the study participants over 50 reported feeling "they have to help their children financially" (p.12).

ACCESSING HEALTH CARE

Patterns of access and use of health care by older women are influenced by the stigma of mental illness, confidentiality concerns, transportation and language barriers, health care costs and the inaccessibility of health information and services. (Similar barriers to accessing and using the available health, social and settlement services, such as language and isolation, have been noted in a number of other chapters: see Chapter 7 on services for women, Chapter 6 on the community interpreter and Chapter 12 on working with women refugees.)

Stigma and Confidentiality

Stigma is generally considered a major barrier that discourages many seniors and their families from seeking care and support for mental illness. The stigma of having a mental illness can have lasting social consequences if the mental health problem is revealed outside the family. Concerns about confidentiality and its potential to have an impact on other family members' welfare means that many elderly immigrants do not seek care immediately or, in some cases, delay care indefinitely. For example, it can affect adult children's and even grandchildren's future marriage prospects within the community. Similar to the study findings in other communities (see for example, Declan & Carlos, 2002), a considerable proportion of the study participants in the recent TMHS report (Beiser et al., 2006) expressed some unwillingness to seek psychological services, and 17 per cent of the study sample noted that "they might not seek help for a health problem because they would be concerned about what others might think" (p. 34).

The perceived concerns about stigma and confidentiality present bigger challenges for those who seek care, supports and services within the community. For example, according to the TMHS findings (Beiser et al., 2006), if the participants had to seek help for mental illness, "51% would choose a Tamil speaking professional; 39% would choose any professional—Tamil or non-Tamil—while 10% specified that they would choose a professional outside their own community." Women were 1.3 times more likely than men to seek a Tamil-speaking service professional over any other service professional (p. 35).

Weather, Transportation and Financial Barriers

As noted earlier in the chapter, older women find weather and transportation to be barriers to seeking help. Because of the difficulties their adult children often face in taking time off work without losing pay, seniors frequently do not ask for their assistance in accompanying them to medical appointments. The TMHS findings (Beiser et al., 2006) revealed that distance and transportation problems prevented older Tamils from getting to a health care provider. These concerns are compounded by language concerns. Owing to the difficulties surrounding communicating their health and medical concerns with health care providers as well as the challenges in finding and coordinating interpreters, some older women have no family physicians and do not undergo regular medical checkups. Often they seek help only during mental health crises situations and for physical health problems by going to walk-in clinics or emergency care settings. Beiser et al. (2006) found that 29 per cent of Tamil study participants reported language difficulties while visiting hospitals. The difficulties were significantly greater for women and for those over 60.

Health Care Costs

Financial concerns about medication expenses and lack of access to health coverage are key influences in seniors' help-seeking patterns. According to Canadian health care policy, immigrant seniors are not eligible to obtain free medication until they reach the Canadian age level for seniors (which is 65). For certain communities—such as Tamil seniors who are considered to be seniors in Sri Lanka at age 55 (and more recently at age 60) and are entitled to pension and other old age benefits at age 55—this policy is of particular concern when coming to Canada.

The elderly might be further restricted from accessing their provincial health care plans if they spend time away from Canada.[4] For example, if an older woman spends seven or more months visiting a child or grandchild in another country, she will lose OHIP coverage in Ontario for the remaining five months of the year. Often the reasons for such lengthy periods away from Canada are due to the exorbitant cost of travel (which can be as much as several thousand dollars), making it impossible to visit children more often and necessitating longer and less frequent visits, as well as the difficulties in physically tolerating long travel as they age. They may feel uncertain of seeing their children or grandchildren again and want to be able to provide support, such as child care for all children (not just the ones in Canada).

The resulting burden of the cost of medication and health care falls on their adult children who do not receive even a tax exemption for medical expenses they pay for their older parents. Because of this, seniors do not tell their children about their health problems, and also avoid buying medication. We know of some older Tamil women who have suffered from late diagnosis and treatment of breast cancer, stroke, heart attack and diabetes because of their reticence to get help for these reasons.

Inaccessiblity of Health Information and/or Services

Canadian radio and television do not air programs that provide linguistically and culturally appropriate and age-specific information on health, health promotion, illness, care and treatment. According to participants in our studies (Guruge, 2007; Kanthasamy, 2005; Shu, 2005), even the available Tamil radio and television programs and newspapers in Canada often do not carry health information or information about existing health services and supports. While there are some programs and services directed toward older adults from different ethnocultural groups—such as social gatherings, educational activities and conferences—these tend to be mainly available in large urban centres and to be offered by agencies as short-term projects. Rarely is there long-term government funding for these kinds of services.

Discussion and Implications

Based on our work experience as well as the available literature, we provide recommendations as well as a list of key strategies for health care professionals, social and settlement workers and policy-makers to address the mental health and illness concerns of older immigrant women who live in Canada.

---

4. However, this concern is not limited to older immigrants.

REDUCING SOCIAL ISOLATION

"Informal" social support from family, friends and communities is associated with better mental health: support helps people to overcome feelings of isolation and cope better with challenges in the new environment. At the same time, intergenerational conflicts, family pressures and reciprocity expectations can have a negative impact on mental health. Restricted access to and use of "formal" social supports and services in the new environment (due to e.g., weather, transportation and language) can also create social isolation for some elderly women.

The following are some strategies to reduce older immigrant women's sense of isolation:

- Assess the availability of supports and resources for older women, and explore strategies to strengthen existing support networks (Han et al., 2007; Pang et al., 2003).
- Expand informal social networks to include members outside the family (Han et al., 2007; Pang et al., 2003) to help older adults build new relationships within their own communities. With emotional, social and practical supports, older adults can be better fortified to overcome other barriers facing them (Lai, 2004).
- Invest in peer support and peer outreach programs, a strategy known to successfully reduce social isolation, especially among more recent newcomer women. (See section on designing outreach programs, page 249.)
- Set up senior-driven drop-in support and social programs for older women that include child care facilities for their grandchildren. (See section on implementing drop-in programs, page 250.)
- Establish linguistically appropriate call centres for seniors who are isolated.
- Address the weather and transportation barriers that older immigrant women face by organizing a funded community bus to take them to and from health and community agencies.
- Organize more community-based social and recreational activities and programs for older women such as community gardens, community kitchens and trips to locations of interest.
- Provide intergenerational social, cultural, recreational and educational programs to bridge intergenerational gaps.
- Conduct further research to explore the interaction between social supports and conflicts, and the kind of social support interventions that might be effective when there is considerable conflict present in social networks.

ADDRESSING FINANCIAL NEEDS

There is strong evidence that higher social and economic statuses are associated with better health (Raphel, 2004). In fact, these two factors seem to be the most important determinants of health (Hyman & Guruge, 2006). For example, income determines quality of living conditions, access to safe housing, and ability to buy sufficient good food (Health Canada, 2002). Immigrants, especially women, are disproportionately poorer than the Canadian-born people, owing to racism, marginalization, gender inequities and the social processes (e.g., lower pay, multiple role burden) that reinforce them (Oxman-Martinez et al., 2000; Vissandjée et al., 1998), all of which can negatively affect their health. The following are some strategies to address financial needs of older women:

- Put in place policies that address the financial needs of older women, as a stable financial status is important for both the mental health and well-being of older women as well as for their health service utilization when dealing with mental illness (Lai, 2004).
- Make changes to the Canadian sponsorship system to eliminate restrictions to elderly people's access to government-funded pension benefits within their first 10 years in Canada.
- Make changes to policies to address barriers older immigrants face in accessing government pensions due to their relatively short employment history in Canada.
- Make speedy improvements to policies governing accreditation of foreign-trained professionals to stop the de-skilling and de-professionalization of immigrants.
- Ensure that each level of government enables women to fully access language classes before and after citizenship confirmation, and that each government level makes the same provisions for those who have obtained permanent residency or refugee status.
- Institute incentives such as training allowances so that women are not placed in a position to choose between earning wages and gaining language training.

ADDRESSING ABUSE AND TRAUMA AS A PRIORITY

Violence against women is a leading public health problem worldwide. The violence takes many forms, such as child abuse, incest, rape, sexual harassment, intimate partner violence and older woman abuse. Such acts can be committed by strangers, but more often they are performed by someone known to the women including family members in the immediate and/or extended family. The following is a list of strategies to address abuse that older women might experience in the post-migration context:

- Reflect on and critically analyze service providers' attitudes and aims regarding current approaches to dealing with women in abusive relationships; for example, health care providers must understand that intimate partner violence occurs among those born in Canada—thus is not unique to "immigrant communities" (Guruge, 2007; Guruge & Humphreys, 2008).
- Advocate for the women and their families as they interface with their new envi-

---

5. This is not an exhaustive list. We refer the reader to Chapter 15 on IPV as well as other more recent literature that specifically explore this topic.

ronment or country, beginning with the needs identified by the women experiencing intimate partner violence (Guruge, 2007; Guruge & Humphreys, 2008).

- Identify a single point of access for information on available resources and
  co-ordinate services and supports to those who need such services.

- Create separate shelters for older women experiencing abuse, and ensure that
  their spiritual, religious, language and dietary needs are met during shelter stay.

- Arrange transportation and escorts for women who require such services to get
  away from an abusive family member.

- Set up linguistically appropriate call centres to provide support and counselling
  for seniors dealing with various forms of abuse.

- Offer one-on-one counselling to older women both in person and on the phone
  to address family stress, intergenerational conflicts and violence perpetrated
  against them.

- Ensure that radio and television programs raise community awareness of intimate partner violence and intergenerational abuse and their impact on older
  women, and that these programs discuss available resources to help women deal
  with abuse.

- Enhance community capacity in dealing with violence and abuse by carefully
  screening and identifying a pool or coalition of trained community leaders to
  actively address violence against women in the community.

- Set up support groups for older women dealing with abuse or its aftermath.
  Older women can benefit from support groups in a number of ways: by decreasing their social isolation; providing them with a forum to share their experiences
  and problem-solve with others dealing with similar problems; improving abuse
  awareness; enhancing their ability to cope; improving self-esteem; and fostering
  feelings of personal growth (Brandl et al., 2003).

- Reduce older immigrant women's financial dependency on their children by
  changing the current government policies that limit the financial situation of
  elderly immigrants (see page 246 on addressing financial needs).

- Acknowledge and celebrate the various ways that older women contribute to
  their own health and well-being and that of their families.

- Establish policies that inform older women's rights within a sponsor-sponsored
  person relationship, and that increase older women's access to such information.

- Direct health promotion programs at entire families to help family members
  together confront the many stresses common among new immigrants and
  enable them to develop coping styles to handle the new stresses.

ADDRESSING BARRIERS THAT LIMIT USE
OF HEALTH AND SOCIAL SERVICES

The barriers to health and social services utilization confronted by older Tamil women
are similar to the ones noted in the literature (see for example Emami et al., 2000;

Hyman & Guruge, 2002; Lai, 2004; Mulvihill & Mailloux, 2000; and Vissandjée et al., 1998). The following are strategies to address these barriers:

- Include evaluative criteria for reducing linguistic, informational, transportation and financial barriers to access to and use of available care and services by older immigrant women when designing new programs and evaluating existing ones.
- Advocate for a health care system that responds to the linguistic needs of its clients.
- Provide all health information in diverse languages: presently, many of the health screening and health promotion campaigns and television and radio programs in most parts of Canada are in English, thus are inaccessible to those who do not speak English.
- Create linkages with family practitioners, lay practitioners and community leaders to help reduce delays in seeking care and facilitate early care and interventions (Williams, 1999).
- Design successful outreach programs as well as drop-in programs to overcome access barriers (see next section).
- Stress the importance of confidentiality with both women and their care providers, including nurses, social workers, physicians and others involved in meeting women's care and settlement needs.
- Ensure that interpreters are professionally trained and skilled in handling complex issues. (See Chapter 6 on this topic.)
- Advocate for leadership in both our public and community sectors to proactively name and work to combat racism, as perceptions and experiences of racial discrimination within the health care system affect access and use of health care services (Beiser et al., 2003; Yee et al., 2006).
- Encourage stakeholders to collaboratively address the many factors—such as age, gender, socioeconomic status and culture—"that intersect and determine the overall health and well-being of consumer survivors from racialized communities" (Yee et al., 2006, p. 3).
- Put in place accountability tools in the form of funding conditions to ensure that service providers maintain their commitment to implementing anti-racism policies.

DESIGNING SUCCESSFUL OUTREACH PROGRAMS

Weather, lack of transportation, limited English and multiple burdens (such as providing child care for grandchildren that limit their time) have been identified as obstacles for immigrant women to get to and use services far away from their homes. As such, it is important to design successful programs that reach out to and efficiently serve people of diverse ethnocultural and linguistic backgrounds. According to Hyman and Guruge (2002), a successful model must:

- demonstrate familiarity with the population's sub demographics

- recognize the needs of the target population
- reveal an understanding of the community's level of readiness to address or deal with concerns or issues of importance to them, or the illnesses associated with stigma
- demonstrate awareness of existing resources and gaps in services
- recognize and incorporate preferred modes of communication
- offer strategies that involve linking with stakeholders within the community
- involve peers in the planning and implementation of outreach programs
- include long-term commitment and financial investment in the success of such programs.

IMPLEMENTING DROP-IN PROGRAMS

Drop-in programs are needed at various community locations to serve older women who are unable to attend programs regularly or at specifically scheduled times. The following are recommendations for implementing these programs:

- Design in collaboration with women's recreational and educational activities that meet their age, gender, social and cultural needs. (Activities such as bingo nights may not be an attractive choice for older women in some communities.)
- Focus subjects to be discussed at drop-in sessions on such topics as health promotion, mental health and well-being and mental illnesses (e.g., healthy family relationships, communication among family members of different generations, understanding and coping with the differences in social, cultural and economic and living conditions between the pre- and post-migration settings and their impact on health and well-being, and living with depression or schizophrenia).
- Create strategies to increase attendance (e.g., set up mechanisms to provide transport assistance and escorts to those who might not be able to plan these in advance).

USING A CLIENT-CENTRED APPROACH

A client-centred approach is essential to addressing the needs of older immigrant women. The following are recommendations for health care professionals to reach this population:

- Appreciate the gender journey that women have endured (Patterson, 2003), and work collaboratively with them to plan support, care and provide treatment based on the individual needs and situations of the women. (Such collaboration might empower women to feel further motivated to deal with the illness or situation more proactively.)
- Consider the diverse needs of women depending on their life stage (i.e., integrate

a life-stage approach to woman-centred care) and have the knowledge and tools to work with seniors.

- Learn about resources that are available in the community and how clients might benefit from them (e.g., shelter or accommodation, food and other basic daily needs, temporary health care or medication assistance, financial assistance, legal assistance for dealing with immigration concerns, ethnocultural organizations and networks that directly connect the women to such services according to their needs).
- Understand the specific context within which care is received "to improve quality of life, cost efficiency of services, and outcomes for elderly immigrant clients" (Weisman et al., 2005, p. 647).

We refer the reader to Chapters 6 and 7 for further strategies for providing linguistically and culturally appropriate services and women-centred care.

BUILDING STRATEGIC PARTNERSHIPS TO OFFER A RANGE OF SERVICES

No one agency is capable of addressing all health, social and settlement concerns. For example, the causes of or risk factors for abuse and solutions for women dealing with abuse at home are interconnected with various forms of violence at the community and societal levels. Therefore, we propose the following recommendations as a starting point:

- Offer a range of services for older women as a "one stop shop" approach to help address their diverse and interconnected health, social and economic needs.
- Improve co-ordination between primary, secondary and tertiary care and services.
- Build research partnerships that involve older women/clients/consumers.
- Build strategic partnerships with diverse communities and stakeholders so that health care professionals can respond effectively and in a timely manner to the changing needs of clients and changing client groups over time.
- Ensure the interdisciplinary collaboration of the many sectors committed to improving Canadian health policy and service delivery. To do so, research, policy and care must be sensitive to women's migration experiences; this goes beyond recognizing cultural diversity (Vissandjée et al., 2007).
- Actively seek and support equal representation and participation of community members on the boards of directors of universities and colleges, hospitals, health councils, and provincial and federal ministries.
- Develop comprehensive and multi-sectoral approaches to promote and sustain the good health of immigrant women; for example, health care agencies and hospitals need to broaden their scope to address determinants of health by co-ordinating services provided by municipal and provincial levels of government.

DEVELOPING SUCCESSFUL HEALTH PROMOTION PROGRAMS

It cannot be assumed that theoretical models and health promotion strategies grounded in majority culture-based research apply equally to subgroups of women for whom social, cultural, linguistic, economic and informational barriers affect their ability to access care and services, and make choices about health care (Hyman & Guruge, 2002). The following are strategies and approaches that might be helpful across communities:

- Use an empowerment philosophy to develop programs that focus on immigrant women's resiliency and capacities to maintain their health and well-being as a way to help the women deal with settlement stresses.
- Incorporate spiritual programs in addition to focusing on recreational, educational and informational sessions on active living when creating health promotion programs.
- Set up health promotion programs in various community locations.
- Adapt health promotion and social programs to the group's "underlying worldview and patterns of social interaction" (Emami et al., 2000, p. 169).
- Incorporate behaviourally focused strategies that have underlying messages of collectivism and ethnic identity (Hyman & Guruge, 2002).
- Involve community leaders and media in innovative approaches to raise awareness of various health promotion strategies and programs in the community, and ensure that programs and interventions are designed and delivered in collaboration with the community (Hyman & Guruge, 2002).
- Develop and implement educational, therapeutic, preventive, health promotional and healing activities that incorporate community leaders' knowledge and expertise (Hyman & Guruge, 2002).
- Encourage and support older women who can take on the role of peer supporters for other older women so that they can together develop and maintain health-promoting practices.
- Involve peers in the planning and implementation of outreach programs and encourage them to take on active roles to:
  (a) change perceived community norms surrounding mental health and illness
  (b) act as a positive social influence
  (c) increase women's awareness of the existing resources
  (d) encourage women to seek and use such resources
  (e) help facilitate transportation to health, social and settlement services.
- Encourage ethnic media to do outreach to educate families about the importance of their role in engaging older women in health promotion activities outside the home (i.e., ensuring that they have time, money and access to transportation for health-promoting activities).
- Increase long-term projects and funding for long-term projects rather than focusing on short-term funding for short-term projects.
- Include comprehensive services that address older women's needs; that is, taking on a social determinants of health approach and ensure access to services (e.g.,

job counselling and training, language and literacy training, family and individual counselling, transportation and child care).

MAKING CHANGES TO POLICIES

"Canada prides itself on having a multicultural identity and in maintaining a universally available health care system. However, health policies and services do not reflect Canada's diverse demographics and do not offer an integrated approach appropriate to the needs and interests of women experiencing migration" (Vissandjée et al., 2007, p. 221). The following are strategies to address these concerns:

- Advocate for an immigration policy that addresses family sponsorship delays and addresses the financial expectations of people who sponsor the elderly.
- Advocate for health policy that addresses medication and health care expenses for seniors.
- Allocate permanent funding for health, social and settlement organizations providing services for older immigrants.
- Provide appropriate housing, nursing homes and shelters for older immigrant women.
- Address safety concerns of seniors living in suburban areas (e.g., accessible sidewalks, well-lit pathways).
- Expect both "mainstream" and ethnocultural media to broadcast appropriate health promotion and illness prevention information in diverse languages, and use evaluation criteria that incorporate such expectations to determine on-going funding for media programs.
- Make it a policy priority to "ensure that women have access to the information to which all Canadian women are entitled, as well as the resources that enable women to contribute to and act upon this knowledge" (Vissandjée et al., 2007, p. 235).
- Develop and systematically use cultural interpretation programs, hire personnel who speak different languages, and make educational materials available in multiple languages.
- Provide formal, mandatory on-going training on diversity and equity to health professionals at all levels and across all disciplines (Betancourt et al., 2002).
- Use public education—through media campaigns—to improve the image and demonstrate the contributions of older immigrant women to Canadian society and its economy.

Conclusion

The concerns noted during our work in the Tamil community are concerns common to older women from other immigrant communities, and in some cases, common to older women who are born in Canada. Given this commonality and the increase in the aging population in Canada, addressing the mental health and well-being of older women and reducing mental health disparities must become a priority for health care professionals. This goal can be realized only by collaborating with health care, social and settlement service providers, as the health of older women is shaped by social determinants of health.

Health care professionals need to focus on health promotion, on strengthening public health education and preventive services, and on eradicating financial, linguistic, transportation and geographic barriers to care and services for older immigrant women. These approaches must be undertaken in a culturally and linguistically appropriate manner and planned by health care professionals along with community members and various key stakeholders. Health care professionals must be committed to dealing with larger societal and systemic barriers such as racism and ageism that continue to affect, both directly and indirectly, the mental health and well-being of older women by limiting their opportunities to fully engage as productive members in society. Immediate research attention is needed to explore whether and how ideas about aging, expectations regarding roles and responsibilities at the inter-personal level, and relationships and affiliations change when older women immigrate to another country, and how these might affect their mental health.

References

Anetzberger, G. (2005). Moving forward on elder abuse and guardianship: Will it take a thesis or a scream? *The Gerontologist, 45,* 279-282.

Aroian, K., Wu, B. & Tran, T. (2005). Health care and social service use among Chinese immigrant elders. *Research in Nursing & Health, 28* (2), 95–105.

Beiser, M. & Hou, F. (2001). Language acquisition, unemployment and depressive disorder among Southeast Asian refugees: A 10-year study. *Social Science & Medicine, 53* (10), 1321–1334.

Beiser, M. (1988). Influences of time, ethnicity, and attachment on depression in Southeast Asian refugees. *American Journal of Psychiatry, 145,* 46–51.

Beiser, M., Simich, L., Pandalangat, N. (2003). Community in distress: Mental health needs and help-seeking in the Tamil community in Toronto. *International Migration, 41* (5), 2003.

Beiser, M., Simich, L., Rummens, J., Pandalangat, N. & Singam, A. (2006). *A community in distress: Report to the community on results of the Tamil mental health community survey.* Unpublished manuscript, University of Toronto.

Betancourt, J.R., Green, A.R. & Carrilo, J.E. (2002). *Cultural Competence in Health Care: Emerging Frameworks and Practical Approaches.* New York: Commonwealth Fund.

Brandl, B. (2007). *Elder Abuse Detection and Intervention: A Collaborative Approach.* New York: Springer.

Brandl, B., Hebert, M., Rozwadowski, J. & Spangler, D. (2003). Feeling Safe, Feeling Strong. Support groups for older abused women. *Violence against Women, 9* (12), 1490–1503.

Chappell, N. (2005). Perceived change in quality of life among Chinese Canadian seniors: The role of involvement in Chinese Culture. *Journal of Happiness Studies, 6* (1), 69–91.

Cohen S. & Willis, T.A. (1985). Stress, social support and the buffering hypothesis. *Psychological Bulletin, 98*, 310–357.

Cuellar, I., Bastida, E. & Braccio, S. (2004). Residency in the United States, subjective well-being, and depression in an older Mexican-origin sample. *Journal of Aging and Health, 16* (4), 447–466.

Declan, T.B., & Carlos, M.G. (2002). Cultural, psychological, and demographic correlates of willingness to use psychological services among East Asian immigrants. *The Journal of Nervous and Mental Disease, 190* (1), 32–39.

Emami, A., Torres, S., Lipson, J. & Ekman, S. (2000). An ethnographic study of a day care center for Iranian immigrant seniors. *Western Journal of Nursing Research, 22* (2), 169–188.

Gorbien, A.B. (2005). Elder abuse and neglect: An overview. *Clinics in Geriatric Medicine, 21* (2), 279–292.

Grewal, S., Bottorff, J. & Hilton, B. (2005). The influence of family on immigrant South Asian women's health. *Journal of Family Nursing, 22* (3), 242–263.

Guruge, S. (2007). *The influence of gender, racial, social, and economic inequalities on the production of and responses to intimate partner violence in the post-migration context.* Unpublished doctoral dissertation, University of Toronto.

Guruge, S. & Humphreys, J. (2008). *Post-migration formal social support needs for women dealing with intimate partner violence.* Manuscript submitted for publication.

Han, H., Kim, M., Lee, H., Pistulka, G. & Kim, K. (2007). Correlates of depression in the Korean American elderly: Focusing on personal resources of social support. *Journal of Cross Cultural Gerontology, 22* (1), 115–127.

Health Canada. (2002). *Population Health.* Available: www.phac-aspc.gc.ca/ph-sp/phdd. Accessed January 9, 2008.

Hyman (2000). Best mechanisms to influence health risk behaviour. [Literature review], prepared for the Ontario Women's Health Council by the University Health Network, Women's Health Program.

Hyman, I. & Guruge, S. (2002). A review of theory and health promotion strategies for new immigrant women. *Canadian Journal of Public Health, 93* (3), 183–187.

Hyman, I. & Guruge, S. (2006). Immigrant women's health. In R. Srivastava (Ed.). *The Health Care Professional's Guide to Clinical Cultural Competence* (pp. 264–280). Toronto: Elsevier Canada.

Hyman, I. (2002). Immigrant and Visible Minority Women. In D.E. Stewart, A. Cheung, L.E. Ferris, I. Hyman, M.M. Cohen & L.J. Williams (Eds.). *Ontario Women's Health Status Report.* Toronto: Ontario Women's Health Council.

Hyman, I., Mason, R., Berman, H., Guruge, S., Manuel, L., Kanagaratnam, P. et al. (2006). Perceptions of and responses to intimate partner violence among Tamil women in Toronto. *Canadian Woman Studies, 25 (1 & 2)*, 145–150.

Hyndman, J. (2003). Aid, conflict, and migration: the Canada-Sri Lanka connection. *The Canadian Geographer, 47* (3), 251–268.

Kandasamy, B. (1995). *Findings of the Tamil community in the City of York.* City of York: York Community Services.

Kanthasamy, P. (2005). *Violence Against Seniors.* Apex Creations, Toronto. A Vasantham Project.

Lai, D. (2004). Depression among elderly Chinese-Canadian immigrants from Mainland China. *Chinese Medical Journal, 117* (5), 677–683.

Marwaha, S. & Livingston, G. (2002). Stigma, racism or choice. Why do depressed ethnic elders avoid psychiatrists? *Journal of Affective Disorders, 72* (3), 257–265.

Morrison, L., Guruge, S. & Snarr, K. A. (1999). Sri Lankan Tamil immigrants in Toronto: Gender, marriage patterns, and sexuality. In G. A. Kelson & D.L. DeLaet (Eds.). *Gender and Immigration* (pp. 144–161). New York: New York University Press.

Mulvihill, M.A. & Mailloux, L. (2000). *Canadian Research on Immigrant and Refugee Women's Health: Linking Research and Policy, First Draft.* Ottawa: Health Canada.

Nathan, Juanita. (2006). Domestic Violence: A Guide to Tamil Community. Apex Creations, A Vasantham Project, funded by Victim Services. Toronto: Ministry of Attorney General's Office.

Oxman-Martinez, J., Abdool, S.N. & Loiselle-Leonard, M. (2000). Immigration, women and health in Canada. *Canadian Journal of Public Health*, 91 (5), 394–395.

Pang, E., Jordan-Marsh, M., Silverstein, M. & Cody, M. (2003). Health-seeking behaviours of elderly Chinese Americans: Shifts in expectations. *The Gerontologist, 43* (6), 864–874.

Patterson, F. (2003). Heeding new voices: Gender-related herstories of Asian and Caribbean-born elderly women. *Affilia, 18* (1), 68–79.

Raphael, D. (2004). Social determinants of health—Canadian perspectives. Toronto: Canadian Scholars' Press.

Shu, K. (2005). *Report on Leadership Training on Prevention of Violence and Abuse.* A Vasantham Project. Unpublished manuscript.

Sohng, K., Sohng, S. & Yeom, H. (2002). Health-promoting behaviors of elderly Korean immigrants in the United States. *Public Health Nursing, 19* (4), 294–300.

Soonthornchaiya, R. & Dancy, B.L. (2006). Perceptions of depression among elderly Thai immigrants. *Issues in Mental Health Nursing, 27,* 681–698.

Statistics Canada (2005). Facts on violence: Elder abuse. Available: www.gov.nf.ca/vpi/facts/elders.html. Accessed December 1, 2007.

Statistics Canada. (2007). A portrait of seniors in Canada—2006. Available: www.statcan.gc.ca/english/freepub/89-519-XIE/89-519-XIE2006001.pdf. Accessed January 22, 2008.

Summers, R.W. & Hoffman, A.M. (Eds.) (2006). *Elder Abuse: A Public Health Perspective.* Washington, DC: American Public Health Association.

Vissandjée, B., Carignan, P., Gravel, S., & Leduc, N. (1998). Promotion de la santé en faveur des femmes immigrant au Québec. *Revue Epidemiologique et Santé Public, 43,* 124–133.

Vissandjée, B., Thurston, W., Apale, A., Nahar, K. (2007). Women's health at the intersection of gender and the experience of international migration. In M. Morrow, O. Hankivsky, & C. Varcoe (Eds.). *Women's Health in Canada. Critical Perspectives on Theory and Policy.* Toronto: University of Toronto Press.

Weisman, A., Feldman, G., Gruman, C., Rosenburg, R., Chamorro, R. & Belozersky, I. (2005). Improving mental health services for Latino and Asian immigrant elders. *Professional Psychology: Research and Practice, 36* (6), 642–648.

World Health Organization. (1998). *Health promotion glossary.* Geneva: Author.

Williams, C. C. (1999). *Ethnoracial Services Task Force Report to the Joint General Psychiatry Program Planning Committee.* Toronto: The Clarke Institute of Psychiatry.

Wyn, R. & Solis, B. (2001). Women's health issues across the lifespan. *Women's Health Issues, 11* (3), 148–159.

Yee, J., Janczur, A., Ocampo, M. & Rahim, C. (2006). Striving for best practices and equitable mental health care access for racialised communities in Toronto. Available: www.accessalliance.ca/index.php?option=com_content&task=view&id=100002&Itemid=28. Accessed January 9, 2008.

Part 5

Highlighting Critical Mental Health Concerns

Chapter 14

Trauma Work with Latin American Women in Canada

EVA SAPHIR

Prologue

In Latin America, it is acceptable to be depressed. In fact, there is an endearing term for it: "depre," as in, "Ai! My depre came upon me again." Or, "I feel very depre." Or, "I am with the depre again." Many may talk to others about their problems; these are "problemitas"—"little problems." People who sit in the park talking to themselves, however, are known as "loquita"—"a little crazy."

What is not acceptable in Latin America is to go to a "doctor" to talk about problems. A doctor could include a psychiatrist, a psychologist, a counsellor of any type—even a priest (unless it is for confession). Someone who goes to a doctor is "loco"—"majorly crazy." This means the person cannot function anywhere, is no longer a real person and may be locked up. Everybody knows someone who is "loca" and "is on drugs forever and acts like a zombie—no longer part of this world."

Many come to a community mental health clinic because their family doctor, community worker or friend has told them that they need help. Sometimes, their first words are, "I am not crazy, you know." At other times, they may say, "I think I am going crazy."

· · ·

In the Hispanic community, a woman is a family's strength. When a woman is unwell, the family suffers. In dealing with mental illness, a woman may feel considerable shame and guilt about being unable to fulfill her role in the family. She also has to deal with the stigma of "craziness" if she seeks help, and the subsequent loss of respect from others (Freire, 2002; Rubio, 2004; Viswanathan et al., 2003).

This chapter focuses on refugee women from Latin America who may find it difficult to orient to their new life in Canada. (Chapter 12 also discusses clinical issues related to primarily Spanish-speaking women from Central and South America.) While, with time, they adjust to life in Canada, the stresses of the resettlement process may bring back past memories that had been buried in the subconscious. Refugee women often have had no time to prepare to leave their home country or to say goodbye to family and friends. They may have left many matters unfinished (Rubio, 2004; Viswanathan et al., 2003). In addition, they may have had single or multiple traumatic experiences, which sometimes culminate in a lifetime of upheaval carefully guarded in secrecy for years. Once in a new country, many wounds may re-open, along with the pain of losing a sense of being functionally competent because they are in a new and alien environment. These experiences can unearth past trauma, leading them to seek care and trauma therapy.

Clients are often surprised that neither the trauma nor the trauma response stop upon arrival in Canada. The expectation of safety, which is the reason for leaving their country, betrays them. They are not completely safe. The immigration process still threatens their life here, as do economic problems, unsuitable housing, inability to speak the language and difficulties in getting needed child care so they can study or work. They need to work through many details necessary for everyday life in an environment where the illusion of safety is challenged at every turn.

Trauma therapy works to harmonize the physical, emotional and cognitive aspects of a person's experience in order to reconstitute a whole person (Ogden & Minton, 2000). In this chapter, I address trauma therapy from my experience as a Latin American mental health clinician and trauma worker. I also discuss techniques that I use in my practice to integrate the context of a client's cultural experience. I use the terms "Hispanic," "Spanish" and "Latin American" interchangeably. I also use the terms "client," "woman" and "refugee woman" interchangeably to refer to women seen in my practice at a mental health clinic. The chapter discusses:

- the social and cultural context of Latin American refugees and immigrants in Canada
- key concepts in working with Latin American women with mental health concerns
- a case study that follows one client through the therapeutic process
- additional therapeutic techniques
- implications for practice.

Hispanic Refugees and Immigrants in Canada: An Overview

Latin America is made up of 21 countries, some of which have been at war with each other. While immigrants from other countries may have a host community to help them settle in a new country, Latin Americans in Canada have come in waves since the 1970s from various countries (e.g., Chile, Guatemala, El Salvador, Argentina, Colombia), and each wave of immigrants often considers the natives of other Spanish-speaking countries as "foreigners." Or, they may come from the same country but claim different political ideologies and, as such, may be suspicious of each other. Consequently, there is little cohesion among diverse Spanish-speaking communities.

Historically, the more established groups have not been interested in helping newcomers whom they may consider to be from different cultures (Rubio, 2004; Viswanathan et al., 2003). It takes many years in Canada to begin to see ourselves as Latin, as a more homogeneous group of immigrants with a common language, instead of as different and disconnected cultures. Non–Spanish Canadians do not tell us apart by country, but more by the "Spanish accent" or the Spanish language, and it is to our benefit politically to stick together as a larger and more visible Hispanic community.

The Hispanic population in Canada grew from 177,000 in 1996 to 217,000 in 2001 (Statistics Canada, 1996, 2001). According to the latest estimates (projection from Statistics Canada, 2001; Kelly, 2004), there are now more than half a million Hispanics in Canada. In the first six months of 2004 alone, there were nearly 12,000 applications for refugee status in Canada; Colombia, Mexico, Costa Rica and Peru are four of the 10 countries with the highest number of applications, accounting for about 30 per cent of the total number of applications for refugee status in Canada (Loarte, 2004a, 2004b).

Many of the immigrants have come during times of political crisis, have experienced trauma and persecution, and have arrived in Canada as refugee claimants. Because many Hispanics come as refugees, they are not fortified with the language skills that they need to help ease the transition into Canadian society. Thirty per cent of Latin American refugees live below the poverty level. The first generation of Hispanics is generally well educated and functioned as professionals in their home countries (Rubio, 2004; Viswanathan et al., 2003); however, lack of English- or French-language skills may lead to unemployment or underemployment in Canada. Other factors such as racism and discrimination may contribute to difficulties in finding employment. Hispanics may be further disadvantaged by the lack of time and/or resources to develop relevant language skills to prepare for the job market, even once they are in Canada. The lack of language skills results in lack of information about resources, rights, opportunities and employability. Women are most affected in these areas because of lack of child care in agencies and organizations providing health and settlement services.

Those who need to flee their countries quickly and cannot arrange immigration and other legal documents may have to wait for several years to be reunited with their families. Navigating the refugee process requires time and money, and those who are unsuccessful remain in emotional and security limbo during the lengthy appeal process. Furthermore, the process of bringing family members, who may also be in danger in the home country, is onerous and expensive. During these times, the family members' lives may be at risk; some people have even been murdered before they were granted a visa to Canada.

Connection to family is one of the strongest values in the Latin community. Traditionally, extended families live close by and receive strong support from each other throughout their lives. The refugee process tears families apart, which often results in social isolation, and loss of identity and social status. These hardships may extend to the second generation (Samaan, 2000).

Working with Latin American Women with Mental Health Concerns

I have organized this chapter around two key concepts: arousal and resourcing. *Arousal*, a physiological response, is the mechanism by which a person prepares to meet a perceived danger. *Resourcing* is the identification of strengths already used by the client, but not necessarily acknowledged by her.

AROUSAL

Arousal helps a person orient to danger and prepare for fight or flight (Ogden & Minton, 2000). In other words, arousal is the physical activation of a whole mind-body response as a result of stress. Stress is any stimulus in the environment to which a living organism responds. All living organisms require a certain amount of arousal to function, which is called an optimal level of arousal (Selye, 1974). A person may have different levels of arousal depending on her or his perception of the intensity of the situation. During times of stress, the arousal threshold lowers and it takes less and less stress to generate a bodily reaction to perceived danger (Ogden & Minton, 2000).

During a stressful situation, the body responds physically and psychologically to the stress. When a crisis endures, this arousal response is repeated and drains the body's ability to manage the stress. Eventually, even images, thoughts, nightmares and memories about a crisis—despite there being no actual present danger—give rise to bodily sensations including rapid heartbeat, sweating, hyperventilation, dizziness and trembling. Sometimes the response can be an unconscious reaction to triggers such as smell, colour or sound, which can bring back memories and intensify responses and the sensations. The client might relive the original situation, and the cyclical pattern continues. She may try to block these sensations and memories, which may increase her level of stress. Avoidance only perpetuates the cycle of arousal and recollection. The client may criticize herself for being weak, incompetent and disabled, which may lead to further escalation of the arousal (Haskell, 2003, 2004; Ogden & Minton, 2000).

The client first responds to arousal either cognitively or physically, but eventually both responses are activated. Cognitive responses may include keeping busy, acting as though they are coping, and taking on more responsibility for the welfare of others. Physical responses may include shaking, sweating, muscle tension and pain. A client may find the physical sensations too overwhelming, which might in the long-run result in numbed feelings, unawareness of physical sensations and lack of appetite. Some of these responses are protective strategies against the extreme discomfort of the experience, and may help a woman cope during and after the original event. For example, a woman being raped may use numbness and dissociation as ways to protect herself from the terror. Therapists need to acknowledge the role these responses may have played in a woman's survival (Haskell, 2003, 2004; Ogden & Minton, 2000).

The therapist may assist the client to deal with the arousal experience by encouraging her to suspend the analysis and judgment that make the event seem real, and to describe the sensations instead. The central task is not to promote relaxation but to encourage a woman to observe and name the sensation and experience it. This helps the woman detach from the frightening images of the trauma. As the focus shifts, the arousal level decreases. In therapy, the aim is to integrate the physical sensations that produce the arousing emotions—which seem to be connected to the memories of trauma—to help disconnect emotions from memory and to give the woman a sense of control over the flashbacks. The new thought "I can manage this" is therefore integrated into the previously arousing and terrifying experience (Ogden & Minton, 2000; Rothschild, 2000). This thought lets the client learn to associate the disturbing responses with the knowledge that these sensations subside if they are observed in this way.

RESOURCING

Resourcing is not about praise, which is generally seen as setting up an expectation to live up to. If a client has a low self-image, she may not accept praise. For example, if I told a client that she was intelligent, she may deflect the praise with something like, "If I were, I wouldn't be in this predicament." Resourcing is about helping the client to recognize what she has already been doing to get through a crisis. The therapeutic strategy is to show her how this action was useful to her at the time and may be useful in the future, but that when she reacts to memories automatically as though she were still in danger, it drains her energy.

THE THERAPEUTIC PROCESS

The process of working with clients involves several steps, including:
- doing initial work
- focusing on present concerns
- addressing further revelations
- taking risks

- dealing with new crises
- following up.

As the following case study will show, this process is not rigid. It is part of an ebb and flow of progress with the client.

Case Study: Dolores

Events or issues presented here are not specific to any one client, but represent a compilation of cases seen in my practice as a mental health clinician over a number of years.

Dolores is in her mid-30s and from a Latin American country that has been in a long civil war. She and her first child came to Canada to join her husband. She was originally referred to me after the birth of her second child. She is now pregnant with her third child. After a pre-assessment, she was seen by the Spanish-speaking staff psychiatrist who prescribed and monitored medication before her current pregnancy. The joint intensive treatment lasted for one year and was tapered off for another year, until Dolores expressed that she was able to deal with her anxieties and would call as needed.

DOING INITIAL WORK

Initial work with a client involves:
- listening and gathering a client history
- creating trust
- resourcing
- managing symptoms.

Listening and Gathering a Client History

At the beginning, in addition to the usual introductions and explanations of confidentiality and legal issues, I go through a short questionnaire to establish a client's past and current status of suicidal thought and intent, sexual and physical abuse, and alcohol and other drug use. The questions are simple, and I present them only after I inform a client that I ask every client these questions. I also clarify that I will not ask for details and that she does not have to answer.

There are advantages to asking these questions early on:
- Asked matter-of-factly, the questions signal that the clinician is not afraid to talk about these topics.
- Explaining that these events are also experienced by others may decrease a client's sense of isolation and need for secrecy.
- These questions present an opportunity to show empathy and admiration for the client's strength in having survived the traumatic situation.
- The questions may open the way for future discussion.

Dolores revealed that she had made a suicide attempt at age 12. She again had strong thoughts about suicide in 1996 when her parents were assassinated in front of her. She was then pregnant with her first child. Her faith and thoughts of her child growing within prevented her from killing herself. She was not currently suicidal. She did not want to answer the question on sexual abuse. I congratulated her for deciding to protect herself in this way.

In her home country, Dolores had worked in a hospital as a nursing assistant. The history she was able to give about the major trauma she had experienced was a quick reference to her parents' assassinations, the murder of a friend, and many phone calls she received that demanded medications or money to buy medications for wounded comrades of the callers. Her parents had worked in the laboratories of the same hospital and had refused to co-operate with the demands. After killing her parents, the persecutors threatened to harm Dolores' child, and kept finding Dolores despite several moves and changed telephone numbers. Because of her state of terror and due to financial constraints, Dolores and her husband agreed that he would go to the United States to establish a home where she and their child could join him. During the two years of waiting to join her husband, Dolores went into hiding with her daughter in the basement of a house, leaving only after dark to get food.

Creating Trust

During the first three sessions, Dolores became hyper-aroused as soon as she began to speak. She repeated phrases like:

> No one can understand what I've been through. I can't talk to anyone because I start to cry. I don't go out because people will start asking me questions and I will break down. I can't go on living like this. I am afraid I am damaging my children and someone will call the Children's Aid and they will take my children away. I keep my curtains closed because they might be watching out for me. I cannot sleep at night because every noise wakes me up jumping. I have nightmares about my parents falling down dead at my feet. My husband says I am crazy.

The goal of these sessions was to create trust and containment for her expressions and to help Dolores differentiate between normal reactions and abnormal events that are not expected to be part of a person's life under ordinary circumstances. The therapy aimed to encourage her to talk about events in her life. She had not been able to speak of the events freely before these sessions.

Resourcing

The process of resourcing made Dolores aware of what was already working for her. This included:
- reframing her feelings as stimuli for healthy protective mechanisms, such as being alert to danger while creating avoidance and safeguarding strategies

- identifying her hyper-arousal as a possible learned response over many years, which was probably useful to her as a first line of defence in past crises (Haskell, 2003, 2004; Ogden & Minton, 2000).

Other resourcing strategies involved:

- giving literature in Spanish on posttraumatic stress disorder and depression
- reassuring Dolores that she was sane, and had been able to protect and care for her child in very difficult situations without the support of her husband for two years
- reaffirming the present (she's here, she's safe, her children are safe and healthy, she does not need to talk about these issues with anyone she doesn't trust)
- assuring her that there would be time to talk when she was ready
- giving hope (acknowledging that it takes time to feel better, but that she has been through the worst)
- using metaphors and images to explain the natural process of arousal in her body (anything that is understood is less scary).

Initial work gives the client a few moments of relief from the discomfort. Subsequent work reinforces the client's ability to manage responses as well as to acknowledge resources.

Managing Symptoms

Dolores had a pattern for handling her hyper-arousal. She would start to cry, her body would stiffen, the fingers of her hands would spread open as far as possible and much energy was spent keeping them apart and rigid. Dolores would grimace and try to extend her neck and the sides of her mouth. She would be very frustrated and apologetic for not being able to stop. When she did manage to speak, she thought that she did not express herself well. It was very important for her to be understood, but she could not put her experience into words that represented what she felt. She would begin a story, then sidetrack to another story in order to explain the first, then sidetrack again to explain the second story. Her bodily agitation undermined her thinking. (Other clients have different patterns; it is useful to notice which patterns each client uses.)

In such situations, a therapist may react by becoming agitated herself. There may be a strong temptation to try to calm *herself* by trying to convince the client to calm down. This, in fact, reinforces to the client that she is not behaving appropriately and that there is some other expectation of her, which she cannot meet.

OBSERVING THE BODY

The therapist works with the client to move to the physical sensations of the body and away from cognition. I asked Dolores to notice sensations in her body by inviting her to pretend that she had a camera behind each eye and to scan her body for sensations, from the inside. For example, I invited Dolores to:

- feel the air on her neck coming from the window behind her
- feel the sensation of her hair on her forehead
- feel the air entering her nostrils dry and perhaps cool, and leaving her nose warm and moist

- feel the sensation of the clothing against different parts of her skin
- feel her chest rise and fall as she breathed
- feel the movement of her shoulders as she breathed

I encouraged Dolores to scan her body and let me know what she sensed.

It is important to differentiate between *sensations* and *feelings* or *emotions*. If Dolores said, "I feel scared," I would ask, "What is happening in your body that tells you that you are scared?" Other questions could include: "What is happening in your body that tells you that you are feeling panic?" "What happens in your body when you think of *x*?" As she disclosed the sensations, I would repeat her description and then ask: "What else do you notice?"

The strategy encourages a client to locate the expressions of thoughts or feelings in the body, and allows her to observe the sensations and events in her body without analysis. In the past, if she had felt butterflies in her stomach or shaking in her hands, she might have interpreted these as "fear," which would have led to associating the fear with memories. Going back to the body serves several purposes:

- It teaches the client to separate bodily experience from the past cognitive memory, which feels beyond control, and to integrate bodily experience within the sphere of what is manageable.
- It helps to promote acceptance and reduce judgment of the bodily experience. An example of a judgmental statement is: "I notice the shaking in my hands and I should not be shaking because it reminds me of the events and I don't want to remember the events."
- Eventually, the client learns that the body is not the enemy; it is a sensory organ. Memories become less upsetting because there is a way to detach from them through observation. It demonstrates to the client that her body remembers how to relax.

Once a client recognizes and observes sensations separately from memories, she learns that the intensity of bodily tensions diminishes. This is the first step in managing the fear of the memories. Once a client understands that bodily responses are natural defensive reactions against real or perceived dangers (Haskell, 2003; Ogden & Minton, 2000; Rothschild, 2000), she is less likely to blame herself. The way out of the automatic response is to practise disconnecting from thinking about and monitoring sensations in the body for short periods of time, for example, while she carries out familiar activities such as riding the streetcar, washing dishes or changing diapers. When flashbacks recur, she will then be able to observe the familiar sensations and distinguish the present from the past. Observing the body is the key to returning to living in the present. Of course, it does not happen at once. Like any learning, it must be encouraged and practised.

Later in this session with Dolores, I reviewed the tensions or pains that she had identified (i.e., headaches, neck aches, stomach aches, stiff shoulders, back pain). She noted that they had lessened or disappeared. When the body disengages from thoughts and emotions, physical sensations diminish. By being with her body and detaching from the memory-body cycle, Dolores was able to relax. The body is a natural entity and, like all things in nature, goes to a lower energy level when it is not disturbed.

For homework, I ask clients to practise identifying and staying with or returning to bodily sensations while doing mundane tasks. For example, a client may notice the feeling of warm water on her body when taking a bath or shower; she may focus on noise outside; or she may explore the sensation of touching a child's face. I suggest 10 minutes of this exercise three times a day. Generally clients do practise this exercise because it gives them a few moments of peace. They report that they feel calmer during the exercise.

STRENGTHENING OBSERVATION WITHOUT ANALYSIS

The next goal is to strengthen a client's ability to observe without analyzing. During the period of clinical assessment and of taking a client's history, the memories and bodily sensations associated with the memories return. At this point, I stop asking questions and guide the client back to bodily awareness. ("Let's stop for a while. What is happening in your body right now?") I repeat the process until a lower arousal state is visible. I ask if she's ready to continue. This slows the process of gathering a client's history, but the client learns that she can manage the strong emotions generated by the painful memories, and that usually helps her feel stronger. Through observation, a client's experience of feeling stronger is repeated many times.

FOCUSING ON PRESENT CONCERNS

Once the hurdle of fear is managed, clients are able to reduce the level of preoccupation with past memories and pay more attention to present issues. For example, Dolores wanted to attend ESL classes, which required that the children go to daycare. Parting from her children was very difficult for Dolores because she feared that if they were not with her, they could be in danger.

Also, as the refugee hearing date neared, the flashbacks and nightmares returned, and Dolores felt that she had lost control again. Clients may get traumatized several times during the refugee process: hearings may be postponed because judges or translators do not show up, or new information is requested by the judge, and hearings get re-scheduled. Because of the flashbacks and nightmares that returned during the months leading to the new hearing dates, Dolores was not able to concentrate on or attend her ESL classes. A teacher and the welfare worker threatened to cut off her benefits if she did not attend classes. The relationship with her husband was tense. He was tired of her being afraid and uncomfortable around people. Also, he had to do all the shopping because she got disoriented when she went out by herself, and was afraid of getting lost. He would yell at her and was short tempered with the kids.

To address some of these concerns, together with the psychiatrist, Dolores and I drafted letters to the school on hospital stationary. Depending on the situation, the letter stated that Dolores was in medical treatment at this clinic and needed to be excused from school until further notice, or would attend classes only as her health permitted. For some women, we may also facilitate an application to the Ontario

Disability Support Program (ODSP), give information about resources for women who have experienced abuse and develop a plan of action in the event that she is lost. On index cards, I wrote Dolores' address, telephone number and some phrases, in English and Spanish, asking people for directions to a phone, to her house, to the hospital, etc. (Chapter 7 discusses issues around navigating services for newcomer women.)

ADDRESSING FURTHER REVELATIONS

In my practice, women have had many traumas. Often they have been abused since childhood. Once the most immediate concerns are brought forth, other traumas come to the forefront. Their situation is comparable to living in a constant earthquake. That they have adapted and survived is a testament to their resilience. This needs to be respected and supported by looking for ways to remind clients of their strengths. As Haskell (2003, 2004) points out, the client's reaction to trauma is neither a dysfunction nor a disorder, but a response to one or many threats (emotional, physical or cognitive) to her survival.

As Dolores lost her fear of being helpless about the memories, other information surfaced. In the course of several sessions, she disclosed her experiences of various forms of violence:

- Her husband had been physically abusive to her when they were living in the United States. Once in Canada, she had shown him literature in Spanish that let him know abuse is against Canadian law. (See Chapter 15 for a discussion on intimate partner violence.)
- Her stepfather had sexually abused her for many years and she wanted him dead.
- Rebels abducted her twin brother when they were 14, and he has not been heard from since.
- She had seen friends from school shot or kidnapped.
- To get to school, she had to walk right against the walls of buildings to be less visible to snipers who were on the roofs near her home. She had to throw herself on the ground when the firing started. She remembered stepping over bodies on the way to school.

I pointed out to Dolores that alertness and fear had been useful in her life; it had trained her to be hyper-alert in times of real danger. Alertness was still somewhat useful to her to function in a new culture. Still, she needed to learn to *choose* when to be alert and when danger had lessened.

TAKING RISKS

As the sessions progressed, Dolores became less fearful and began to risk new experiences. Often clients see themselves as cowardly for having taken so long to get to this point. This is when it is helpful to introduce the concept of heroism by noting the saying "Heroism is not about going into battle without fear, but about going into battle *despite* fear." In the case of therapy, heroism is about recognizing and facing the illusion of apparent mortal danger presented by the memories, and realizing that they are not a real threat to life. While it is difficult to rapidly change an emotion, a decision to act, despite the emotion, is always possible. The outcome of this risk is emotional growth.

Dolores tried several things over the course of therapy:

- She joined a group for women who had experienced abuse. This helped her to feel less isolated by hearing other women's stories and seeing how much some of them had grown. She learned more parenting skills and made new friends.
- She returned to school part time when her husband was working nights, so she could leave the children with him in the afternoons.
- She went shopping during daylight hours.

DEALING WITH NEW CRISES

As Dolores became more confident, her husband became more verbally aggressive, and one night he also became physically abusive to her. After she called 911, the police arrived at her home and arrested him. Her social service benefits were reduced because he was no longer living at home. (Social service benefits are allotted based on the number of people in the family, not on the needs of those people. If the husband leaves, the amount is reduced by the husband's allotment.) There would be a court date, and she was worried about what this would do to their refugee claim. Because of the restraining order against the husband, the couple could not communicate.

Dolores experienced guilt, shame and fear about being in charge and making decisions; about the need to take the kids with her wherever she went; about her loneliness, since she could not communicate with her husband; and about her confusion.

During therapy, Dolores was able to coherently tell me what had happened. She was tearful, but not self-critical about being tearful. She showed much less of the grimaces, hand tensions and verbal tangents that were prominent during the initial sessions. I pointed this out to her. She was able to acknowledge her progress.

She learned to manage her arousal but did not yet have the focus and energy to do so consistently. After a consultation with the team's Spanish-speaking psychiatrist, Dolores began to take medication that made it easier for her to focus and balance her energy level to more consistently manage the hyper-arousal. The psychiatrist explained how the medication worked and its possible side-effects. Dolores also received written information in Spanish.

Dolores went to court to show support for her husband. I delivered messages between her and her husband because they were not allowed to communicate directly. The process of his return to the family took almost a year. Six months after her husband had been arrested, Dolores said, "I feel stable."

FOLLOWING UP

The emotional stability experienced by clients is not consistent. In particular, flashbacks and nightmares return in difficult and stressful times connected with the refugee process (e.g., when they receive a letter about a hearing date or about the cancellation of a hearing date or as they await a written decision from immigration, which can take months). If an application is rejected, the panic and helplessness increase as arrangements for the review are put in place.

The question of separation from the therapist becomes more of a concern as clients begin to feel better. Clients have had enough "termination," abandonment and loss. I do not "terminate" sessions with clients. The clients themselves manage the separation. When the time seemed right, I asked Dolores, "Do you think that you still need to see me weekly, can you manage less often or do you want to call me when you want another appointment?" Dolores opted to see me every two weeks at first, then once a month, then as needed.

In the "as-needed" stage, she called me twice in six months and I saw her twice after each call. The issues were about the resurging pain of a yet another hearing postponement and the anxiety of awaiting a response that was two months overdue.

Other Techniques

Additional tools may be used in working with the body. These tools are based on many practice models (e.g., Adlerian, sensorimotor, action and commitment, and cognitive therapies). I incorporate these into my practice at my discretion, in keeping with my own philosophy and experience. They include:

- working with impulses
- working with reframing
- working without forcing change.

I inform clients upfront that some tools may not work and I have other tools that we can try. In doing so, I also demonstrate risk-taking to clients.

WORKING WITH IMPULSES

As clients become more skilled and comfortable about monitoring their body, it may be possible to guide them to identify impulses that may be present when the body is relaxed and that would not otherwise be noticeable. A client may have been unable to complete defence movements at the time of an attack, which can create tension in the body (Ogden & Minton, 2000). Being able to complete defence movements relieves the tension.

An exercise to illustrate this can be done by standing in a doorway with your arms at your sides. Slowly raise both arms and press the back of your hands against the sides of the door frame as hard as possible for about 30 seconds. Relax your arms and step outside or inside the door. Without apparent volition, your arms will rise on their own, completing the movement that would have been exerted by your muscles without the barrier of the frame.

I asked a client to focus on her body and describe the sensations. After a while, I asked her to notice any impulse or desire to move any part of her body. I instructed her not to move anything yet, only to notice any part that may want to start moving. She noted that her hands wanted to make fists. I asked her to move one hand slowly into a fist, then the other hand and to notice what happened in the rest of her body as she did this. She noted that her body started to tense and have more energy. She began to tense different parts of her body—her arms, legs, shoulders and abdomen—to move as the impulse led, one part at a time. At this point, she felt the impulse to hit. I put a pillow against the back of my chair and moved the chair in front of her, pressing my knee onto the seat to secure the chair. I invited her to try a punch. She did hesitantly at first, but with encouragement (and a bit of cheerleading), the hits got stronger, her face flushed, her body focused on the pillow. She started to breathe hard and I made a grunting sound as she punched and exhaled air. I invited her to let the sound out from her diaphragm and include whatever words wanted to come out. What came out over and over again was, "It's not my fault!" When she had exhausted this need and stopped, she felt stronger, more energized and more relaxed.

When a person is not able to fight back, the feeling of helplessness may become programmed as an automatic response to stress. Hence, whenever the person is stressed, she feels that her body becomes helpless (Ogden & Minton, 2000). By disconnecting the body-mind cycle, the person can help the body reorganize this programming to more appropriate defensive impulses. Conscious movement may reprogram the body and change cognition (Rothschild, 2000). Inviting the client to move in different ways (e.g., slouched vs. erect, forward vs. backward, swinging the arms vs. holding the arms stiffly at one's sides) also helps the client note how movements affect emotions and to practise the body awareness that is used in managing flashbacks.

WORKING WITH REFRAMING

Another client, in an agitated state, said that she did not see any sense in her life because she always had to suffer. The only thing that kept her from ending her life was that she had a young child. I pointed out how impressed I was by her deep mothering instinct, especially when she, herself, had not had such a mother. She mentioned that her grandmother was a role model. Now she was remembering at least one good thing in her life, and we were able to start a list of other good things. As she made the list, she noticed that her body was more relaxed.

WORKING WITHOUT FORCING CHANGE

A client who arrived at my office paced back and forth in the waiting room while she waited for me. At one point, she went outside to smoke. When she entered my office, she was too agitated to sit. She said her whole body felt like she had a spring inside that had to keep moving. She paced, did little jumps, rubbed her hands, shook her arms and apologetically explained that she could never sit still, not even at home.

I assured her that she could keep moving while we talked and that it did not bother me at all. While sitting, she rocked back and forth rapidly and jiggled her legs. She was in constant motion. I asked her to notice her body and the sensations as she moved—for example, the air moving by her face, her thighs moving up and down, her feet bouncing off the floor, her hands under her thighs stabilizing her. After she was able to describe a few things on her own, I asked her if she was willing to try an experiment. She agreed. I asked her to stay conscious of the sensations in her body and then stop the moving for a few seconds. She stopped and then started again. She said that it was intolerable; she could not breathe and felt very warm.

I congratulated her on the natural intelligence and instinct to keep herself calm by moving. I explained that some people might not be able to tolerate as much tension as she has, but that she manages it by rocking, jiggling and moving. I suggested that she do the observing exercise while she is moving and note her bodily sensations—in the streetcar, at home, anywhere. She began to understand that her movement was a coping strategy, not a weakness. Within three sessions, the movements had lessened by half.

Implications for Practice

There are several ways to apply and expand on the themes discussed in this chapter:
- use the client's language where possible
- recognize commonalities between cultures
- ask questions and make suggestions
- be flexible
- suspend judgment
- do your own work
- maintain your balance.

USE THE CLIENT'S LANGUAGE WHERE POSSIBLE

Context is important in understanding a client, and treatment in the person's mother tongue facilitates trust and expression. The appendix at the end of this chapter lists terms for sensory motor experience in both Spanish and English. Tools like this can be helpful in fostering a client's comfort to confide in her therapist.

RECOGNIZE COMMONALITIES BETWEEN CULTURES

Cultures have more commonalities than differences. All cultures encourage family ties, value spiritual connections, create social and moral norms and apply social pressures to conform to certain roles. The treatment of trauma is most directly connected to people's:

- perceived risk to life and the duration of this peril
- previous history of trauma and/or other mental health issues
- strategies and successes in surviving previous trauma (having been able to defend themselves in this or another crisis)
- past problem-solving experiences
- having a purpose for living
- past or existing support systems
- willingness to seek help
- resilience and flexibility
- curiosity versus fear of the unknown
- acceptance, respect and expectations for themselves
- relationship with and level of trust in their therapist (Haskell, 2003, 2004).

ASK QUESTIONS AND MAKE SUGGESTIONS

A therapist's curiosity helps to create a co-operative therapeutic process. The therapist might suggest a technique: "I wonder what would happen if we try *x*." "Are you willing to try this and see what happens?" If it doesn't seem to produce the therapist's expected result, then that is itself a learning experience, and a way to model risk-taking for the client.

BE FLEXIBLE

A therapist's flexibility has to do with having many tools at hand. In my practice, I have used aspects of sensorimotor, developmental, cognitive, solution-focused and Adlerian psychotherapy, among many other approaches. Many tools and techniques can be incorporated into most theoretical orientations used in trauma therapy. Psychodrama and writing are excellent tools to encourage expression. Movement and music are very helpful in expressing nonverbal ideas and can be interpreted through various lenses. Art therapy is also a method of doing therapy. Art therapy in itself can be cognitive, psychoanalytical and solution-focused. Regardless of the name of the theoretical lens or the tools used, trauma therapy involves understanding the experience of being human and seeing the client from many theoretical points of view. It helps to go to as many workshops as possible, and to read articles and books. The more tools in your therapy toolbox, the more flexible you can be with the individual and the situation. The learning never stops. "Instinctual therapy" is merely a process of quickly choosing from many options.

SUSPEND JUDGMENT

Being able to suspend judgment and to reframe are essential. If a client says: "After the assault, I went home, got my father's gun, went looking for him and shot him," this is not the time to tell her that murder is illegal and against whatever holy book she may believe in. The natural follow-up would be to find out if there have been other times in her life when she acted impulsively. Reframing might focus on her dedication to her purpose and consider other times when she had practised such dedication. Another natural follow-up might be to try to enlist this dedication to her healing and surviving in this new culture.

DO YOUR OWN WORK

Working with women with a history of trauma can present difficulties for the therapist—the possibility of *vicarious traumatization* (McCann and Pearlman, 1990) and the potential for *counter-transference* (emotion felt by a therapist toward a client). (Note that "vicarious traumatization" has replaced the term "burnout" in describing the reactions of therapists who listen to horrendous stories of human abuse.) The therapist must have his or her own source of therapy to understand the difficulties and fears associated with making changes and taking risks. It is a humbling experience, and humility is a good starting point for a therapist. Therapists must have the experience of having worked through difficult issues in their own lives and the courage to be comfortable with their imperfections.

Clinical supervision is usually provided in the workplace. It provides not only a door back to a humanity outside the trauma, but also the grounding contact with a source of reassurance and guidance and an opportunity to refocus self-awareness. It is akin to decompression. Where this is not available in the workplace, a clinician must request an outside supervisor or join a peer supervision group. Another option is to find (and pay for) a private source of supervision.

MAINTAIN YOUR BALANCE

A trauma therapist who has no conscious life outside work is also a traumatized person. There is an increasing focus on the effect of working with traumatized clients on mental health workers, including the effect of vicarious traumatization. McCann and Pearlman (1990) suggest that:

[A]ll therapists working with trauma survivors will experience lasting alterations in their cognitive schema, having significant impact on the therapist feelings, relationships and life. Whether these changes are ultimately destructive to the helper and to the therapeutic process depends largely on the extent to which the therapist can engage in a parallel process to that of the victim client, the process of integrating and transforming these experiences of horror . . . (p. 134)

This "parallel process" simply refers to reconnecting with life outside the horror; it is a mandatory part of therapists' work. Taking responsibility for your own mental health is a professional duty that is not often taken into account in preparation for this work and often not recognized in the workplace.

Reconnecting with life is a personal task that is every bit as important as any other professional duty. Although once one leaves work other tasks and responsibilities often take priority, renewal (or reconnecting with oneself) is essential between the professional and the private interpersonal tasks. This renewal space may be called "solitude." Renewal can be done anywhere and need only take a few seconds, but it is best when practised regularly. The exercises, described in this chapter, of reconnecting with the body serve this purpose. Although an hour a day would be ideal, this is generally not practical and having an unrealistic goal increases anxiety. Even a five-minute sit a day will start the connection.

This practice of solitude can be continued anywhere—while washing dishes, in the subway, at a concert, in the car, while changing diapers, etc. One simply turns part of one's consciousness to observing one's own bodily sensations. The other step in this process is consciously labelling this experience as a pleasurable event. A follow-up exercise is to notice two additional things every day that are pleasurable and to consciously label these as pleasurable. Examples may be as fleeting as smelling a rose, noticing a shadow, holding a baby or finding a penny.

Conclusion

The examples of clients discussed in this chapter could be women from any culture. While a person's particular background is important in understanding a client, there are commonalities in people from all cultures, and the treatments for trauma discussed in this chapter are also applicable outside the Latin American community.

APPENDIX 14-1

Vocabulary for Sensorimotor Experience / Palabras para Describir Experiencias del Cuerpo*

ENGLISH	SPANISH
achy	dolorido
airy	ligero, sutil
blocked	bloqueado, obstruido
breathless	falta de aliento
bubbly	burbujeando
chills	escalofrio
clammy	pegajoso
congested	amontonado, congestionado
cool	fresco
dense	denso, compacto, espeso
dizzy	mareado
dull	entorpecido
electric	electrico
energized	con energia
faint	debil, apagado
flaccid	flacido, blando
fluid	fluido, como liquido
flushed	sentirse colorado, con flujo
flutters	batir rapidamente, tremulos
frozen	congelado
fuzzy	velloso, cubierto de peluza
goosebumps	carne de gallina
heavy	pesado
itchy	pinchando, picazon
jerky	tironeado, sacudido, saltado, espasmo, contraccion, tiron
jumbly	mezclado, revuelto
jumpy	saltando
light	liviano
moist	humedo
nauseous	con nausea
numb	sintiendo nada, entumecido, paralizado
paralyzed	paralizado
pounding	martillando
pressure	presion
prickly	espinoso, punzante, pinchante
puffy/bloated	hinchado
radiating	hechando rayos
shaky	temblorozo
sharp	cortante, agudo
shivery	tiritando, temblando
shudder	temblor
spinning	girando, dando vueltas
stringy	fibroso, como cuerda o cordon
suffocating	ahogando
sweaty	sudando
tense	tieso, tenso
throbbing	pulsando, latiendo, palpitando
tight	firme, apretado
tingly	sentir hormigueo
tremble	temblor
vibration	vibracion, vibrando
warm	caluroso
wobbly	instable, temblequeando

* Compiled in English by Pat Ogden (1999), in *Trauma Recovery Manual*. Boulder, CO: Sensorimotor Psychotherapy Institute. Translated to Spanish by Eva Saphir.

References

Freire, G.M. (2002). Hispanics and the politics of health care. *Journal of Health and Social Policy, 14* (4), 21–35.

Haskell, L. (2003). *First Stage Trauma Treatment: A Guide for Mental Health Professionals Working with Women.* Toronto: Centre for Addiction and Mental Health.

Haskell, L. (2004). *Women, Abuse and Trauma Therapy: An Information Guide.* Toronto: Centre for Addiction and Mental Health.

Kelly, K. (2004). Visible minorities: A diverse group. *Canadian Social Trends, 37,* 2–8. Ottawa: Statistics Canada.

Loarte, A. (2004a). Analisis de las tasas de aceptacion de las demandas de refugio de hispanos en Canada en la primera mitad del 2004. Message posted to http://groups.yahoo.com/group/eleccion/messages/18590?threaded=1&m=e&var=1&tidx=1.

Loarte, A. (2004b). Hispanos solicitan más refugio en Canadá durante el 2004. Message posted to http://groups.yahoo.com/group/eleccion/messages/18470?threaded=1&m=e&var=1&tidx=1.

Ogden, P. (1999). *Trauma Recovery Manual.* Boulder, CO: Sensorimotor Psychotherapy Institute.

Ogden, P. & Minton, K. (2000). Sensorimotor psychotherapy: One method for processing traumatic memory. *Traumatology, 6* (3), 1–20.

McCann, L. & Pearlman, L.A. (1990). Vicarious traumatization: A framework for understanding the psychological effects of working with victims. *Journal of Traumatic Stress, 3* (1), 131–149.

Rothschild, B. (2000). *The Body Remembers: The Psychophysiology of Trauma and Trauma Treatment.* New York: W.W. Norton & Company.

Rubio, F. (2004). *Social Inclusion: The Basis of and Possible Effects of Social Inclusion and Exclusion on the Hispanic Community in Toronto.* Unpublished paper, Hispanic Development Council, Toronto.

Samaan, R.A. (2000). The influences of race, ethnicity and poverty on the mental health of children. *Journal of Health Care for the Poor and Underserved, 11* (1), 100–110.

Selye, H. (1974). *Stress without Distress.* Toronto: McClelland and Stewart.

Statistics Canada. (1996). *1996 Census: Mother Tongue, Home Language and Knowledge of Languages.* Cited in *The Daily* (1997, December 2). Available: www.statcan.ca/Daily/English/971202/d971202. htm. Accessed January 5, 2008.

Statistics Canada. (2001). *Population by Selected Ethnic Origins, by Provinces and Territories.* Available: www40.statcan.ca/l01/cst01/demo26a.htm?sdi=population. Accessed January 5, 2008.

Viswanathan, L., Shakir, U., Chung, T. & Ramos, D. (2003). *Social Inclusion and the City: Considerations for Social Planning.* Toronto: Alternative Planning Group. Available: www.hispaniccouncil.net/id11.html. Accessed January 5, 2008.

Chapter 15

Intimate Partner Violence among Immigrant and Refugee Women

ROBIN MASON AND ILENE HYMAN

The 1979 United Nations' *Convention on the Elimination of All Forms of Discrimination against Women* and, later, the 1993 *Declaration on the Elimination of Violence against Women* acknowledged that women experience multiple forms of violence over the course of their lives. Any form of violence "violates, impairs, or nullifies women's enjoyment of their human rights and fundamental freedoms" (Astbury, 2005). While women experience multiple forms of violence ranging from everyday acts of misogyny and discrimination to rape as an act of war, the most common form of violence occurs between intimate partners.

Intimate partner violence (IPV) has been defined by the U.S. Centers for Disease Control and Prevention as the experience or threat of physical or sexual violence and/or psychological/emotional abuse by current or former spouses and/or non-marital partners (Saltzman et al., 1999). In essence, IPV is a repetitive, escalating form of violence perpetrated by someone the victim trusts. Although IPV can occur between same sex partners as well as heterosexual ones, most frequently IPV takes the form of male-perpetrated violence against women (Tjaden & Thoennes, 2000). In this chapter, we will discuss IPV in the context of heterosexual relationships and immigration.

Since 1990, Canada has accepted approximately 230,000 immigrants per year, or about 0.7 per cent of the Canadian population (Kessel, 1998). Women comprise just over half (51 per cent) of all people who immigrate to Canada each year, and immigrant women represent 18 per cent of all women living in Canada (Chard et al., 2000). As discussed elsewhere in this book, immigrant women are not a homogenous group.

They vary in terms of country of origin, length of stay, "visibility" (e.g., racial visibility), category of migration, socio-economic status, knowledge of host country languages and hence employment opportunities, and degree of assimilation—all of which affect their life circumstances, health and help-seeking. Naturally, within any cultural group, individuals will also vary considerably from one another.

This chapter begins with a literature review on IPV with a specific focus on immigrant and refugee women. It includes information on the etiology of IPV, risk and protective factors, prevalence, health impacts and barriers to help-seeking. The chapter concludes with implications for mental health professionals for identifying, assessing, responding and preventing IPV.

Etiology

Different etiological theories have been proposed to explain IPV. At the individual level, psychological theories attribute blame to the victim or the perpetrator. However, there has been little empirical support for the claim that personality disorders in either the perpetrator or victim predispose individuals to violent behaviours (Gelles, 1993). Other theories, such as the family violence theory (Straus et al., 1980) and the subculture of violence theory (Wolfgang & Ferracuti, 1982), implicate the role of witnessing violence and the presence of social values and norms that perpetuate gender inequality in the etiology of violence.

Social structural theories relate the occurrence of violence to social structures as opposed to individual or family structures. At sociological and structural levels, feminist theories and status inconsistency theories predominate. According to the feminist perspective, gender inequality and male domination underlie violence against women (Dobash & Dobash, 1979). It is hypothesized that violence stems from women's traditionally devalued and inferior role in the family and wider society. There is some research to support this perspective. For example, partner abuse appears to be more common in patriarchal societies where cultural values, including social mores and religious beliefs, dictate male dominance in gender relationships, condone violence against women and create separate codes of conduct for men and women (Sugarman & Frankel, 1996; Yick & Agbayani-Siewert, 1997). Further, male-perpetrated partner abuse is reportedly more common in couples where men hold more traditional beliefs about gendered roles than their wives (Raj & Silverman, 2002), which may be a feature in communities of recent immigrants. Cross-cultural studies have also found that in trying to conform to idealized notions of wife and mother and adapting to changes in life circumstances that follow migration, immigrant women may experience and tolerate more violence than women in the majority population (Bui & Morash, 1999).

According to theories of status inconsistency, the family is a power system with members having differing amounts of resources. Those who are threatened by their lack of resources, or perceive their status to be inconsistent with social norms, may use violence as a strategy to compensate for lack of power (Campbell, 1992; Goode, 1971;

Yick, 2001). Status inconsistency frequently occurs after migration as post-migration stressors such as poverty, underemployment, minority status, discrimination, isolation and role reversals affect the power dynamics between men and women (Bui & Morash, 1999; Narayan, 1995; West, 1998; Yick, 2001).

However, existing theories may not capture the realities of IPV in immigrant and refugee couples. In feminist theory, the focus is largely on factors that underlie the occurrence of violence—namely, gender inequality and male domination—but does not consider what happens at the level of the couple and what happens when couples migrate. For example, couples who migrate from traditional societies where patriarchal ideologies prevail may find themselves forced to confront more egalitarian notions of male-female relations. Theories of status inconsistency take change into consideration but have largely focused on the negative aspects of change on the power dynamics between men and women, rather than positive factors such as resiliency that may reduce the risk of IPV in immigrant and refugee couples.

Risk and Protective Factors

Factors associated with IPV have been well established in the literature and have been described as multifactorial and multi-level (Jewkes, 2002; Jewkes et al., 2002). In the ecological model proposed by the World Health Organization, risk factors at one level are mediated by those at other levels. Individual-level factors include socio-demographic characteristics such as young age, low income, lack of academic achievement or opportunity, witnessing or experiencing violence as a child, substance use problems and social isolation. Family-level factors include marital conflict, poor family functioning, male dominance, and the presence or absence of children. Community-level factors include support networks, community norms regarding violence, levels of unemployment, availability of weapons, and male and female attitudes toward violence. Societal-level factors include legislation on weapons and women and children's rights (World Health Organization, 2002).

There is a small but growing body of literature on risk factors associated with IPV in immigrant populations. Most of the research has focused on the negative effects of *change* following migration. For example, post-migration changes in income and status, gender roles and traditional supports have been associated with an increased risk of marital conflict and IPV (Krulfeld, 1994; Min, 2001; Morash et al., 2000; Tang & Oatley, 2002).

Less research has examined protective factors associated with marital conflict and IPV. Our research on post-migration changes in marital relationships following migration in the Ethiopian community in Toronto identified several positive changes following migration (Hyman et al., 2004). Newcomer couples reported improvements in communication and levels of intimacy following migration. Although dependency rooted in economic, psychological and social support has been identified as a key factor influencing IPV (Raj & Silverman, 2002), for some couples, the greater reliance on one another in the absence of traditional supports (i.e., family and friends) led to increased closeness (Hyman et al., 2004). These findings contribute new knowledge on risk and protective factors associated with IPV in immigrant and refugee communities. However, as this study did not directly examine the effect of these changes on IPV, further research is critical in this area.

Prevalence

According to the 1993 Statistics Canada Violence against Women Survey (Statistics Canada, 1993), 10 per cent of Canadian women 18 years of age and over experienced violence in the 12 months preceding the survey and 51 per cent had experienced physical or sexual assault since age 16. Spousal abuse from husbands or common-law partners was reported by 25 per cent of respondents reporting abuse. Data from the 1999 General Social Survey on Victimization, a national, cross-sectional telephone survey, indicated that an estimated eight per cent of Canadian women who were married or living common-law experienced violence committed by their partner on at least one occasion during the previous five-year period (Statistics Canada, 2000). The 2004 version of the General Social Survey (GSS) using the same survey methods and questions reported a one per cent change in prevalence with seven per cent of Canadian women experiencing violence on at least one occasion.

Less is known about the prevalence of IPV among Canadian immigrant and refugee women (Cohen et al., 2002; Cohen & Maclean, 2003). Reports suggest that immigrant women in Canada experience slightly lower rates of IPV compared to Canadian-born women and that there are no significant differences in rates of IPV between visible minority and non-visible minority women (Cohen & Maclean, 2003). However, little research has examined the prevalence of IPV within sub-groups of immigrant women or assessed whether prevalence rates change over time.

Recently, data from the 1999 GSS were used to examine the effect of immigrant length of stay in Canada on IPV while controlling for socio-cultural and other factors associated with IPV. Although the GSS should be used cautiously and has been critiqued for both failing to capture the full extent of violence against women in Canada and for excluding particular groups of racialized women (Jiwani, 2000), analyses by Hyman et al. (2006) found that the crude prevalence of IPV was similar in recent and non-recent immigrant women. However, after controlling for socio-cultural and other factors associated with IPV, the risk of IPV was significantly lower among recent immigrant women compared to their non-recent counterparts. The issue, however, is complex. No studies have specifically examined differences in prevalence rates between immigrant and refugee women.

Added complications arise when it is recognized that, despite attempts to develop common definitions of IPV, differences persist in the definition and/or acknowledgment of what constitutes abuse across settings and circumstances. This poses a significant problem in determining the numbers of women who experience abuse within the context of an intimate relationship (Backman, 1998). Further, complications arise in assessing prevalence since not all abused women acknowledge or define their experiences with their partners as abusive. The extremes of the definition of abuse may be easy to identify but language limits our ability to label grey areas (Burge, 1998). When aggression does not fall into accepted views of abuse, women may not have the language to describe it and ask for help. Immigrant and refugee women may particularly struggle to name and define their experiences as abusive due to different understandings and experiences about normative male-female relations and familial roles, differing customs and beliefs governing acceptable and unacceptable behaviours, and varying levels of familiarity with concepts of abuse. In fact, correctly identifying, naming and labelling abuse as abuse is a significant step in the journey to begin to be less controlled by the abuser (Anderson, 2003).

We speculated that prevalence rates did increase with length of stay as immigrant women learned to recognize acts as abusive and developed the language to identify and speak about their experiences. However, this was not borne out in our study with Tamil women; they recognized acts of abuse but experienced significant barriers in deciding to disclose or seek help. In particular, community prohibitions on separation and divorce, and the associated stigma and isolation of women who leave their marriage, create insupportable conditions for many women. Furthermore, in a community that believes in arranged marriages, the future hopes and marital prospects for children of women who are separated or divorced are compromised.

Health Impacts

The impacts of IPV are well established and include physical, psychological, social and economic consequences.

Women with a history of IPV report 60 per cent higher rates of all health problems than do women with no history of abuse (Campbell et al., 2002). IPV victims report ongoing health problems, such as chronic pain, gastrointestinal disorders and irritable bowel syndrome, which can interfere with or limit daily functioning (Heise & Garcia-Moreno, 2002). IPV can also affect reproductive health and can lead to pelvic pain, sexual and gynecological disorders, unwanted pregnancy, premature labour and birth, and sexually transmitted diseases including HIV/AIDS (Heise et al., 1995; Plichta & Abraham, 1996; Schei, 1990; Schei & Bakketeig, 1989).

In addition to physical injuries and chronic conditions, IPV is associated with poor mental health, symptoms of posttraumatic stress disorder (PTSD), depression and anxiety (Coker et al., 2002; Jaffe et al., 1986). In fact, depression is considered to be the most pervasive negative mental health outcome, with severity of abuse significantly correlated to severity of depression (Dienemann et al., 2000). People are most likely to become depressed when they experience feelings of loss and defeat, especially in situations involving an intimate tie and situations that engender feelings of entrapment and humiliation and losses of autonomy, control and self-esteem (Resnick et al., 1997).

According to Astbury (2005), knowledge is growing on the defining social variables and critical characteristics of situations that trigger depression. At least one study has shown that stigma can be a determinant of emotional distress (Bennetts et al., 1999). Women with a history of IPV are also more likely to adopt behaviours that present further health risk, such as alcohol or other substance use problems, and increased risk of suicide attempts (Coker et al., 2000).

In terms of social consequences, women in violent relationships have been found to be restricted in the way they gain access to services, take part in public life and receive emotional support from friends and relatives (Heise & Garcia-Moreno, 2002). Therefore, women who have experienced IPV are more likely to have health problems, encounter spells of unemployment and receive welfare (Lloyd & Taluc, 1999). In addition to affecting women's health and well-being, researchers report that children who witness IPV are at greater risk of developmental problems, school failure, violence against others and low self-esteem. They are also more likely to develop psychiatric disorders and other psychopathologies (Appleyard & Osofsky, 2003; Nelson et al., 2004).

IPV also entails enormous costs to society in terms of health, law enforcement, community and legal services. Estimates for the annual cost for medical treatment of all forms of violence against women in Canada range from $408 million Cdn (Greaves et al., 1995) to $1.5 billion Cdn (Day, 1995). Women who have been abused are known to use health services at rates higher than do women who have not been abused, including higher rates of physician visits, emergency room visits and hospitalizations (Kernic et al., 2000; Moeller et al., 1993; Wisner et al., 1999). Women who have been emotionally abused report more symptoms and somatic disturbances and make more medical visits than non-abused women (Wagner & Mongan, 1998).

Less is known about the consequences of IPV among immigrant and refugee women. The forms of violence experienced by immigrant women may include those from the social context (i.e., racism) and may be amplified by pre-existing belief systems. The erosion of self-esteem accompanying IPV may be compounded in women who aren't fluent in English or French and who have lost traditional support networks. Add to this the effects of part-time, temporary and low-paid employment on self-esteem, and the health impacts of IPV may be difficult to disentangle from other aspects of immigrant women's experience. Nonetheless, one might surmise that the adverse health effects are similar to those experienced by non-immigrant women, although they may be exacerbated by longer delays in disclosure of the abuse (Astbury et al., 2000) and by experiences of violence beyond the context of the intimate relationship. Sexual assault, abduction, sexual abuse, harassment and/or the obligation to grant sexual favours in return for food or necessary legal papers during the migration process may be associated with posttraumatic stress disorder and may further complicate the experience of IPV for refugee women (Oxman-Martinez et al., 2000). However, there has been little empirical research in this area.

Barriers to Help-Seeking

Despite the serious adverse impact of IPV on women's health, studies suggest that many women do not seek help from health care providers and community services (Henning & Klesges, 2002). Findings from the 1999 General Social Survey on Victimization suggested that only half of Canadian women experiencing IPV sought help from social services (Du Mont et al., 2005). It is likely that many factors influence women's decisions to disclose and/or seek help, including severity and frequency of abuse, fear, shame, availability and accessibility of help, and impact on children (Coker et al., 2000; Kaukinen, 2002; Yoshioka et al., 2003). Women who experience IPV may also rely more heavily on informal sources of support (e.g., from family and friends) than formal sources of support (Kaukinen, 2002; Kershner & Anderson, 2002).

When we conducted a literature review on access and barriers to help-seeking for immigrant women, we found relatively little research on help-seeking for IPV among immigrant and refugee women. Reports using focus groups and key informant data consistently suggest that immigrant and refugee women in Canada underuse medical and legal services, shelters and hotlines compared to abused women in the majority population (MacLeod & Shin, 1993; Smith, 2004). This has been attributed to multiple and intersecting barriers that immigrant women face in accessing help. These barriers include those encountered by women in the majority population as well as legal, contextual and cultural barriers (Bui, 2003; MacLeod, 1992; Musisi & Muktar, 1991; Raj & Silverman, 2002; Smith, 2004). The following sections discuss each of these barriers.

LEGAL

Immigrant women often arrive in Canada as dependants of their spouses or as individuals sponsored by their family or spouse. Abusive spouses often use sponsorship obligations to assert power and control within the family (Jiwani, 2001). Women who are visitors (international students, temporary workers, tourists) and wives of visitors are also vulnerable because they have no legal or permanent status in Canada while their immigration applications are being processed. Women without refugee or landed immigrant status do not have access to health care, social assistance or subsidized housing (Jiwani, 2001). According to MacLeod and Shin (1993), even in cases where women sponsored their husbands, fear of deportation, of having children taken away, of jeopardizing potential applications for citizenship and of not being able to sponsor extended family members deterred immigrant women from seeking help.

CONTEXTUAL

Barriers that relate to the immigrant context include lack of knowledge of services, lack of language-specific services or resources, lack of culturally appropriate services, racism and fears of becoming involved with the Canadian legal system as a result of experience with repressive regimes in the country of origin (Moussa, 1993; Raj & Silverman, 2002). Several studies highlight the need for more staff training on minority issues and culturally sensitive practice methods, including the use of culturally consistent ideology and language (Huisman, 1996; Loue & Faust, 1998; West, 1998; Yick, 1999). Resources available to women who experience IPV may vary greatly according to culture and class (Agnew, 1998).

CULTURAL

There are many different definitions and starting points for a discussion about culture, which the *Merriam-Webster Dictionary* (2006) defines as:

> a: . . . the integrated pattern of human knowledge, belief, and behavior that depends upon the capacity for learning and transmitting knowledge to succeeding generations b: the customary beliefs, social forms, and material traits of a racial, religious, or social group . . . c: the set of shared attitudes, values, goals, and practices that characterizes an institution or organization.

Cultural barriers are those social constructs, such as patriarchal ideology and family values/filial piety, collectivism and religious beliefs, that may make it difficult for abused women to seek help.

Patriarchal ideology refers to the accompanying set of beliefs that justifies and maintains a system of social organization of male domination over women (Sugarman & Frankel, 1996). In patriarchal communities, the husband is culturally accepted as ruler of the family, regarded as the formal authority and permitted to use force to ensure the compliance of his wife and children (Haj-Yahia, 1998). Traditional gender roles may keep women isolated and dependent, reducing their options for separation and/or remarriage (Raj & Silverman, 2002).

In collectivist communities, values emphasizing family ties, harmony and order prevail and individuals are taught to subordinate the self to the interests of the family and community (Ho, 1990). Women are also taught that the intact family is best for children (Bui & Morash, 1999). As a result, many women are reluctant to disclose incidents of abuse for fear of being ostracized or stigmatized or of having their children ostracized or stigmatized (Smith, 2004). Among Mexican women, concern for the well-being of children was a more important deciding factor in whether to stay or leave an abusive relationship than were resident status, money concerns or language barriers (Acevedo, 2000). Our research in the Tamil community in Toronto also finds that Tamil women believe that the presence of children should influence a woman's response to IPV—that is, whether or not she should tolerate the abuse (Hyman et al., 2006; Mason et al., in press).

For many immigrant communities, religion is central to maintaining their cultural identity. Religious beliefs may also dictate responses to IPV (Smith, 2004). Although within any religion individuals vary in their practices from those who are more liberal to those who rigidly adhere to religious tracts, the writings from several religions (e.g., Catholicism, Confucianism, Islam) emphasize the sacred nature of the marriage bond while reinforcing male superiority and dominance (Sorenson, 1996).

In order to respond appropriately to the needs of immigrant and refugee women who experience IPV, barriers, including legal, contextual and cultural barriers, must be addressed.

Implications for Mental Health Professionals

Since women who experience IPV use health services more frequently than women who have not been abused, health professionals have a critical role to play in identifying, assessing, responding to and preventing IPV. Given the complexity and intersecting issues facing immigrant women who experience IPV, health professionals need to be knowledgeable about IPV in general, willing to learn about the specific meanings of IPV within a woman's cultural context, respect her expertise and be able to work collaboratively with her and others (e.g., other health professionals, police, child protection workers) to determine appropriate actions. As in any clinical encounter with a client from a background different from the clinician's own, clinicians must be aware of their own biases and guard against ethnocentrism.

IDENTIFICATION AND ASSESSMENT

Many health-related accreditation bodies in North America recommend screening female patients for IPV (see Clark & Du Mont, 2003; Waalen et al., 2000). According to epidemiological definitions, the word "screening" is used to indicate a test that can detect a target condition even when there are no apparent symptoms *and* when early detection is likely to lead to a favourable health outcome (Lilienfeld & Lilienfeld, 1980). Thus, both detection and a positive response to a given, available treatment need to be present to meet the criteria for screening. Pap smears are a common illustration of a screen for cervical cancer. However, screening for IPV differs from conventional screening in a number of significant ways:

- Not all individuals experiencing ipv can be detected because the individuals themselves choose whether or not to disclose the abuse.
- When screening for IPV, early detection does not necessarily lead to early treatment and a better health outcome because the condition is the result of another person's actions.
- Women who experience IPV may not acknowledge or understand that their relationship is abusive. Coming to that recognition may in itself be a long-term process.

Despite being significantly different from most other conditions for which screening is appropriate, health care professionals continue to use the word *screening* to describe the act of asking individuals about ipv.

Whether called screening or assessment, health care professionals should be alert for cues that indicate where a woman is in her journey and should develop appropriate strategies to respond to and support the woman's decision in whatever action she is willing to pursue.

Many different tools are being used to identify women who have experienced ipv. Most tools rely on direct inquiry using a single question or a series of questions, such as, "How do you and your partner resolve arguments? Have you ever been hurt, physically or psychologically, by someone close to you?" Some tools include an introductory statement, for example, "No matter how well couples get along, there are times when they have spats or fights because they're in a bad mood or tired, or for some other reason. They also use many different ways of trying to settle their differences." Other tools are framed in ways that let women know their experiences may be common; for example, "Because violence is so common in women's lives and because there is help available for women being abused, I now ask every patient about domestic violence." Few studies have examined the validity, reliability or acceptability of screening tools in other languages and with non-English-speaking populations and no research has been conducted on newcomer women's preferences regarding methods of screening. Studies on breast and cervical cancer screening suggest that cultural factors such as gender of physician, embarrassment and modesty influence women's preferences. This was true in studies examining barriers to breast and cancer screening among Chinese and Vietnamese women (Hyman et al., 2003; McPhee et al., 1996).

 Since there is insufficient evidence for the universal screening of all women for ipv, *indicator-based screening* is often used. Indicator-based screening refers to maintaining a heightened level of suspicion to red flags or indicators of risk for ipv. For example, abused women may report elevated levels of anxiety, depression, suicide attempts and posttraumatic stress disorder (Carlson et al., 2002; Golding, 2002) and use more sedatives and sleeping pills than women who have not experienced ipv (Groeneveld & Shain, 1989). Other suggestive red flags include cancelled appointments, especially if the partner has made the call; frequent or early prescription renewals; frequent "accidents" causing injury; a partner who does not want her to be seen alone; and an unexplained exacerbation of an existing chronic condition. In addition, women with unemployed partners and or partners with an alcohol or other drug problem may be at increased risk of ipv (Wathen et al., 2007). Women who are in abusive relationships become increasingly vulnerable during life cycle phases such as pregnancy and postpartum periods. Health care providers should be alert for cues that may suggest increased violence; for example, the woman may express fear of going home, she may worry about her own safety and that of her infant or she may have such obvious signs as bruising, scratches or bleeding.

Mental health professionals need to be aware of well-documented patient and professional-related barriers to identifying IPV:

- Not all women recognize certain behaviours as abusive (Chang, 2001; Zink et al., 2004). Immigrant and refugee women in particular may struggle to name and define their experiences as abusive due to different understandings and experiences about normative male-female relations and familial roles, differing customs and beliefs governing acceptable and unacceptable behaviours, and varying levels of familiarity with concepts of abuse.

- Women who experience IPV are reluctant to disclose for many reasons. These include denial, shock, shame, embarrassment, lack of trust in the doctor, fear of retaliation, financial constraints, protection of the abuser, fear the police will be informed and fear of losing child custody (AMA Council on Scientific Affairs, 1992; Loring & Smith, 1994; Mazza et al., 1996; Rodriguez et al., 1999; McCauley et al., 1998; Peckover, 2003; Rodriguez et al., 1998). Immigrant and refugee women may experience additional barriers to disclosure including previous experiences of violence and trauma, fear of losing their immigrant status or a breakdown of their sponsorship agreement, lack of familiarity with the dominant language and culture, loss of status for the family, stigma and community censure (Bauer et al., 2000; Canadian Council on Social Development, 2001; MacLeod & Shin, 1993; Rodriguez et al., 2001).

- Health professionals themselves may be reluctant to identify women who experience IPV. Studies suggest that lack of training, time constraints, incomplete knowledge of prevalence and treatment, and lack of interest and sympathy are key issues contributing to health care provider reluctance in asking about IPV. Sugg and Inui (1992) identified several additional barriers to screening, including fear of opening a "Pandora's box," discomfort with screening patients of a similar educational or economic background to themselves, fear of offending a patient or violating her privacy and frustration with patients' lack of willingness to take action.

Nonetheless, a recent review of the literature reported that between 43 per cent and 96 per cent of women who are asked direct questions about IPV agreed that such questions were acceptable and important to ask in health care settings so that those needing help receive it (Ramsay et al., 2002). Similar results were found in two American qualitative studies of Latina, Asian and African-American women (Rodriguez et al., 1998, 2001). In fact, most women disclosed IPV when asked (Rodriguez et al., 1998) and reported that being asked helped them recognize the issue, reduced their sense of isolation and secrecy, validated their feelings and initiated a process of change (Chang & Martin, 2001).

RESPONDING TO DISCLOSURE

Studies on women's desired responses following disclosure suggest they want health professionals to ask direct questions about IPV, listen and validate the woman's experience, express concern, and be non-judgmental and supportive (Bacchu et al., 2002; Bauer & Rodriquez, 1995; Campbell & Campbell, 1995; Levin, 1992; Rodriguez et al., 1996). However, while the act of disclosing abuse to a health professional may be considered an intervention in that it can reduce isolation and validate women's experiences (Gerbert et al., 1996, 1999; Krasnoff & Moscati, 2002), many experts agree that the effective management of IPV requires more than simple identification (Garcia-Moreno, 2002; Glass et al., 2001; Waalen et al., 2000). Therefore, health professionals need to be aware of recommended procedures following the disclosure of IPV, including documentation, risk assessment, safety planning, mandatory reporting and providing referrals. The next sections discuss each of these procedures.

Documentation

Once a disclosure has been made, health care professionals are responsible for documenting the encounter according to the guidelines established by the governing college. Documentation serves many purposes, including creating a historical record for medico-legal purposes, chronicling the development or change of existing or new conditions, and creating a venue for developing treatment plans. In cases of IPV, careful documentation is a key component of an effective health care response (Collège des Médecins du Québec, 2005; Ferris et al., 1997), and the record may be subpoenaed for court proceedings in criminal or family court proceedings.

As with any chart, clear, legible notes and the date and time of day are required. Factual information should be included and conjecture or summary statements avoided. Terms or phrases that suggest or imply doubt about the patient's reliability, such as "the patient claims . . . " or "the patient alleges . . . " (Isaac & Pualani, 2001), should be avoided. When possible, the patient or client's own words should be used. When feelings of personal responsibility or guilt are expressed and are documented, the notes should also include reference to how common such feelings are in women who experience IPV (MacDonald, 2005). When English is not the patient's first language, or if the interview is conducted through an interpreter, it is also important to note this. For obvious reasons, family members should not be used as interpreters.

Risk Assessment

Risk assessments are used to appraise the present level of risk for injury or homicide. The individual's own sense of safety should not be the sole criteria for assuming she is not in danger, as women often underestimate the risk they face. To conduct a risk assessment, practitioners should inquire about any escalation in severity or in frequency of violence, the presence of a gun or other weapon in the home, or changes to other circumstances (e.g., a recent or impending separation, threats uttered, increased alcohol or other drug use). The presence of any of these factors may indicate the need for immediate action including providing referrals to local shelters and legal counsel. Often completing a risk assessment with a client allows her to appraise her situation differently; at minimum, it informs her of the gravity of the issue to the practitioner. (For an example of a risk assessment tool, see www.dangerassessment.org.)

Health professionals should also assess all women disclosing IPV for depression and suicide risk (Cherniak et al., 2005).

Safety Planning

Safety planning is a critical part of the clinical encounter for women who disclose IPV. Health professionals need to work with women to think through the details of what would be done and where help could be found should there be further episodes of violence. For example, measures that can be taken to prepare for further violence may include developing a code with children or neighbours to let them know that police assistance is required. During violent episodes, safety can be increased by making as much noise as possible, by avoiding conflict in rooms with a single exit or rooms where there are weapons available such as the kitchen, where there could be knives. Many organizations advise women to prepare a suitcase and leave it at a friend's home along with important papers, a change of clothes and special comfort items for children if she must leave during a crisis. When developing a safety plan for an immigrant woman, there may be additional issues to consider. For example, she may not be fluent in English, know her neighbours or have any friends apart from her husband and his friends. Safety plans may need to consider strategies to counter her isolation and to deal with possible community stigma about separation and divorce.

Mandatory Reporting

In Canada there is no mandate to report IPV to the police or other authorities unless children are involved. Although the duty to report IPV to child protection services varies from province to province, in all jurisdictions when there are concerns about a child's safety and well-being, a report must be made to the appropriate child protection agency. In Ontario, for example, there is a duty to report any situation involving a child under 16 years where there are "reasonable grounds" to suspect physical, sexual and/or emotional abuse; neglect; and/or risk of harm. Therefore, in Ontario children may be considered to be "at risk" of emotional harm and in need of protection when they have witnessed IPV.

Referral

Studies exploring women's desired responses from health professionals following disclosure suggest that women want referrals to shelters, counselling, and social and legal services (Bacchu et al., 2002; Bauer & Rodriguez, 1995; Campbell & Campbell, 1995; Levin, 1992; Rodriguez et al., 1996) as well as to organizations that provide advocacy, job training and financial support (Petersen et al., 2003). Less is known about immigrant and refugee women's desired responses; however, in a study of Canadian women fluent in neither English nor French, focus group participants emphasized the desire for practical referrals and sources of help (MacLeod & Shin, 1993). Health care professionals should be knowledgeable about resources from which they can make appropriate selections of agencies that are best suited to respond to a woman's situation. (See Chapter 7 for a discussion of services for women who have immigrated to Canada).

PREVENTION

When considering primary prevention of IPV in the general population or immigrant communities, it is important to recognize the need for prevention at the level of the individual, couple, community and society.

Primary prevention of IPV can be considered at each of the same levels as proposed in the ecological model of violence (World Health Organization, 2002) and discussed in the section on risk and protective factors on page 281.

Individual

Until recently, most interventions for IPV have largely focused on the individual. These included reactive interventions, such as crisis management, emergency care, shelters and criminal justice against perpetrators. Proactive primary prevention measures at this level would also include early diagnosis and treatment of psychological or personality disorders, addictions and substance abuse, early intervention in order to minimize either children's aggression or victimization and supportive parenting programs in order that children are raised in violence-free families.

Couple

At the level of the relationship, primary prevention interventions include early education about healthy relationships, culturally appropriate couples' counselling, and strengthening the couples' connections to the community to ensure there is adequate social support and to minimize the risk of women's isolation. Service providers should ideally work in partnership with community-based organizations to develop culturally appropriate education and counselling strategies. Providers should also work to establish programs for young men and women about healthy dating relationships, responsible fatherhood programs and programs to steer boys away from violence.

Community

At the community level, primary prevention includes working toward strong socially supportive and safe communities with adequate income levels and minimal unemployment amongst its members. When added to other immigrant-related stressors, financial hardship can undermine healthy relationships. Interventions designed to help Canadian employers recognize international training, work experience and expertise would help to alleviate some of the stress facing immigrant couples. Providing recreational facilities, including parks and playgrounds that support ongoing interactions among community members and allow for the early detection of things going amiss, may also be considered a primary prevention. Service providers should work with ethnocultural community organizations to develop and support community-based initiatives to reduce and prevent IPV. These should include developing, supporting and/or maintaining community capacity building; gathering information on culturally appropriate responses to IPV; and developing community-specific messages about IPV.

Public education and media campaigns need to be developed and targeted to specific communities, using imagery and messages that are acceptable to community members. For example, an Australian study found that in contrast to the images frequently used in violence prevention campaigns, racialized women did not want to see negative images of battered women; rather, they wanted an increased emphasis on positive values and to see images of happy families demonstrating strong family units, community, and social ownership of the issue (Moore et al., 2002). A violence-prevention project conducted by the Family Service Association of Toronto with four newcomer communities highlighted the need for community-specific media messages and dissemination strategies. For example, one community used a short film that was shown in movie theatres, another developed print materials in the form of a booklet and another chose to use public service announcements on the radio.

Society

In the broader social context, we must work to ensure that immigrant women are not triply victimized by their race, gender and immigration status. One priority is to educate policy-makers about the ramifications of existing legislation that makes it impossible for some women to leave abusive relationships. Additionally, we must work toward formal policies and informal values, both locally and nationally, that condemn violence against women. We must ensure that for those who do experience IPV or other forms of violence, there is culturally sensitive, appropriate and timely access to services, including legal counsel. Ultimately, it is not just an individual but also a collective responsibility to prevent IPV and its often devastating consequences.

Conclusion

This chapter looked at various aspects of IPV—from examining possible causes, to assessing the prevalence of this form of violence, to looking at barriers to women seeking help and, perhaps most importantly, determining how health professionals can help.

Identifying women who have experienced IPV is only the first step. Once mental health professionals know that a woman has experienced violence from a partner or someone else she trusts, they need to assess whether she is safe. And they need to provide the woman with referrals to services that help to support newcomer women.

While reports indicate that immigrant women in Canada may not experience IPV to quite the same extent as Canadian-born women, this may reflect a difficulty newcomer women have in disclosing histories of abuse. We need to not only help women to tell their stories, but find ways to prevent this kind of violence from occurring.

References

Acevedo, M. (2000). The role of acculturation in explaining ethnic differences in the prenatal health-risk behaviors, mental health, and parenting beliefs of Mexican American and European American at-risk women. *Child Abuse & Neglect, 24,* 111–127.

Agnew, V. (1998). *In Search of a Safe Place: Abused Women and Culturally Sensitive Services.* Toronto: University of Toronto Press.

American Medical Association Council on Scientific Affairs. (1992). Violence against women: Relevance for medical practitioners. *Journal of the American Medical Association, 267* (23), 3184–3189.

Anderson, D.J. (2003). The impact on subsequent violence of returning to an abusive partner. *Journal of Comparative Family Studies, 34* (1), 93–112.

Appleyard, K. & Osofsky, J.D. (2003). Parenting after trauma: Supporting parents and caregivers in the treatment of children impacted by violence. *Infant Mental Health Journal, 24* (2), 111–125.

Astbury, J.A. (2005). Women's mental health: From hysteria to human rights. In S. Romans & M.V. Seeman (Eds.), *Women's Mental Health* (pp. 377–392). Philadelphia: Lippincott Williams & Wilkins.

Astbury, J., Atkinson, J., Duke, J.E., Easteal, P.L., Kurrie, S.E., Tait, P.R. et al. (2000). The impact of domestic violence on individuals. *The Medical Journal of Australia, 173* (8), 427–431.

Bacchu, L., Mezey, G. & Bewley, S. (2002). Women's perceptions and experiences of routine enquiry for domestic violence in a maternity service. *British Journal of Obstetrics and Gynaecology, 109,* 9–16.

Backman, R. (1998). Incidence rates of violence against women: A comparison of the redesigned National Crime Victimization Survey and of the 1985 National Family Violence Survey. Available: http://new.vawnet.org/category/Main_Doc.php?docid=385. Accessed January 15, 2008.

Bauer, H.M. & Rodriquez, M.A. (1995). Letting compassion open the door: Battered women's disclosure to medical providers. *Cambridge Quarterly of Healthcare, 4,* 459–465.

Bauer, H., Rodriguez, M., Quiroga, S. & Flores-Ortiz, Y. (2000). Barriers to health care for abused Latina and Asian immigrant women. *Journal of Health Care for the Poor and Underserved, 11,* 33–44.

Bennetts, A., Shaffer, N., Manopaiboon, C., Chaiyakul, P., Siriwasin, W., Mock, P. et al. (1999). Determinants of depression and HIV-related worry among HIV-positive women who have recently given birth, Bangkok, Thailand. *Social Science & Medicine, 49* (6), 737–749.

Bui, H. (2003). Help-seeking behavior among abused immigrant women. *Violence against Women, 9,* 207–239.

Bui, H.N. & Morash, M. (1999). Domestic violence in the Vietnamese immigrant community: An exploratory study. *Violence against Women, 5,* 769–795.

Burge, S.K. (1998). How do you define abuse? Practice commentary. *Archives of Family Medicine, 7,* 31–32.

Campbell, J.C. (1992). Prevention of wife battering: Insights from cultural analysis. *Response, 14,* 18–24.

Campbell, J. & Campbell, D. (1995). The influence of abuse on pregnancy intention. *Women's Health Issues, 5,* 214–223.

Campbell, J., Jones, A., Dienemann, J., Kub, J., O'Campo, P., Gielen, A.C. et al. (2002). Intimate partner violence and physical health consequences. *Archives of Internal Medicine, 162* (10), 1157–1163.

Canadian Council on Social Development. (2001). *The Progress of Canada's Children.* Ottawa: Canadian Council on Social Development.

Carlson, B.E., McNutt, L-A., Choi, D.Y. & Rose, I.M. (2002). Intimate partner abuse and mental health: The role of social support and other protective factors. *Violence against Women, 8* (6), 720–745.

Chang, J. (2001, October). *When health care providers ask about intimate partner violence: A description of outcomes from the perspective of female survivors.* Abstract presented at the 129th annual meeting of the American Public Health Association, Atlanta, GA.

Chang, J. & Martin, S. (2001). What happens when health care providers ask about intimate partner violence? A description of consequences from the perspectives of female survivors. *Journal of the American Medical Women's Association, 58,* 76–81.

Chard, J., Badets, J. & Howatson-Lee, L. (2000). *Women in Canada: A Gender-Based Statistical Report.* Ottawa: Statistics Canada.

Cherniak, D., Grant, L., Mason, R., Moore, B. & Pellizzari, R. (2005). Intimate partner violence consensus statement. *Journal of Obstetricians and Gynaecologists of Canada, 27,* 365–383.

Citizenship and Immigration Canada. (2005). *You Asked about Immigration and Citizenship.* Ottawa: Minister of Public Works and Government Services. Available: www.cic.gc.ca/enGLIsh/pdf/pub/youasked.pdf. Accessed January 5, 2008.

Clark, J. & Du Mont, J. (2003). Intimate partner violence and health. *Canadian Journal of Public Health, 94,* 52–63.

Cohen, M. & Maclean, H. (2003). Violence against Canadian women. In M. Desmeules, D. Stewart, A. Kazanjian, H. Maclean, J. Payne & B. Vissandjée (Eds.), *Women's Health Surveillance Report: A Multidimensional Look at the Health of Canadian Women.* Ottawa: Canadian Institute for Health Information. Available: www.phac-aspc.gc.ca/publicat/whsr-rssf/pdf/CPHI_WomensHealth_e.pdf. Accessed January 15, 2008.

Cohen, M., Schei, B., Ansara, D., Gallop, R., Stuckless, N. & Stewart, D.E. (2002). A history of personal violence and postpartum depression: Is there a link? *Archives of Women's Mental Health, 4,* 83–92.

Coker, A., Davis, K., Arias, I., Desai, S., Sanderson, M., Brandt, H. et al. (2002). Physical and mental health effects of intimate partner violence for men and women. *American Journal of Preventive Medicine, 23,* 260–268.

Coker, A., Smith, P., Bethea, L., King, M.R. & McKeown, R. (2000). Physical health consequences of physical and psychological intimate partner violence. *Archives of Family Medicine, 9,* 451–457.

Collège des Médecins du Québec. (2005). *La tenue des dossiers par le médecin en centre hospitalier de soins généraux et ̣ialisés: Guide d'exercice.* Available: www.cmq.org/DocumentLibrary/Uploaded Contents/CmsDocuments/Guide-tenue-dossiers-hosp.pdf. Accessed January 15, 2008.

Day, T. (1995). *The Health-Related Costs of Violence against Women in Canada.* London, ON: Centre for Research on Violence against Women.

Dienemann, J., Boyle, E., Baker, D., Resnick, W., Wiederhorn, N. & Campbell, J. (2000). Intimate partner abuse among women diagnosed with depression. *Issues in Mental Health Nursing, 21,* 499–513.

Dobash, R.E. & Dobash, R. (1979). *Violence against Wives: A Case against the Patriarchy.* New York: Free Press.

Du Mont, J., Forte, T., Cohen, M., Hyman, I. & Romans, S. (2005). Changing help-seeking rates for intimate partner violence in Canada. *Women & Health, 41* (1), 1–19.

Ferris, L., McMain-Klein, M. & Silver, L. (1997). Documenting wife abuse: A guide for physicians. *Canadian Medical Association Journal, 156,* 1015–1022.

Garcia-Moreno, C. (2002). Dilemmas and opportunities for an appropriate health-service response to violence against women. *Lancet, 359* (9316), 1509–1514.

Gelles, R. (1993). Through a sociological lens: Social structure and family violence. In R. Gelles & D. Loseke (Eds.), *Current Controversies on Family Violence* (pp. 31–46). Newbury Park, CA: Sage.

Gerbert, B., Bronstone, A., Pantilat, S., McPhee, S., Allerton, M. & Moe, J. (1999). When asked, patients tell: Disclosure of sensitive health-risk behaviors. *Medical Care, 37*, 104–111.

Gerbert, B., Johnston, K., Caspers, N., Bleecker, T., Woods, A. & Rosenbaum, A. (1996). Experiences of battered women in health care settings: A qualitative study. *Women & Health, 24*, 1–17.

Glass, N., Dearwater, S. & Campbell, J. (2001). Intimate partner violence screening and intervention: Data from eleven Pennsylvania and California community hospital emergency departments. *Journal of Emergency Nursing 27* (2), 141–149.

Golding, J. (2002). Intimate partner violence as a risk factor for mental disorders: A meta-analysis. *Journal of Family Violence, 14*, 99–132.

Goode, W.J. (1971). Force and violence in the family. *Journal of Marriage and the Family, 33*, 624–636.

Greaves, E., Hankivsky, O. & Kingston-Riechers, J. (1995). *Selected Estimates of the Costs of Violence against Women.* London, ON: Centre for Research on Violence against Women and Children.

Groeneveld, J. & Shain, M. (1989). *Drug Abuse among Victims of Physical and Sexual Abuse: A Preliminary Report.* Toronto: Addiction Research Foundation.

Haj-Yahia, M.M. (1998). Beliefs about wife beating among Palestinian women: The influence of their patriarchal ideology. *Violence against Women, 4* (5), 533–558.

Heise, L. & Garcia-Moreno, C. (2002). *Violence by Intimate Partners: World Report on Violence and Health.* Geneva: World Health Organization.

Heise, L., Moore, K. & Toubia, N. (1995). *Sexual Coercion and Reproductive Health: A Focus on Research.* New York: Population Council.

Henning, K. & Klesges, L. (2002). Utilization of counseling and supportive services by female victims of domestic abuse. *Violence and Victims, 17*, 623–636.

Ho, C.K. (1990). An analysis of domestic violence in Asian American communities: A multicultural approach to counseling. *Women & Therapy, 9* (1–2), 129–150.

Huisman, K. (1996). Wife battering in Asian American communities: Identifying the needs of an over-looked segment of our society. *Violence against Women, 2*, 260–283.

Hyman, I., Cameron, J.I., Singh, M. & Stewart, D.E. (2003). Physician-related determinants of cervical cancer screening among Chinese and Vietnamese women in Toronto. *Journal of Health Care for the Poor and Underserved, 14* (4), 489–502.

Hyman, I., Forte, T., Du Mont, J., Romans, S. & Cohen, M.M. (2006). The prevalence of intimate partner violence in immigrant women in Canada. *American Journal of Public Health, 96* (4), 654–659.

Hyman, I., Guruge, S., Mason, R., Stuckless, N., Gould, J., Tang, T. et al. (2004). Post-migration changes in gender relations among Ethiopian immigrant couples in Toronto. *Canadian Journal of Nursing Research, 36*, 74–89.

Hyman, I., Mason, R., Berman, H., Guruge, S., Kanagaratnam, P., Manuel, L. et al. (2006). Perceptions of and responses to intimate partner violence among Tamil women in Toronto. *Canadian Woman Studies, 25* (1 & 2), 145–150.

Isaac, N. & Pualani, E. (2001). *Documenting Domestic Violence: How Health Care Providers Can Help Victims.* Washington, DC: National Institute of Justice.

Jaffe, P., Wolfe, D.A., Wilson, S. & Zak, L. (1986). Emotional and physical health problems of battered women. *Canadian Journal of Psychiatry, 31* (7), 625–629.

Jewkes, R. (2002). Intimate partner violence: Causes and prevention. *Lancet, 359*, 1423–1429.

Jewkes, R., Levin, J. & Penn-Kekana, L. (2002). Risk factors for domestic violence: Findings from a South African cross-sectional study. *Social Science & Medicine, 55*, 1603–1617.

Jiwani, Y. (2000). The 1999 General Social Survey on spousal violence: An analysis. *Canadian Woman Studies, 20* (3), 34–40.

Jiwani, Y. (2001). *Intersecting Inequalities: Immigrant Women of Colour, Violence and Health Care.* Vancouver: The FREDA Centre for Research on Violence against Women and Children.

Kaukinen, C. (2002). The help-seeking of women violent crime victims: Findings from the Canadian Violence against Women Survey. *International Journal of Sociology and Social Policy, 22,* 5–44.

Kernic, M.A., Wolf, M.E. & Holt, V.L. (2000). Rates and relative risk of hospital admission among women in violent intimate partner relationships. *American Journal of Public Health, 90* (9), 1416–1420.

Kershner, M. & Anderson, J. (2002). Barriers to disclosure of abuse among rural women. *Minnesota Medicine, 83,* 32–37.

Krasnoff, M. & Moscati, R. (2002). Domestic violence screening and referral can be effective. *Annals of Emergency Medicine, 40,* 485–492.

Krulfeld, R.M. (1994). Changing concepts of gender roles and identities in refugee communities. In L. Camino & R.M. Krulfeld (Eds.), *Reconstructing Lives, Recapturing Meaning: Refugee Identity, Gender and Culture Change* (pp. 71–96). Washington, DC: Gordon and Breach Publishers.

Levin, S.B. (1992). *Hearing the Unheard: Stories of Women Who Have Been Battered.* Unpublished dissertation, The Union Institute, Cincinnati. Cited in Sleutel, M.R. (1998). Women's experiences of abuse: A review of qualitative research. *Issues in Mental Health Nursing, 19* (6), 525–539.

Lilienfeld, A.M. & Lilienfeld, D.E. (1980). *Foundations of Epidemiology* (2nd ed.). New York: Oxford University Press.

Lloyd, S. & Taluc, N. (1999). The effects of male violence on female employment. *Violence against Women, 5,* 370–392.

Loue, S. & Faust, M. (1998). *Intimate Partner Violence among Immigrants: Handbook of Immigrant Health.* New York: Plenum Press.

MacDonald, S. (2005, June). *Documenting woman abuse.* Paper presented at the Woman Abuse Council of Toronto Conference, Toronto.

MacLeod, L. (1992). *Counselling for Change: Evolutionary Trends in Counselling Services for Women Who Are Abused and for Their Children in Canada.* Ottawa: National Clearinghouse on Family Violence.

MacLeod, L. & Shin, M.Y. (1993). *"Like a Wingless Bird": A Tribute to the Survival and Courage of Women Who Are Abused and Who Speak Neither English nor French* (Report No. H72-21/110-1994E). Ottawa: Minister of Supply and Services Canada.

Mason, R., Hyman, I., Berman, H., Guruge, S., Kanaganatram, P., Manuel, L. "Violence is an international language": Tamil women's perceptions of Intimate Partner Violence. *Violence Against Women* (in press).

Mazza, D., Dennerstein, L. & Ryan, V. (1996). Physical, sexual and emotional violence against women: A general practice-based prevalence study. *Medical Journal of Australia, 164* (1), 14–17.

McCauley, J., Yurk, R., Jenckes, M. & Ford, D. (1998). Inside "Pandora's Box": Abused women's experiences with and perceptions of clinicians and health services. *Journal of General Internal Medicine, 13,* 549–555.

McPhee, S.J., Bird, J.A., Ha, N.T., Jenkins, C.N.H., Fordham, D. & Le, B. (1996). Pathways to early cancer detection for Vietnamese women: Suc khoe la vang! (Health is gold!). *Health Education Quarterly, 2,* s60–s75.

Merriam-Webster On-Line. (2006). Definition of culture. Available: www.m-w.com/dictionary/culture. Accessed January 15, 2008.

Min, P. (2001). Changes in Korean immigrants' gender role and social status, and their marital conflicts. *Sociological Forum, 16*, 301–320.

Moeller, T.P., Bachmann, G.A. & Moeller, J.R. (1993). The combined effects of physical, sexual, and emotional abuse during childhood: Long-term health consequences for women. *Child Abuse & Neglect, 17*, 623–640.

Moore, M., Lane D. & Connolly, A. (2002). *One NESB size does not fit all! What makes a health promotion campaign "culturally appropriate"?* Available: www.mmha.org.au/mmhaproducts/synergy/2002Autumn/OneSizeDoesNotFitAll. Accessed January 5, 2008.

Morash, M., Bui, H.N. & Santiago, A.M. (2000). Cultural-specific gender ideology and wife abuse in Mexican-descent families. *International Review of Victimology, 7*, 67–91.

Moussa, H. (1993). The social construction of women refugees: A journey of discontinuities and continuities. *Dissertation Abstracts International, 53* (12-A), 4213.

Musisi, N. & Muktar, F. (1991). *Exploratory Research: Wife Assault in Metropolitan Toronto's African Immigrant and Refugee Community.* Toronto: Canadian African Newcomer Aid Centre of Toronto.

Narayan, U. (1995). "Male-order" brides: Immigrant women, domestic violence and immigration law. *Hypatia, 10*, 104–119.

Nelson, H.D., Nygren, P., McInerney, Y. & Klein J. (2004). Screening women and elderly adults for family and intimate partner violence: A review of the evidence for the U.S. Preventive Services Task Force. *Annals of Internal Medicine, 140* (5), 387–396.

Oxman-Martinez, J., Abdool, S.N. & Loiselle-Leonard, M. (2000). Immigration, women and health in Canada. *Canadian Journal of Public Health, 91*, 394–395.

Peckover, S. (2003). I could have done with a little more help: An analysis of women's helpseeking from health visitors in the context of domestic violence. *Health & Social Care in the Community, 11*, 275–282.

Petersen, R., Moracco, K.E., Goldstein, K.M. & Clark, K.A. (2003). Women's perspectives on intimate partner violence services: The hope in Pandora's box. *Journal of the American Medical Women's Association, 58*, 185–190.

Plichta, S.B. & Abraham, C. (1996). Violence and gynecologic health in women <50 years old. *American Journal of Obstetrics and Gynecology, 174* (3), 903–907.

Raj, A. & Silverman, J. (2002). Violence against immigrant women: The roles of culture, context, and legal immigrant status on intimate partner violence. *Violence against Women, 8*, 367–398.

Ramsay, J., Richardson, J., Carter, Y., Davidson, L. & Feder, G. (2002). Should health professionals screen women for domestic violence? Systematic review. *British Medical Journal, 325*, 314–318B.

Resnick, H.S., Acierno, R. & Kilpatrick, D.G. (1997). Health impact of interpersonal violence. 2: Medical and mental health outcomes. *Behavioral Medicine, 23* (2), 65–78.

Rodriguez, M.A., Bauer, H., Flores-Ortiz, Y. & Szkupinski Quiroga, S. (1998). Factors affecting patient-physician communication for abused Latina and Asian immigrant women. *Journal of Family Practice, 47*, 309–311.

Rodriguez, M.A., Bauer, H., McLoughlin, E. & Grumbach, K. (1999). Screening and intervention for intimate partner abuse: Practices and attitudes of primary care physicians. *Journal of the American Medical Association, 282*, 468–474.

Rodriguez, M.A., Quiroga, S.S. & Bauer, H.M. (1996). Breaking the silence: Battered women's perspectives on medical care. *Archives of Family Medicine, 5*, 153–158.

Rodriguez, M., Sheldon, W., Bauer, H. & Perez-Stable, E. (2001). The factors associated with disclosure of intimate partner abuse to clinicians. *Journal of Family Practice, 50*, 338–344.

Saltzman, L.E., Fanslow, J.L., McMahon, P.M. & Shelley, G.A. (1999). *Intimate Partner Violence Surveillance: Uniform Definitions and Recommended Data Elements.* Atlanta, GA: National Center for Injury Prevention and Control.

Schei, B. (1990). Psychosocial factors in pelvic pain: A controlled study of women living in physically abusive relationships. *Acta Obstetricia et Gynecologica Scandinavica, 69,* 67–71.

Schei, B. & Bakketeig, L.S. (1989). Gynaecological impact of sexual and physical abuse by spouse: A study of a random sample of Norwegian women. *British Journal of Obstetrics and Gynaecology,* 96 (12), 1379–1383.

Smith, E. (2004). *Nowhere to Turn? Responding to Partner Violence against Immigrant and Visible Minority Women.* Ottawa: Canadian Council on Social Development.

Sorenson, S.B. (1996). Violence against women: Examining ethnic differences and commonalities. *Evaluation Review, 20* (2), 123–145.

Statistics Canada. (1993). *Violence against Women Survey* (Report No. 11-001E). Ottawa: Government of Canada.

Statistics Canada. (2000). *General Social Survey Cycle 13 Victimization* (Report No. 12M0013GPE). Ottawa: Government of Canada.

Straus, M., Gelles, R. & Steinmetz, S. (1980). *Behind Closed Doors: Violence in the American Family.* Garden City, NY: Anchor Press/Doubleday.

Sugarman, D.B. & Frankel, S.L. (1996). Patriarchal ideology and wife-assault: A meta-analytic review. *Journal of Family Violence, 11,* 13–40.

Sugg, N.K. & Inui, T. (1992). Primary care physician's response to domestic violence: Opening Pandora's box. *Journal of the American Medical Association, 267* (23), 3157–3160.

Tang, T. & Oatley, K. (2002, August). *Transition and engagement of life roles among Chinese immigrant women.* Poster Presentation at the American Psychological Association Annual Convention, Chicago, IL.

Tjaden, P. & Thoennes, N. (2000). *Extent, Nature, and Consequences of Intimate Partner Violence: Findings from the National Violence against Women Survey* (NCJ 181867). Washington, DC: U.S. Department of Justice.

United Nations. (1979). *Convention on the Elimination of All Forms of Discrimination against Women.* Available: www.un.org/womenwatch/daw/cedaw/text/econvention.htm. Accessed January 4, 2008.

United Nations. (1993). *Declaration on the Elimination of Violence against Women. Grand Assembly Resolution 48/104.* Available: www.unhchr.ch/Huridocda/Huridoca.nsf/0/42e7191fae543562c1256ba7 004e963c/$FILE/G0210428.doc. Accessed January 4, 2008.

Waalen, J., Goodwin, M.M., Spitz, A.M., Petersen, R. & Saltzman, L.E. (2000). Screening for intimate partner violence by health care providers: Barriers and interventions. *American Journal of Preventive Medicine, 19,* 230–237.

Wagner, P.J. & Mongan, P.F. (1998). Validating the concept of abuse: Women's perceptions of defining behaviors and the effects of emotional abuse on health indicators. *Archives of Family Medicine, 7,* 25–29.

Walker, L. (1979). *The Battered Woman.* New York: Harper and Row.

Wathen, N., Jamieson, E., Wilson, M., Daly, M., Worster, A., Macmillan, H. (2007). Risk indicators to identify intimate partner violence in the emergency department. *Open Medicine, 1* (2), E113–122.

West, C.M. (1998). Lifting the "political gag order." In J.L. Jasinski & L.M. Williams (Eds.), *Partner Violence: A Comprehensive Review of 20 Years of Research* (pp. 184–209). Thousand Oaks, CA: Sage Publications.

Wisner, C.L., Gilmer, T.P., Saltzman, L.E. & Zink, T.M. (1999). Intimate partner violence against women: Do victims cost health plans more? *Journal of Family Practice, 48*, 439–443.

Wolfgang, M. & Ferracuti, F. (1982). *The Subculture of Violence*. Thousand Oaks, CA: Sage Publications.

World Health Organization. (2002). *World Report on Violence and Health*. Geneva: Author.

Yick, A. (1999). Domestic violence in the Chinese American community: Cultural taboos and barriers. *Family Violence and Sexual Assault Bulletin, 15*, 16–23.

Yick, A.G. (2001). Feminist theory and status inconsistency theory: Application to domestic violence in Chinese immigrant families. *Violence against Women, 7*, 545–562.

Yick, A.G. & Agbayani-Siewert, P. (1997). Perceptions of domestic violence in a Chinese American community. *Journal of Interpersonal Violence, 12*, 832–846.

Yoshioka, M., Gilbert, L., El-Bassel, N. & Baig-Amin, M. (2003). Social support and disclosure of abuse: Comparing South Asian, African American, and Hispanic battered women. *Journal of Family Violence, 18*, 171–180.

Zink, T., Elder, N., Jacobson, J. & Klostermann, B. (2004). Medical management of intimate partner violence considering the stages of change: Precontemplation and contemplation. *American Family Medicine, 2*, 231–239.

Chapter 16

Postpartum Depression among Immigrant Women

PAOLA ARDILES, CINDY-LEE DENNIS AND LORI E. ROSS

The purpose of this chapter is to provide a review of the current literature on postpartum depression among immigrant women, and to provide recommendations for practice based on the principles of mental health promotion. We compare postpartum depression to postpartum mood disorders, which also include postpartum anxiety, psychosis and obsessive-compulsive disorder. The literature in this area uses multiple terms such as "postpartum depression" or "postnatal depression" and, as is the case with other mental health issues, postpartum depression is sometimes referred to as a condition, a mental state, an illness or a disorder.

To address some of the complex issues that are involved when working with immigrant women in the context of postpartum depression, we use a health promotion framework that emphasizes psychosocial risk and protective factors associated with mental health issues, in combination with a broader social determinants of health approach (Canadian Mental Health Association [CMHA], 2000). This type of approach allows the examination of factors such as acculturation, discrimination, the role of the extended family, and rituals and traditions, which may play an important part in determining maternal mental health in immigrant women.

Research on Postpartum Depression among Immigrant Women

WHAT IS POSTPARTUM DEPRESSION?

For some women, childbirth can represent a time of great vulnerability to psychological problems, with postpartum mood disorders representing the most frequent maternal complication following delivery (Stocky & Lynch, 2000). Psychological problems around childbirth can vary in severity from the early maternity blues ("baby blues") to postpartum psychosis, a serious state affecting less than one per cent of mothers (Evins & Theofrastous, 1997). Postpartum depression is a condition often associated with the disabling symptoms of low mood, emotional instability, sleep problems, confusion, anxiety, guilt and suicidal thinking (Beck, 1992). Frequently exacerbating these symptoms are low self-esteem, inability to cope, feelings of incompetence and loneliness (Beck, 1992; Mills et al., 1995; Righetti-Veltema et al., 1998; Ritter et al., 2000). The rate of onset of postpartum depression is greatest in the first 12 weeks postpartum (Cooper & Murray, 1998), and the illness usually lasts longer when symptoms are more severe and when treatment is delayed (England et al., 1994). Up to 50 per cent of mothers not receiving care and treatment will remain clinically depressed at six months postpartum (Kumar & Robson, 1984; Whiffen & Gotlib, 1993), with an estimated 25 per cent of cases of untreated postpartum depression continuing past the first year (Carpiniello et al., 1997).

Postpartum depression is a major health issue for women from diverse cultural backgrounds (Affonso et al., 2000). Research studies have yielded varying prevalence rates, ranging from three per cent to more than 25 per cent of women in the first year following delivery. A meta-analysis of 59 studies reported an overall prevalence of major postpartum depression to be 13 per cent within the first 12 weeks postpartum (O'Hara & Swain, 1996). While national Canadian statistics are unknown, a recently completed study of 645 mothers in British Columbia found the prevalence of depressive symptoms at four and eight weeks postpartum to be 9.1 per cent and eight per cent respectively (Dennis, 2004).

Most prevalence studies have included samples of predominantly Caucasian women or homogeneous samples in their native countries (Dennis, 2003a). As such, little is known about the prevalence of postpartum depression among immigrant women. Research suggests that women from non-western and western cultural communities experience postpartum mood problems at approximately the same rates (O'Hara, 1994). However, there is emerging evidence for higher rates of postpartum depressive symptoms in immigrant women than in native-born women (Zelkowitz et al., 2004).

PRESENTATION AND DETECTION OF POSTPARTUM DEPRESSION

The presentation or symptom profile of depression can vary from woman to woman. In addition, women from some groups may have more physical or somatic complaints (e.g., sleep disturbances, fatigue, loss of appetite) while others may have more emotional or affective symptoms (e.g., sadness, feelings of guilt, crying) of depression. Somatization is a common way to express depression among Asian and African cultures, while complaints of sadness, together with guilt, are more characteristic of depression in western cultures (Bashiri & Spielvogel, 1999). This difference could lead to difficulties in screening for and diagnosing depression in non-western populations if western-developed tools are being used. However, recent international research has found no consistent differences in somatization of depression between diverse groups of women (Small et al., 2003; Simon et al., 1999). For example, one recent study of post-partum depression in Vietnamese, Turkish and Filipino women living in Australia found no consistent difference in rates of somatization between these immigrant groups and Australian-born women (Small et al., 2003). In fact, some research findings indicate that variables other than ethnicity and culture, including whether or not some-one had a consistent relationship with a health care provider, were better predictors of which depressive symptoms an individual reported (Simon et al., 1999).

The Edinburgh Postnatal Depression Scale (EPDS; Cox et al., 1987) is currently the most widely used instrument to assess for postpartum depression and identify mothers at higher risk (Beck, 2001). Although the scale has been translated into various languages (e.g., Chinese, German, Greek, French, Arabic, Czech, Dutch, Hebrew, Hindi), the translated scales may provide unreliable results due to words or phrases that cannot be literally translated into another language. The questions may carry slightly different meanings in translation; for example, when translating the statement in the EPDS "Things have been getting on top of me." Further, because of potential cross-cultural differences in expression of depressive symptoms, appropriate cut-off scores may vary for different populations. For example, a cut-off score of 12/13 has been repeatedly validated and recommended for detecting postpartum depression (Cox et al., 1987) and a score of 9/10 has been recommended for assessing a risk for developing postpartum depression in community-based screening in North America (Murray & Carothers, 1990; Zelkowitz & Milet, 1995). However, a cut-off of 9/10 was most appro-priate at six weeks postpartum for detecting postpartum depression among a group of women from Hong Kong (Lee et al., 1998); a cut-off of 8/9 was suitable for screening among a group of Japanese mothers (Okano et al., 1998), and a cut-off of 9/10 was suggested for Vietnamese women (Matthey et al., 1997). It is also possible that the Chinese women participants, like their Vietnamese counterparts, were reluctant to reveal unhappiness or distress in the early postpartum period to an interviewer; the women seemed less constrained in responding to a self-report questionnaire. Using a clinical diagnostic interview, Yoshida et al. (1997) found similar depression rates among Japanese women living in England and Japan. The authors also commented that the difference in cut-off scores between various populations might be due to the exclusion of somatic symptoms in the EPDS, since some women might voice physical problems about themselves or their infant rather than expressing mental and psychological concerns directly.

These findings indicate the need to be cautious about the appropriateness of the use of screening tools to assess populations other than the one in which the scale was developed and the potential need to combine screening tools with other assessment procedures and clinical judgment (Ross et al., 2005).

POSTPARTUM DEPRESSION RISK FACTORS

Research suggests a multifactorial etiology (causation) for postpartum depression (Ross et al., 2004). Research to date also suggests that risk factors for postpartum depression are generally consistent across different ethnocultural groups. For example, prenatal depression and a lack of social support have been found to be risk factors among Lebanese women in Beirut (Chaaya et al., 2002), Mexican-American women in the United States (Martinez-Schallmoser et al., 2003) and Indian women in Goa (Patel et al., 2002). Similarly, in a cross-cultural study incorporating 11 countries (France, Italy, Sweden, Ireland, Uganda, Japan, Austria, United States, Switzerland, Portugal, United Kingdom), a lack of social support was consistently found to be a significant postpartum depression risk factor (Oates et al., 2004). While acknowledging diversity within ethnocultural groups, some research has also pointed to a link between having a baby girl and postpartum depression among women in Hong Kong and India (Lee et al., 2000; Patel et al., 2002; Rodrigues et al., 2003). One study found that some women might be at increased risk for other adverse outcomes, such as relationship deterioration (including marital violence) and problems with in-laws (Patel et al., 2002), which can be linked to postpartum depression. Other possible risk factors include lack of practical support from the baby's father, a poor relationship with in-laws and family conflicts (Danaci et al., 2002; Lee et al., 2004; Oates et al., 2004; Rodrigues et al., 2003). There is a strong link between a lack of social or partner support and postpartum depression (Beck, 2001; O'Hara & Swain, 1996). Additional research is warranted to better understand risk factors for postpartum depression in diverse ethnocultural groups in order to create appropriate interventions and policies that are applicable for women of diverse ethnocultural backgrounds.

Immigrant status in itself can be a risk factor for postpartum depression. For example, in a Canadian sample of 1,559 women screened through two community health centres at six weeks postpartum, recent immigrant mothers, particularly those who had given birth to a second child, were at higher risk of developing postpartum depression than Canadian-born women (Zelkowitz & Milet, 1995). Among 1,337 Turkish women who had given birth in the previous six months, being an immigrant was a significant risk factor (Danaci et al., 2002). Similar findings were noted in a prospective study of 327 Jewish Jerusalem women (Dankner et al., 2000). In a random sample of 288 women from a community cohort at 26 weeks' pregnancy, immigrant status was the only significant demographic predictor of postpartum depression identified by either *univariate* or *multivariate* analysis (techniques of analysis involving one or more statistical variables at a time), with Russian immigrants to Israel having more than twice the risk as Israeli-born mothers had (Glasser et al., 1998). Furthermore, in a recent Canadian multifactor-ial predictive study (a study involving several factors simultaneously used to predict the outcome) of 594 women, immigrant women were five times more likely to develop depressive symptoms in the early postpartum period compared to Canadian-born mothers in the same period (Dennis et al., 2004).

While scant research has been conducted as to why these women are at risk, research with general immigrant populations has demonstrated a link between the acculturation process and depression (Aroian & Norris, 2002; Bhugra, 2004; Constantine et al., 2004; Dennis, 2003b; Dennis et al., 2004; Hovey, 2000; Miller & Chandler, 2002; Oh et al., 2002; Vega et al., 1987; Williams & Berry, 1991). However, the relationship between acculturation, acculturative stress and postpartum depression has not been widely explored. One study that examined the impact of acculturation on maternal mood in 15 new Hmong mothers (mothers from an ethnic group in southeast Asia and China) who had immigrated to the United States within the past two to 21 years found that almost half of the women participants were clinically depressed or anxious, with less-acculturated mothers tending to be at higher risk (Foss, 2001).

Research also suggests that social support and socio-economic status may lessen the potential negative consequences of acculturative stress (Hovey, 2000; Williams & Berry, 1991). Lack of social support and low socio-economic status are significant risk factors for postpartum depression (Beck, 2001). Lack of support may be a particular concern for immigrant women. For example, in an Australian study that examined the mental health of a cohort of Filipino- and Australian-born mothers, Filipino-born mothers had smaller social networks at the birth of their child and reported more symptoms of anxiety and depression at their first postpartum clinic visit and at a five-year follow-up than did their Australian counterparts (Alati et al., 2004). Another key factor associated with immigration and the post-migration context can be stresses associated with acculturation. In adapting to their host country, immi-grant women face many challenges, such as learning a new language, adapting to unfamiliar customs and social interaction, and dealing with new rules and laws. These processes and changes can lead to an increased risk for depression (Constantine et al., 2004; Williams & Berry, 1991).

Some immigrant women (especially recent immigrants of colour) may face a "triple jeopardy" of simultaneously belonging to various marginalized groups (Vissandjée et al., 2001). They can experience ethnic or racial prejudice, systemic sexism and discrimination because of their immigrant status. Results from a recent qualitative study revealed that immigrant women in Canada often feel discriminated against as immigrants *and* as mothers (Ross et al., 2007). Specifically, some participants noted that Canadian society was unfriendly toward mothers and small children, and reported that on occasion they have felt discriminated against in public when people judged that their baby was crying too loudly or that their stroller was in the way (Ross et al., 2007).

Western society has created unrealistic expectations about mothers (Berggren-Clive, 1998) and motherhood (Nicolson, 1990) that place women at risk for mental health problems during the postpartum period. Pervasive in both professionals and lay people is the myth that motherhood is equated with total fulfilment and happiness (Berggren-Clive, 1998; Nicolson, 1990). When mothers experience a conflict between the expectations and the realities of motherhood (Beck, 2002), they might become disillusioned and despairing. Immigrant mothers in Canada have reported similar concerns regarding the social expectations and internalizations of the "perfect mother" role (Ross et al., 2007), as depicted on television programs and in magazines—standards that might be hard to achieve in real life.

Finally, attitudes and beliefs held by health and social service providers may have an impact on the care they deliver to immigrant mothers. For instance, the Western health system based on the biomedical approach emphasizes the role of personal responsibility for health care. By emphasizing the responsibility of the woman, some health care providers neglect to pay attention to the social conditions (e.g., housing, child care and nutrition) that immigrant woman deal with in the post-migration context that might affect their physical and mental health. Negative stereotypes about immigrant women, dismissal of their health concerns, and lack of sensitivity to racism in Canadian society at large may be contributing factors to postpartum depression among immigrant women, and need to be addressed in future research.

POSTPARTUM PRACTICES AND RITUALS AS PROTECTIVE FACTORS

Research-based evidence suggests that postpartum practices and rituals play a role in protecting women against postpartum depression (Bashiri & Spielvogel, 1999; Lee et al., 2004; Stewart & Jambunathan, 1996). In many communities around the world, special practices and customs impose structure, meaning and support in the perinatal period and promote the successful transition to motherhood (Stuchbery et al., 1998). These postpartum rituals have been studied to varying degrees among Arabic (Hundt et al., 2000; Nahas & Amasheh, 1999), Chinese (Cheung, 1997; Chu, 2005; Davis, 2001; Holroyd et al., 1997; Lee et al., 1998), Japanese (Yoshida et al., 2001), Malaysian (Kit et al., 1997), Taiwanese (Huang & Mathers, 2001) and Thai (Kaewsarn et al., 2003) women. The practices included different aspects of organized support to the mother from female relatives: practices include providing social support, regulating the mother's diet to promote her long-term health, enforcing certain hygiene practices (such as avoiding showers that could make her cold) and restricting her physical activity. These are typically performed during the first 40 days after childbirth (Hundt et al., 2000; Matthey et al., 2002).

While initially some speculated that postpartum depression was a "culture-bound phenomenon" present only in Western societies in which no structured rituals allow for recognition of the vulnerability and special status of a new mother (Stern & Kruckman,

1983), more recent international research has established that postpartum depression is present in diverse communities around the world (e.g., see Affonso et al., 2000), and that the relationship between various postpartum rituals and postpartum depression is more complicated than previously believed. While these rituals may protect some women against postpartum depression, others may find that the rituals create added stress and even isolation for the new mother, thus making her more prone to postpartum depression. How the woman responds will be affected by whether she wants to follow the rituals or whether they are imposed on her. (Posmontier & Horowitz, 2004).

There is some contemporary evidence of a potential protective effect of postpartum rituals on mental health. For example, a study of Jewish women living in Jerusalem found a decreasing trend for postpartum depression among the more religious and orthodox sections of that society (Dankner et al., 2000). The researchers suggested that postpartum depression may develop less frequently, or is easier to cope with, in religious women because of the more cohesive social structure, emphasis on rituals and greater community support. However, further research is needed to study if "traditional" postpartum practices isolate some women or contribute to a feeling of lack of personal control over their own and their babies' lives. For example, in a qualitative study involving in-depth interviews with 20 Hong Kong Chinese women to examine their perceptions of stress and support in "doing the month" (*Tso-Yueh-Tzu*), four central themes were identified: feeling bound by the environmental constraints; having difficulties in following the prescriptions of the rituals; having conflicts with relatives who want to impose unwanted rituals; and wanting to have more control over caring for her own baby (Leung et al., 2005). The researchers found that the practice was not necessarily protective and supportive to all women in the study, and raised the question of how women can adapt the ritual to accommodate modern life.

Similarly, in an Australian study of 102 Chinese immigrant women that investigated practices they had followed in the first six weeks postpartum (Matthey et al., 2002), the majority (90.2 per cent) had adhered to some form of practice, with the most frequent being eating warm "yang" food (e.g., eggs, poultry, meat, potatoes) (78 per cent), staying at home for one month (55 per cent) and using warm water for washing themselves (19 per cent). Of note was that 18 per cent of these women felt ambivalent about following such practices, with the impression being that the adoption of such practices was more a result of family or in-law expectations than the wishes of the woman. Of the 9.8 per cent who did not follow any form of postpartum practices, only half felt ambivalent or negative about not doing so. There was no relationship between the women's mood at six weeks postpartum and how she felt about following or not following such practices. This research indicates that childbirth traditions, rituals and practices can also be a source of stress, particularly for those who do not have enough support or resources to adhere to or participate in practices believed important to health. Inability to participate in cultural traditions might be perceived as a failure of the mother, which might also lead to future symptoms of depression.

Participating in childbirth rituals or traditions may also have implications for the detection and treatment of postpartum depression. Based on their research with women in China and the practice of "doing the month," Lee and colleagues (1998) have speculated that the tangible support a new mother initially received may actually mask a depression by preventing her from expressing feelings of sadness or anxiety, or may simply postpone the onset of depressive symptoms.

Providing Postpartum Depression Services to Immigrant Women

As a result of the many barriers immigrant women face in accessing appropriate mental health care, many immigrant women with postpartum depression may go undiagnosed, untreated and uncared for. (See Chapter 4 for a detailed discussion of the social determinants of depression on women's mental health.) Special care must therefore be taken to ensure that postpartum depression services are accessible, acceptable and effective for immigrant women. Health care workers in Canada must be prepared to deliver culturally appropriate care to manage postpartum depression. However, before adopting any specific strategy to work with immigrant mothers, it is important to recognize that culture, as a determinant of health, also intersects with gender, education, age and other variables such as socio-economic circumstances (Anderson et al., 2005). In the following section, we describe a number of strategies used at St. Joseph's Health Centre in Toronto to provide care to immigrant women dealing with postpartum depression.

A MODEL OF CULTURALLY APPROPRIATE POSTPARTUM CARE

The St. Joseph's Maternal Support Program has been an integral part of the St. Joseph's Women's Health Centre since its inception in 1989. This centre provides a spectrum of integrated services addressing the needs of a culturally and socio-economically diverse population. The program is led by a registered nurse and social worker, and uses multiple approaches to provide holistic, client-centred care to immigrant mothers (and their families). The services are offered in diverse languages. The staff work collaboratively with professional interpreters, physicians, health units and community agencies, and are often involved in research projects with academic institutions. They also share their work through community-based presentations and conferences.

Support groups are offered to women dealing with issues related to social isolation or a lack of understanding by family members, while individual psychotherapy is provided to address psychological issues that might be difficult to address or disclose in groups, such as traumatic experiences or feelings of resentment toward the infant. The program provides couple therapy to deal with relational issues, such as the distribution of infant care and domestic tasks, or communication problems. The program also offers telephone support to mothers who are unable to travel to the centre due to various factors, such as geographical distance or an ill infant. Peer support is offered by women who have previously used the services and have received training to take on the supportive role to other mothers who are isolated in the community. The program recognizes the importance of child care and provides free child care. In addition, the St. Joseph's Women's Centre provides employment opportunities for local community members.

The development of these services arose from the recognition that although the clients were from different cultural and socio-economic backgrounds, they shared many experiences in adapting to motherhood. A unique aspect of the program is its integration of a broader perspective to care that examines the socio-political and cultural context of motherhood.

STRATEGIES FOR WORKING WITH IMMIGRANT WOMEN

The following section highlights strategies based on mental health promotion principles aimed at delivering postpartum care to immigrant women. In 1996, an international workshop was held in Toronto, which gave rise to the definition of mental health promotion as "the process of enhancing the capacity of individuals and communities to take control over their lives and improve their mental health. Mental health promotion uses strategies that foster supportive environments and individual resilience while showing respect for culture, equity, social justice, interconnections and personal dignity" (Centre for Health Promotion, 1997).

Delivering Culturally Appropriate Care
Participate actively in diversity and cultural competency training and in designing culturally appropriate care. Workplaces can integrate cultural competency policies and practices at various levels including the planning and delivery of services. For example, professionals working in the mental health area are encouraged to receive ongoing training to deliver culturally appropriate care. This does not imply that all health professionals will have knowledge about every cultural tradition or speak every language. Culturally appropriate care suggests that awareness as well as incorporation of the concerns and issues faced by immigrant mothers—such as language barriers, lack of social support, change in socio-economic status, lack of access to certain care and services owing to their citizenship status and racism, and acculturative stress—are important. It is also salient that health professionals working with new immigrant mothers be aware of other contextual factors that may have an impact on psychological adjustment to a new country such as their experience of trauma prior to migration (CMHA, 2000). (Chapter 14 addresses trauma work with Latin American women, but is also relevant for women from any culture who have experienced violence.)

Health professionals should be aware of the ways in which their personal characteristics, such as communication style, attitudes and beliefs affect how they provide postpartum care. For instance, health professionals' knowledge about the complexities of issues around postpartum depression, as well as their own attitudes toward immigrant women and mothers will determine the type of care they deliver.

An example of how workplaces can implement cultural competency education for mental health professionals is provided by the Canadian Mental Health Association (2000) in its publication *Building Bridges: Mental Health Education Workshops for Immigrants and Refugees*. This guide discusses cross-cultural mental health and the impact of migration stress, as well as effects of racism on the mental health of immigrants and ethnic minorities. Many health care institutions are beginning to offer diversity training in-house or online.

Addressing Language Barriers

Use trained and certified cultural interpreters. Ideally, mothers should be assessed for postpartum depression without family members present. If a mother is not proficient enough to understand, read and speak in English, interpreters who are culturally competent should be incorporated in the assessment and care planning (Bashiri & Spielvogel, 1999). Every health professional must become skilled in using interpretation services and protocols (Chapter 6 on the community interpreter discusses the intricacies of cultural and language interpretation). It is also important to disseminate information about the Canadian health care system, particularly as it relates to maternal and infant care (i.e., labour and delivery practices, vaccinations), postpartum depression, treatment choices and support services. Such information should be provided in multiple languages and through diverse channels such as pamphlets, brochures, educational videos, web pages and radio.

Creating Supportive Environments

Help a new immigrant mother to establish connections with other members of her community/communities. An important initial step in supporting immigrant women is to help them navigate an unfamiliar health care system. Health professionals should familiarize themselves with community-based services for new mothers, fathers and families. Referring women to other community and social services may also be pivotal in their obtaining resources that provide comprehensive and supportive care. Immigrant mothers often welcome the support of health professionals who share their language and culture. However, there can also be many negative aspects to these strategies. As noted in Chapter 7 on resources for women, not all immigrant communities will have ethnocultural-specific supports for new mothers and their families. Furthermore, relying solely on ethno-specific services may lead to further stigmatization and isolation. Due to concerns about confidentiality, some women may also not want to participate in specific programs if they know other women from their community will be present.

Addressing Life Context and Determinants of Health

Take into account the context of the everyday lives of the mothers when implementing programs and policies. Social determinants affecting women's mental health should be considered when developing postpartum programs. (See Chapter 4 for a discussion of the social determinants of depression.) Many of the strategies for working with women experiencing general depression can also be effective when working with postpartum mothers. However, there are some specific issues that require attention. For instance, it is key that services for mothers include providing child care and transportation costs. In addition, pregnancy and childbirth may be a time when traditional gender roles are accentuated. Partners and family members may hold unrealistic expectations about motherhood and may exert additional pressure on a new mother by criticizing her appearance or untidiness or success in caring for the baby. Partners and family members thus need to talk, prior to the birth, about what is reasonable to expect from the mother. Information about postpartum depression should also be provided to both women and their family members to clarify the seriousness of postpartum depression as well as to reduce the potential stigma associated with seeking treatment. Otherwise, the woman's depressive symptoms might be dismissed as the "blues."

Building Partnerships within the Organization and Beyond

Work in multidisciplinary teams within one's own workplace and build partnerships with external agencies. Collaborative work is more effective in addressing the complex issues (e.g., employment, health care, legal issues and housing) that affect the mental health of postpartum immigrant women. By working together toward common goals, different organizations and stakeholders can build on unique competencies and perspectives. For instance, health professionals can develop postpartum depression education campaigns in partnership with ethnocultural community agencies, which often have established ties with community members through various outreach programs. Furthermore, health professionals can work toward generating policies and making organizational change to create healthy environments that support postpartum mothers. In particular, hospital policies on the postpartum units related to breastfeeding, discharge times and number of visitors allowed can significantly shape the experience of a new mother in the immediate postpartum period. Immigrant women may practice postpartum rituals that often incorporate dietary restrictions, rest and seclusion, and hygiene practices.

Using Multiple Approaches and Levels

Use a combination of methods (i.e., education, policy change, community development, collaboration) and work at multiple levels (i.e., individual, family, community, organizational, societal) to provide comprehensive care. Adopting multiple approaches will also allow health professionals to be more responsive to new information or evidence. For example, if research reveals that involving partners in the treatment of postpartum depression is an effective strategy, postpartum programs should aim to involve partners. Programs could work directly with families by delivering information sessions aimed at raising awareness about postpartum depression.

In addition, health professionals can work to increase their own understanding about the community's needs around postpartum issues (i.e., the degree of accessibility, usefulness and relevance of the services provided). Apart from improving existing services, evaluating the effectiveness and people's satisfaction with existing programs may also help with the planning and implementation of new programs that address maternal preferences and promote evidence-based practice. Health professionals can also make use of the local media to advocate for postpartum care in their community.

It can also be beneficial to invite reporters from the local newspapers to various health care settings to hear from the immigrant mothers themselves. At the individual level, health professionals must work on developing a relationship with the immigrant mother. Many of the issues related to dealing with postpartum depression in the post-migration context are complex: health professionals cannot expect women to disclose sensitive information without initially building trust and respect, which can sometimes take a considerable amount of time.

Conclusion

In this chapter we have outlined both common experiences and factors as well as culturally or contextually specific factors that health care professionals might address when working with immigrant women in the postpartum period. Although a number of successful strategies such as working with cultural interpreters, providing peer support and conducting psychoeducational sessions can be useful when working with immigrant mothers experiencing postpartum depression, each mother is unique. For instance, the support from the extended family may play a prominent role for some women coping with postpartum depression, and, in other cases, the role of religion may have a significant impact on a woman's healing strategy.

It is crucial to understand the context in which immigrant mothers live in Canada. Awareness of how broader determinants of health, such as discrimination, poverty and social isolation, may contribute to stress and the development of postpartum depression is vital. These diverse aspects and unique concerns should be addressed in planning effective and innovative postpartum interventions for immigrant women in the community. Incorporating a holistic approach to health by considering the different aspects of a mother's physical, social, emotional and spiritual health is critical to delivering culturally competent postpartum care.

References

Affonso, D.D., De, A.K., Horowitz, J.A. & Mayberry, L.J. (2000). An international study exploring levels of postpartum depressive symptomatology. *Journal of Psychosomatic Research, 49* (3), 207–216.

Alati, R., Najman, J. & Williams, G.H. (2004). The mental health of Filipino-born women 5 and 14 years after they have given birth in Australia: A longitudinal study. *Health Sociology Review, 13* (2), 145–156.

Anderson, J.M., Reimer Kirkham, S., Waxler-Morrison, N., Herbert, C., Murphy, M. & Richardson, E. (2005). In N. Waxler-Morrison, J.M. Anderson, E. Richardson & N.A. Chambers (Eds.), *Cross-Cultural Caring: A Handbook for Health Professionals* (2nd ed.; pp. 245–269). Vancouver: University of British Columbia Press.

Aroian, K.J. & Norris, A. (2002). Assessing risk for depression among immigrants at two-year follow-up. *Archives of Psychiatric Nursing, 16* (6), 245–253.

Bashiri, N. & Spielvogel, A.M. (1999). Postpartum depression: A cross-cultural perspective. *Primary Care Update for Ob/Gyns, 6* (3), 82–87.

Beck, C.T. (1992). The lived experience of postpartum depression: A phenomenological study. *Nursing Research, 41* (3), 166–170.

Beck, C.T. (2001). Predictors of postpartum depression: An update. *Nursing Research, 50* (5), 275–285.

Beck, C.T. (2002). Postpartum depression: A metasynthesis. *Qualitative Health Research, 12* (4), 453–472.

Berggren-Clive, K. (1998). Out of the darkness and into the light: Women's experiences with depression after childbirth. *Canadian Journal of Community Mental Health, 17* (1), 103–120.

Bhugra, D. (2004). Migration and mental health. *Acta Psychiatrica Scandinavica, 109* (4), 243–258.

Canadian Mental Health Association. (2000). *Building Bridges: Mental Health Education Workshops for Immigrants and Refugees.* Toronto: CMHA Toronto Branch.

Carpiniello, B., Pariante, C.M., Serri, F., Costa, G. & Carta, M.G. (1997). Validation of the Edinburgh Postnatal Depression Scale in Italy. *Journal of Psychosomatic Obstetrics & Gynecology, 18* (4), 280–285.

Centre for Health Promotion. (1997). Proceedings from the International Workshop on Mental Health Promotion, University of Toronto. In C. Willinsky & B. Pape (Eds.), *Mental Health Promotion: Social Action Series.* Toronto: Canadian Mental Health Association National Office.

Chaaya, M., Campbell, O.M., El Kak, F., Shaar, D., Harb, H. & Kaddour, A. (2002). Postpartum depression: Prevalence and determinants in Lebanon. *Archives of Women's Mental Health, 5* (2), 65–72.

Cheung, N.F. (1997). Chinese zuo yuezi (sitting in for the first month of the postnatal period) in Scotland. *Midwifery, 13* (2), 55–65.

Chu, C.M. (2005). Postnatal experience and health needs of Chinese migrant women in Brisbane, Australia. *Ethnicity & Health, 10* (1), 33–56.

Constantine, M.G., Okazaki, S. & Utsey, S.O. (2004). Self-concealment, social self-efficacy, acculturative stress, and depression in African, Asian, and Latin American international college students. *American Journal of Orthopsychiatry, 74* (3), 230–241.

Cooper, P.J. & Murray, L. (1998). Postnatal depression. [See comments.] *British Medical Journal, 316* (7148), 1884–1886.

Cox, J.L., Holden, J.M. & Sagovsky, R. (1987). Detection of postnatal depression: Development of the 10-item Edinburgh Postnatal Depression Scale. *British Journal of Psychiatry, 150*, 782–786.

Cox, J.L., Murray, D. & Chapman, G. (1993). A controlled study of the onset, duration and prevalence of postnatal depression. *British Journal of Psychiatry, 163*, 27–31.

Danaci, A.E., Dinc, G., Deveci, A., Sen, F.S. & Icelli, I. (2002). Postnatal depression in Turkey: Epidemiological and cultural aspects. *Social Psychiatry & Psychiatric Epidemiology, 37* (3), 125–129.

Dankner, R., Goldberg, R.P., Fisch, R.Z. & Crum, R.M. (2000). Cultural elements of postpartum depression: A study of 327 Jewish Jerusalem women. *Journal of Reproductive Medicine, 45* (2), 97–104.

Davis, R.E. (2001). The postpartum experience for Southeast Asian women in the United States. *American Journal of Maternal Child Nursing, 26* (4), 208–213.

Dennis, C.-L. (2003a). The detection, prevention, and treatment of postpartum depression. In D. Stewart, E. Robertson, C.-L. Dennis, S. Grace & T. Wallington (Eds.), *Postpartum Depression: Critical Literature Review and Recommendations.* Toronto: Toronto Public Health.

Dennis, C.-L. (2003b). The effect of peer support on postpartum depression: A pilot randomized controlled trial. *Canadian Journal of Psychiatry, 48* (2), 115–124.

Dennis, C.-L. (2004). Can we identify mothers at risk for postpartum depression in the immediate postpartum period using the Edinburgh Postnatal Depression Scale? *Journal of Affective Disorders, 78* (2), 163–169.

Dennis, C.-L., Janssen, P.A. & Singer, J. (2004). Identifying women at-risk for postpartum depression in the immediate postpartum period. *Acta Psychiatrica Scandinavica, 110* (5), 338–346.

England, S.J., Ballard, C. & George, S. (1994). Chronicity in postnatal depression. *European Journal of Psychiatry, 8* (2), 93–96.

Evins, G.G. & Theofrastous, J.P. (1997). Postpartum depression: A review of postpartum screening. *Primary Care Update for Ob/Gyns, 4* (6), 241–246.

Foss, G.F. (2001). Maternal sensitivity, posttraumatic stress, and acculturation in Vietnamese and Hmong mothers. *American Journal of Maternal Child Nursing, 26* (5), 257–263.

Glasser, S., Barell, V., Shoham, A., Ziv, A., Boyko, V., Lusky, A. et al. (1998). Prospective study of postpartum depression in an Israeli cohort: Prevalence, incidence and demographic risk factors. *Journal of Psychosomatic Obstetrics and Gynecology, 19* (3), 155–164.

Holroyd, E., Katie, F.K., Chun, L.S. & Ha, S.W. (1997). "Doing the month": An exploration of postpartum practices in Chinese women. *Health Care for Women International, 18* (3), 301–313.

Hovey, J.D. (2000). Psychosocial predictors of depression among Central American immigrants. *Psychological Reports, 86* (3 Pt. 2), 1237–1240.

Huang, Y.C. & Mathers, N. (2001). Postnatal depression: Biological or cultural? A comparative study of postnatal women in the UK and Taiwan. *Journal of Advanced Nursing, 33* (3), 279–287.

Hundt, G.L., Beckerleg, S., Kassem, F., Abu Jafar, A.M., Belmaker, I., Abu Saad, K. et al. (2000). Women's health custom made: Building on the 40 days postpartum for Arab women. *Health Care for Women International, 21* (6), 529–542.

Kaewsarn, P., Moyle, W. & Creedy, D. (2003). Traditional postpartum practices among Thai women. *Journal of Advanced Nursing, 41* (4), 358–366.

Kit, L.K., Janet, G. & Jegasothy, R. (1997). Incidence of postnatal depression in Malaysian women. *Journal of Obstetrics and Gynaecology Research, 23* (1), 85–89.

Kumar, R. & Robson, K.M. (1984). A prospective study of emotional disorders in childbearing women. *British Journal of Psychiatry, 144*, 35–47.

Lee, D., Yip, A., Leung, T. & Chung, T. (2000). Identifying women at risk of postnatal depression: Prospective longitudinal study. *Hong Kong Medical Journal, 6* (4), 349–354.

Lee, D., Yip, S., Chiu, H., Leung, T., Chan, K., Chau, I. et al. (1998). Detecting postnatal depression in Chinese women: Validation of the Chinese version of the Edinburgh Postnatal Depression Scale. *British Journal of Psychiatry, 172*, 433–437.

Lee, D.T., Yip, A.S., Leung, T.Y. & Chung, T.K. (2004). Ethnoepidemiology of postnatal depression: Prospective multivariate study of sociocultural risk factors in a Chinese population in Hong Kong. *British Journal of Psychiatry, 184*, 34–40.

Leung, S.K., Arthur, D. & Martinson, I.M. (2005). Perceived stress and support of the Chinese postpartum ritual "doing the month." *Health Care for Women International, 26* (3), 212–224.

Martinez-Schallmoser, L., Telleen, S. & MacMullen, N.J. (2003). The effect of social support and acculturation on postpartum depression in Mexican American women. *Journal of Transcultural Nursing, 14* (4), 329–338.

Matthey, S., Barnett, B.E. & Elliott, A. (1997). Vietnamese and Arabic women's responses to the

Diagnostic Interview Schedule (depression) and self-report questionnaires: Cause for concern. *Australian and New Zealand Journal of Psychiatry, 31* (3), 360–369.

Matthey, S., Panasetis, P. & Barnett, B. (2002). Adherence to cultural practices following childbirth in migrant Chinese women and relation to postpartum mood. *Health Care for Women International, 23* (6–7), 567–575.

Miller, A.M. & Chandler, P.J. (2002). Acculturation, resilience, and depression in midlife women from the former Soviet Union. *Nursing Research, 51* (1), 26–32.

Mills, E.P., Finchilescu, G. & Lea, S.J. (1995). Postnatal depression: An examination of psychosocial factors. *South African Medical Journal, 85* (2), 99–105.

Murray, L. & Carothers, A.D. (1990). The validation of the Edinburgh Postnatal Depression Scale on a community sample. *British Journal of Psychiatry, 157*, 288–290.

Nahas, V. & Amasheh, N. (1999). Culture care meanings and experiences of postpartum depression among Jordanian Australian women: A transcultural study. *Journal of Transcultural Nursing, 10* (1), 37–45.

Nicolson, P. (1990). Understanding postnatal depression: A mother-centered approach. *Journal of Advanced Nursing, 15* (6), 689–695.

Oates, M.R., Cox, J.L., Neema, S., Asten, P., Glangeaud-Freudenthal, N., Figueiredo, B. et al. (2004). Postnatal depression across countries and cultures: A qualitative study. *British Journal of Psychiatry: Supplement, 46*, s10–16.

Oh, Y., Koeske, G.F. & Sales, E. (2002). Acculturation, stress, and depressive symptoms among Korean immigrants in the United States. *Journal of Social Psychology, 142* (4), 511–526.

O'Hara, M.W. (1994). Postpartum depression: Identification and measurement in a cross-cultural context. In J. Cox & J. Holden (Eds.), *Perinatal Psychiatry: Use and Misuse of the Edinburgh Postnatal Depression Scale* (pp. 145–168). London: The Royal College of Psychiatrists.

O'Hara, M. & Swain, A. (1996). Rates and risk of postpartum depression: A meta-analysis. *International Review of Psychiatry, 8*, 37–54.

Okano, T., Nomura, J., Kumar, R., Kaneko, E., Tamaki, R., Hanafusa, I. et al. (1998). An epidemiological and clinical investigation of postpartum psychiatric illness in Japanese mothers. *Journal of Affective Disorders, 48* (2–3), 233–240.

Patel, V., Rodrigues, M. & DeSouza, N. (2002). Gender, poverty, and postnatal depression: A study of mothers in Goa, India. *American Journal of Psychiatry, 159* (1), 43–47.

Posmontier, B. & Horowitz, J.A. (2004). Postpartum practices and depression prevalences: Technocentric and ethnokinship cultural perspectives. *Journal of Transcultural Nursing, 15* (1), 34-43.

Righetti-Veltema, M., Conne-Perreard, E., Bousquet, A. & Manzano, J. (1998). Risk factors and predictive signs of postpartum depression. *Journal of Affective Disorders, 49* (3), 167–180.

Ritter, C., Hobfoll, S.E., Lavin, J., Cameron, R.P. & Hulsizer, M.R. (2000). Stress, psychosocial resources, and depressive symptomatology during pregnancy in low-income, inner-city women. *Health Psychology, 19* (6), 576–585.

Rodrigues, M., Patel, V., Jaswal, S. & de Souza, N. (2003). Listening to mothers: Qualitative studies on motherhood and depression from Goa, India. *Social Science & Medicine, 57* (10), 1797–1806.

Ross, L.E., Ardiles, P., Mamisachvili, L., Mancewicz, G., Rabin, K., Stuckless, N. et al. (2007). *Understanding the Role of Culture in Postpartum Mood Problems: A Pilot Project.* Unpublished manuscript.

Ross, L.E., Dennis, C.-L., Robertson Blackmore, E. & Stewart, D.E. (2005). *Postpartum Depression: A Guide for Front-Line Health and Social Service Providers.* Toronto: Centre for Addiction and Mental Health.

Ross, L.E., Sellers, E.M., Gilbert Evans, S.E. & Romach, M.K. (2004). Mood changes during pregnancy and the postpartum period: Development of a biopsychosocial model. *Acta Psychiatrica Scandinavica, 109* (6), 457–466.

Simon, G.E., VonKorff, M., Piccinelli, M., Fullerton, C. & Ormel, J. (1999). An International Study of the Relation between Somatic Symptoms and Depression. *New England Journal of Medicine, 341* (18), 1329–1335.

Small, R., Lumley, J. & Yelland, J. (2003). How useful is the concept of somatization in cross-cultural studies of maternal depression? A contribution from the Mothers in a New Country (MINC) study. *Journal of Psychosomatic Obstetrics and Gynaecology, 24* (1), 45–52.

Stern, G. & Kruckman, L. (1983). Multi-disciplinary perspectives on post-partum depression: An anthropological critique. *Social Science & Medicine, 17* (15), 1027–1041.

Stewart, S. & Jambunathan, J. (1996). Hmong women and postpartum depression. *Health Care for Women International, 17* (4), 319–330.

Stocky, A. & Lynch, J. (2000). Acute psychiatric disturbance in pregnancy and the puerperium. *Baillière's Best Practice & Research: Clinical Obstetrics & Gynaecology, 14* (1), 73–87.

Stuchbery, M., Matthey, S. & Barnett, B. (1998). Postnatal depression and social supports in Vietnamese, Arabic and Anglo-Celtic mothers. *Social Psychiatry & Psychiatric Epidemiology, 33* (10), 483–490.

Vega, W.A., Kolody, B. & Valle, J.R. (1987). Migration and mental health: An empirical test of depression risk factors among immigrant Mexican women. *International Migration Review, 21* (3), 512–530.

Vissandjée, B., Weinfeld, M., Dupere, S. & Abdool, S. (2001). Sex, gender, ethnicity and access to health care services: Research and policy challenges for immigrant women in Canada. *Journal of International Migration and Integration, 2* (1), 55–75.

Whiffen, V.E. & Gotlib, I.H. (1993). Comparison of postpartum and nonpostpartum depression: Clinical presentation, psychiatric history, and psychosocial functioning. *Journal of Consulting and Clinical Psychology, 61* (3), 485–494.

Williams, C.L. & Berry, J.W. (1991). Primary prevention of acculturative stress among refugees: Application of psychological theory and practice. *American Psychology, 46* (6), 632–641.

Yoshida, K., Marks, M.N., Kibe, N., Kumar, R., Nakano, H. & Tashiro, N. (1997). Postnatal depression in Japanese women who have given birth in England. *Journal of Affective Disorders, 43* (1), 69–77.

Yoshida, K., Yamashita, H., Ueda, M. & Tashiro, N. (2001). Postnatal depression in Japanese mothers and the reconsideration of "Satogaeri bunben." *Pediatrics International, 43* (2), 189–193.

Zelkowitz, P. & Milet, T.H. (1995). Screening for post-partum depression in a community sample. *Canadian Journal of Psychiatry, 40* (2), 80–86.

Zelkowitz, P., Schinazi, J., Katofsky, L., Saucier, J.F., Valenzuela, M., Westreich, R. et al. (2004). Factors associated with depression in pregnant immigrant women. *Transcultural Psychiatry, 41* (4), 445–464.

Part 6

Conclusion

Chapter 17

Future Directions

ENID COLLINS AND SEPALI GURUGE

During migration and resettlement, immigrant women deal with myriad experiences involving social isolation, downward social and economic mobility, discrimination, poverty, language difficulties and other challenges that not only affect their mental health but also create barriers to their accessing and using mental health services. In spite of adversity, immigrant women demonstrate incredible resiliencies and resourcefulness in overcoming challenges and contributing to their own health and well-being, that of their families, communities and Canadian society at large. Removing socio-economic, political and policy barriers could only help them to succeed further.

Contributors to this book highlight the need to change the way mental health services are offered, and to eliminate systemic barriers to women's access to these services. Based on the work presented in this book and the literature, this final chapter highlights some directions for future research, education, practice and policy development. It is our hope that mental health professionals, students, policy-makers and researchers can glean some insights from these recommendations and further develop directions for shaping mental health care for immigrant women.

Research

While there is a growing body of research on immigrant women in Canada, a number of gaps still exist. Finding answers to the following questions is a beginning step to addressing these gaps.

AREAS FOR FUTURE RESEARCH

Mental Health Status

- What are the determinants of mental health? How is mental health defined and understood? How do these determinants differ for young girls, adolescent girls, adult and older women?
- What is the mental health and illness status of recently arrived immigrant and refugee women, and how does this change over time?
- What is the impact of pre-migration experiences on the long-term mental health and illness of refugee women compared to immigrant women?

Risk Factors and Health Consequences

- How is acculturation linked to the adoption of "risky behaviours" such as alcohol and other drug use? Do these risky behaviours contribute to the deterioration of the health of immigrant girls and women over time and, if so, how?
- What are the prevalence rates and risk and protective factors of intimate partner violence (IPV) in the post-migration context, and how do they differ from those in the pre-migration context? Do rates of IPV vary between women who are sponsored by their husbands and women who arrive alone, unsponsored or as independent immigrants, and if so, how?
- What are the health, social and economic impacts of IPV among immigrant women? What is the cumulative effect of various forms of violence (including rape, sexual assault, childhood abuse, racism and workplace bullying) that women have encountered over their lives?
- What are the common and unique risk factors for postpartum depression across communities? Are they different or similar in pre- and post-migration settings and, if so, how?
- How do social support needs of immigrant women change over time? What are the cost, conflict and reciprocity concerns associated with any support they may be given? How do these concerns affect their health in the post-migration context?
- What are the key mental health concerns among newcomer girls and youth? How do these concerns affect their ability to navigate peer relationships and relationships across the generations?
- What are the experiences and unique concerns of newcomer girls living in rural areas and how do these concerns affect their mental health? What are their experiences of racism, sexism and heterosexism and how are they different or similar to what newcomer girls and youth experience in urban settings? How do these experiences affect their success in education and employment?
- What are the experiences of immigrant women who are lesbian, bisexual or transgendered in accessing the mental health care system in Canada? What care, support and resources must be put in place to address their care concerns and improve their experiences?

- What is the impact of immigration on the health of older women? What are the issues of relevance to older immigrant women in Canada in the context of mental health and illness, and how does their health status change over time? What social and economic resources must be put in place to ensure their good health?

Resiliencies

- What personal, social and economic resources allow refugee women to deal with adversity they might have faced prior to migration, during border crossing and/or in the post-migration context in Canada?
- What are the "health-promoting knowledge and behaviors that can be learned from immigrants and refugees?" (Mulvihill et al., 2001, p.14). How can these behaviours be supported and/or further enhanced?
- What are the diverse ways that immigrant women mobilize resources to succeed in education and employment?
- How do immigrant women contribute to the well-being and success of their family members?
- What can we learn from the supports and strengths that exist within extended family units in pre-migration contexts and how can we incorporate what we have learned to improve intergenerational family relationships in the post-migration context?

GUIDELINES FOR ENGAGING IN RESEARCH

- Work in interdisciplinary health research teams.
- Incorporate methods and strategies based on social justice and equity.
- Apply reflexive, collaborative and inclusive approaches to research with participants.
- Use theoretical perspectives, conceptual frameworks and research methodologies that enable women to have a voice in creating knowledge.
- Incorporate gender-based analysis and diversity analysis into research so as to develop gender-sensitive and culturally relevant models and health care practices and interventions (Mulvihill et al., 2001).
- Involve women in the research process to strengthen their awareness of their own abilities and resources and support their efforts to mobilize for change.
- Collaborate with health, social and settlement service providers in the community to address research areas of importance to local communities such as homelessness and violence (Sherkin, 2004).
- Partner with academics and community groups that use innovative models in research on the health needs and concerns of racialized communities.
- Make available on websites and/or in refereed journal publications the findings of research undertaken by various non-governmental organizations (Gagnon et al., 2004).

- Create mechanisms by which results of research on immigrant women's mental health and illness can become accessible to the women themselves.

Education

Mental health professionals in Canada are educated in a range of disciplines, each with its own professional culture and specific knowledge and skills. Canadian curricula in health disciplines, including nursing, medicine, social work and psychiatry, have historically incorporated an understanding based on the biomedical model and relied primarily on North American and Eurocentric perspectives. In recent years, some educators have begun to respond to the changing context of practice, and to the changing demographics of clients, by using innovative strategies to prepare students to become competent practitioners to face new realities in mental health practice. However, these changes are occurring slowly across disciplines and educational programs.

Next, we present recommendations for changes in curricula and guidelines for faculty in professional disciplines and educational institutions.

RECOMMENDATIONS FOR CHANGES TO CURRICULA CONTENT

- Include in curricula critical conceptual and theoretical frameworks to help students examine how the context within which women access care and support influences their mental health.
- Include in curricula opportunities for students to learn about the impact of various forms of discrimination on women's lives, and explore meaningful anti-oppression strategies in working with diverse groups of women.
- Focus on holistic approaches to dealing with mental health and illness: assessment and treatment strategies must address the physical, mental, spiritual, social-cultural, economic, political and historical contexts of immigrant women's lives.

RECOMMENDATIONS FOR FACULTY IN PROFESSIONAL DISCIPLINES

- Examine one's own power and privilege in relation to students of diverse ethnocultural backgrounds.
- Expand one's knowledge of changing communities and social and systemic issues that influence the lives of people in diverse communities, and the mental health concerns and issues that are relevant to them.
- Create opportunities for students in mental health settings to learn in multi-disciplinary teams.

- Incorporate outreach into teaching and practicum as a way to develop collaborative partnerships with diverse communities.
- Negotiate learning experiences in clinical settings where students have opportunities to listen to the voices and experiences of immigrant women.
- Develop collaborative research and teaching models that allow faculty to engage women in creating and sharing knowledge of their experiences during migration and resettlement in supportive, non-threatening environments.

RECOMMENDATIONS FOR EDUCATIONAL INSTITUTIONS

- Demonstrate a shift in value from emphasizing primarily North American and Eurocentric knowledge and practice based on the medical model, to equally recognizing many ways of knowing.
- Allocate resources to prepare students to become competent mental health practitioners who can provide effective and appropriate care to women of all backgrounds.
- Implement mentoring and support for newcomer students to graduate from professional (educational) programs.
- Incorporate strategies to address lower rates of admissions to graduate schools from racialized communities, especially in practice disciplines.
- Develop anti-racist curricula and create a safe space for students to talk about racism.
- Ensure that faculty members represent the diverse demographics of students.

Practice

Mental health professionals who work with women in various practice settings are in key positions to recognize both the common and unique experiences of immigrant women and to implement proactive strategies that promote the mutual rights and obligations of women consumers and professionals. Provided next are few key recommendations for mental health professionals and mental health agencies.

RECOMMENDATIONS FOR MENTAL HEALTH PROFESSIONALS

Learning, Training and Self-Reflection
- Learn about the Canadian immigration system, structure and policies, and their impact on women's mental health.
- Participate actively in ongoing diversity training, culture competence and anti-oppression work.
- Engage in ongoing self-reflection. Examine one's own values, beliefs, power and privilege to identify how they may influence the way one practices, including how

they might prevent women from receiving optimum care; understand the power and privilege mental health professionals hold within the therapeutic relationship.
- Become comfortable with asking about and documenting abuse, conducting risk assessments and safety planning, following through reporting guidelines and policies, and making appropriate referrals to respond to the needs of women who are dealing with various forms of violence in their lives.
- Obtain appropriate supervision to address the effects of vicarious traumatization.
- Seek care and support to deal with the effect of various forms of violence on one's own life.

Women's Strengths
- Support women to find their voice by helping them to recognize that they are experts on their own lives.
- Explore with women how their unique experiences affect their mental health; for example, being uprooted from their homes, communities and countries; multiples losses; social isolation; oppression; discrimination; poverty and violence.
- Develop strategies that enable women to identify, draw from and build on their learning from past experiences as well as recognize their strengths and accomplishments.

Inclusive and Holistic Approaches
- Encourage holistic practice models that consider the totality of women's experience by, for example, hearing and validating the impact of sexism, racism and heterosexism on women's mental health (Shashiah & Yee, 2006).
- Involve women in developing and managing their treatment plan. For example, explore with women any requests they might have about using alternative therapies.
- Develop holistic approaches that view the mind, body and spirit as an integrated whole. Acquire knowledge and incorporate into care women's spirituality and expressions of spirituality.
- Include people whom women want to involve in their care and treatment, such as family, friends or people from the community. (Mental illness is stigmatized in most communities, so women may be cautious in their choice of people who they wish to participate in their care.)
- Create programs with women that enable them to connect with others who share similar experiences, voice their concerns collectively, and rebuild new and supportive social networks.

TOWARD SYSTEMIC CHANGE

- Develop strategies to collectively confront systemic racism, sexism and heterosexism.
- Consider the context of women's everyday lives when planning care and treatment. Consider "what major accessibility and capacity needs of immigrant and

refugee women do existing health and social services not successfully meet?" (Mulvihill et al., 2001, p. 14). With knowledge of immigrant women's needs, one can then work to address the gaps in services.

- Collaborate with groups and community-based agencies that provide services to immigrant women such as those providing legal, housing, employment and recreation services.
- Lobby for organizations that are committed to social justice and equity and challenge practices that are discriminatory, oppressive and/or create barriers to equitable care.

RECOMMENDATIONS FOR MENTAL HEALTH PROMOTION SERVICES PROVIDERS

- Take a holistic approach to mental health promotion by considering physical, mental, social, emotional and spiritual aspects of women's lives.
- Build on women's strengths and resilience by advocating for policies that create supportive environments and are conducive to mental health promotion.
- Involve stakeholders at multiple levels, including the individual, family and community, as well as within organizations and the larger society to address the diverse needs of women and put in place the supports and resources women require to engage in mental health promotion activities.
- Engage in community-based and ethnic media–based campaigns to raise awareness of rights, responsibilities, laws and customs of Canadian citizens.
- Develop collaborative working relationships with communities to develop innovative strategies to address such issues as stigma related to violence. Strategies could, for example, involve engaging men, women and youth in education about intimate partner violence.
- Work with educators, guidance counsellors, teachers and principals to develop curricula and after-school programs based on anti-oppression frameworks.

RECOMMENDATIONS FOR MENTAL HEALTH AGENCIES/INSTITUTIONS

- Promote multidisciplinary teamwork within organizations and encourage input from all mental health team members who participate in women's care.
- Promote organizational changes that reflect the needs of diverse mental health consumers by, for example, including cultural interpretation and education programs and material in languages common to consumers; by ensuring interpreters have training in issues related to mental health and follow ethical and confidentiality guidelines; and by removing barriers to women's access to care.
- Demonstrate a commitment to promoting equity and inclusive services and

workplaces (e.g., by providing funding for anti-racism strategies), which means doing more than adopting anti-racist terminology (Shahsiah & Yee, 2006).

- Promote workplace policies and practices that are equitable (Collins, 2004).
- Engage in supportive alliances with communities and build on their strengths to develop and maintain community-based mental health promotion programs.

Policy

A clear link exists between research, practice, education and policy. It is important that mental health professionals develop partnerships with communities to identify policies that affect the availability of and access to care, supports and services for women of all backgrounds. Presented here are a few ideas. (We refer the reader to other chapters of this book as well as other works—including Mulvihill et al., 2001— for further ideas.)

ENSURING MULTIPLE VOICES

- Incorporate the voices, interests and aspirations of women in policy development by consulting and working with women to develop mental health promotion strategies across sectors. For example, some women may be advocates for child care, others for promoting safe neighbourhoods, while still others may be interested in recreational facilities for themselves and their families.
- Establish forums that are "built upon the use of inclusive language and directly networked with health and social policy researchers" (Vissandjée et al., 2007, p. 234).
- Put in place mechanisms such as the establishment of committees made up of a cross-section of community leaders to consult and advise on existing policies and the development of new ones.

SUPPORT AND FUNDING

- Increase allocation of funding and resources for community-based health promotion and illness prevention programs.
- Increase allocation of funding from all levels of government to improve the capacities of various "immigrant-serving organizations" and ethno-racial agencies to meet the settlement needs of women.
- Acknowledge, support and provide designated funding to guidance counsellors, settlement workers and others providing assistance to mothers who have been separated from their children and/or who are working to address issues arising from reunification with their children (Bernhard et al., 2005).

- Strengthen government-supported programs for skills development, employment training, leadership training and further education to meet the unique needs of women arriving in Canada under its specific immigration criteria and categories.
- Provide funding and support programs to bring about zero tolerance of discrimination in workplaces.

ACCESS

- Develop standards for training cultural interpreters in collaboration with mental health professionals, educators, policy-makers and professional organizations to support women's access to appropriate care.
- Make available services and programs such as transportation and drop-in programs to increase older immigrant women's access to health and settlement services for their health and well-being.
- Design and deliver "community based health care, home care, and early childhood education programs to ensure against over-reliance on [older women] as a source of unpaid caregivers" (Mulvihill et al., 2001, p. 22).
- Increase the number of language training programs across geographical settings and facilitate immigrant women's participation in such programs by providing child care, opportunities for social interaction and financial incentives.

ADDRESSING SYSTEMIC BARRIERS

- Create policies to address the ongoing delays and devaluation of professional skills and qualifications of immigrant women and the persistence of labour market inequities (Vissandjée et al., 2007).
- Put in place policies to address the financial needs of older immigrant women.
- Encourage collaboration among agencies, institutions and hospitals to improve accessibility and quality of services, ensuring that they are provided seamlessly and in non-stigmatizing ways.
- Institute ways to address school policies and programs that may contribute to the marginalization of girls and youth from racialized communities.
- Create speedy changes to address the ongoing delays in processing immigration family sponsorship applications.
- Ensure strategies are put in place to inform every woman of her rights within a sponsor-sponsored relationship. Put in place policies to address the immigration and/or legal concerns and needs of women dealing with IPV.

Final Thoughts

While Canada's mental health system has served the needs of consumers for decades, the system needs to change to reflect the needs of immigrant groups who now constitute a significant percentage of the population. Urgent changes are needed in the delivery of mental health services including mental health promotion, care and treatment to ensure effective and relevant services to immigrant women. For this to occur, mental health practitioners need to collaborate and work innovatively with women consumers, their communities, and various stakeholders at the local, provincial and national levels of government as well as academic and policy partners. Mental health professionals must look to and use frameworks and strategies that help to address inequalities, oppression and marginalization and that enable immigrant women to build on their strengths and give voice to their experiences.

References

Bernhard, J., Landholt, P. & Goldring, L. (2005, July). Transnational, multi-local motherhood: Experiences of separation and reunification among Latin American families in Canada. *CERIS Working Paper No. 40. Toronto: CERIS.* Available: www.ceris.metropolis.net. Accessed January 28, 2008.

Collins, E. (2004). Career mobility among immigrant registered nurses in Canada: Experiences of Caribbean women. Unpublished doctoral thesis, University of Toronto.

Gagnon, A.J., Tuck, J. & Barkun, L. (2004). A systematic review of questionnaires measuring the health of resettling refugee women. *Health Care for Women International, 25* (2), 111–149.

Gerrish, K., Husband, C. & Mackenzie, J. (1996). *Nursing for a Multi-ethnic Society.* Buckingham: Open University Press.

Hyman, I. & Guruge, S. (2007). Immigrant women's health. In R. Srivastava (Ed.). *The Health Care Professional's Guide to Cultural Competence* (pp. 264–280). Toronto: Mosby, Elsevier.

Lo, H. & Pottinger, A. (2007). Mental health practice. In R. Srivastava (Ed.). *The Health Care Professional's Guide to Cultural Competence* (pp. 247–261), Toronto: Mosby, Elsevier.

Martinez-Schallmoser, L., Telleen, S. & MacMullen, N.J. (2003). The effect of social support and acculturation on postpartum depression in Mexican American women. *Journal of Transcultural Nursing, 14* (4), 329–338.

Mulvihill, M., Mailloux, L. & Atkin, W. (2001). Advancing policy and research responses to immigrant and refugee women's health in Canada. Prepared for the Centres of Excellence in Women's Health. Winnipeg: Canadian Women's Health Network.

Shahsiah, S. & Yee, J. (2006, November). Striving for Best Practices and Equitable Mental Health Care for Racialised Communities in Toronto. Available: www.accessalliance.ca. Accessed February 1, 2008.

Sherkin, S. (2004). Community-based research on immigrant women: Contributions and challenges. *CERIS Working Paper No. 32. Toronto: CERIS.* Available: http://ceris.metropolis.net. Accessed January 28. 2008.

Vissandjée, B., Thurston, W., Apale, A. & Nahar, K. (2007). Women's health at the intersection of gender and the experience of international migration In M. Morrow, O. Hankivsky & C. Varcoe (Eds.). *Women's Health in Canada: Critical Perspectives on Theory and Policy* (pp. 221–243). Toronto: University of Toronto Press.

About the Editors

SEPALI GURUGE, RN, BScN, M.Sc., PhD. Associate Professor, School of Nursing, Ryerson University, Toronto, Canada

Sepali's nursing experience includes practice, teaching, research and consultation at several major hospitals in Toronto. Her teaching and research interests are in the areas of women's health, immigrants' health, mental health and violence against women throughout the migration process. She obtained her education in Sri Lanka, in the former Soviet Union and in Canada. Sepali's doctoral dissertation in nursing from the University of Toronto explored the influence of gender, racial, social and economic inequalities on the production of and responses to intimate partner violence in the post-migration context. Her post-doctoral work in nursing at the University of Western Ontario focused on the health effects of partner violence. Sepali has published and presented papers both nationally and internationally, and is presently engaged in international research on women's health with colleagues in Sri Lanka, Ethiopia, "mainland" United States and Hawaii.

ENID COLLINS, RN, MS, M.Ed., EdD. Professor Emeritus, School of Nursing, Ryerson University, Toronto, Canada

Enid brings to this project a range of perspectives as an immigrant woman, a nurse and an educator. Before coming to Canada, she completed a diploma as a registered nurse at the Kingston Public Hospital School of Nursing in Jamaica. She later did undergraduate and graduate work in Canada and the United States. Enid's work in nursing leadership, practice and education spans many areas, including maternal child health nursing, community health nursing, women's health and transcultural health. She has long been an advocate, mentor and role model for women in nursing and health care. Enid completed her doctoral work in sociology and equity studies at the Ontario Institute for Studies in Education. Her doctoral dissertation examined career mobility among Caribbean women who were registered nurses in Canada.

About the Authors

DIANA ABRAHAM, MSW, is an immigrant from Guyana and a former senior consultant with the Ontario Ministry of Citizenship and Immigration. At the ministry, her responsibilities included developing training programs for spoken language interpreters who assist women to access services for victims of domestic violence. She has been actively involved in the movement to advance the recognition of standards for the practice of community interpreters and is currently a PhD candidate at the Faculty of Environmental Studies at York University.

PAOLA ARDILES, MHSc., immigrated to Canada as a child from Latin America in the '70s. Paola is a certified cultural interpreter and has facilitated support groups for new mothers and newcomers to Canada. Her research focuses on women's health, with an emphasis on immigrant health issues. She is a co-investigator in a qualitative study examining the role of ethnocultural factors in postpartum depression (PPD). Paola has facilitated workshops across Ontario and co-produced a training video on PPD for health and social service providers working with diverse populations. She has a master's degree in health promotion from the University of Toronto.

B. KHAMISA BAYA, MA, is currently doing a doctorate in development studies in the Department of Political Science at the University of Toronto, where she is doing her thesis on Sudanese refugees. Khamisa was born in Sudan and is the co-founder of Ani-Sa'a: The Association of Sudanese Women in Research and Development. Her work has focused on immigrant women's health and her interests are mainly in the areas of women's health, gender, equity and refugees.

SILVANA BAZET, Clinical Member, Ontario Society of Psychotherapists, is a psychotherapist in private practice in Toronto who specializes in issues related to sexual orientation, ethno-racial identity, migration and gender identity, working from anti-oppression and relational perspectives. Silvana is also an educator, developing and facilitating numerous workshops on these topics at conferences and community agencies. She is a Latin American lesbian who has been doing community and social justice work for more than 20 years.

HELENE BERMAN, RN, PhD, is an associate professor of nursing at the University of Western Ontario and Scotiabank Chair for the Centre for Research and Education on Violence Against Women and Children. Her research focuses on the intersections of culture, health and violence in children's lives. She has led several national studies on subtle and explicit forms of violence experienced by girls and young women. Helene is past chairperson of the Alliance of Canadian

Research Centres on Violence and co-editor of *In the Best Interests of the Girl Child,* a report funded by Status of Women Canada.

SARAH BUKHARI, MA, is co-founder of Ani-Sa'a: The Association of Sudanese Women in Research and Development and does volunteer community development work within the Sudanese community in Ontario. Currently director of program development at a non-profit organization, she is pursuing her interests in community development, literacy, race relations and social justice. Sarah holds a master's in political science from the American University in Cairo.

AGATHA CAMPBELL, MSW, RSW, completed her secondary schooling in the Caribbean, where she grew up. She later immigrated to Canada and, while working full time, completed her undergraduate degree at York University. She then did her master's at Wilfred Laurier University. Agatha currently works as a social worker in child welfare. She has a keen interest in attachment, separation and reunification resulting from personal and professional experiences.

CINDY-LEE DENNIS, PhD, is an associate professor at the Lawrence Bloomberg Faculty of Nursing at the University of Toronto and holds a Canada Research Chair in Perinatal Community Health. She is the principal investigator of two large, multi-site randomized controlled trials related to the prevention and treatment of postpartum depression (PPD) and is a co-investigator on six other research projects. Cindy-Lee has published more than 50 peer-reviewed articles on diverse maternal and infant health outcomes including the detection, prevention and treatment of PPD. She has also co-authored a bestselling book on postpartum depression and has completed five Cochrane systematic reviews on this topic.

FARZANA DOCTOR, MSW, RSW, is a consultant and trainer specializing in diversity and clinical issues related to working with marginalized populations. She is also a psychotherapist in private practice, specializing in working with individuals and couples from an anti-oppression perspective. Farzana has co-authored books, book chapters and articles on working with lesbian, gay, bisexual, transgender and transsexual people with substance use and depression concerns, and on counselling lesbian and bisexual women of colour. She has been an instructor at the University of Toronto and Ryerson Faculties of Social Work. Farzana authored a novel, *Stealing Nasreen* (Inanna, 2007). She received her master's from Carlton University in 1993.

ZORINA FLAMAN, RN, MHS, CSPI, was born in the Caribbean and completed her initial nursing training in England. After doing her undergraduate degree at York University, Zorina undertook her master's through Athabasca University while working full time. Presently, Zorina works at a pediatric hospital in Toronto as a certified poison information specialist and is associated with the *Diversity in Action Initiative* at the same hospital. Zorina is interested in working with immigrant women and their children, poison prevention, health promotion and diversity.

DIANA L. GUSTAFSON, RN, BA, M.Ed., PhD, has had an interest in social justice since her youth. Long before she had labels for feminism and anti-oppression, Diana was concerned about equity. That commitment infused her work as a nurse, clinical specialist and educator, and is a recurring theme in her research, teaching and community work. Diana brings her disciplinary roots in health, education, sociology and women studies to her current position as associate professor of social science and health with the Division of Community Health and Humanities at the Faculty of Medicine at Memorial University in St. John's, Newfoundland.

ILENE HYMAN, PhD, has expertise in the area of health and its determinants for immigrant and racialized populations. She has been involved in several research studies examining intimate partner violence in newcomer communities including studies of prevalence, risk factors and help-seeking behaviour. Ilene is an assistant professor in the Department of Public Health Sciences at the University of Toronto and is affiliated with CERIS—The Ontario Metropolis Centre.

YASMIN JIWANI, PhD, is an associate professor in the Department of Communication Studies at Concordia University. Prior to moving to Montreal, she was the principal researcher and co-ordinator of the BC/Yukon Centre for Research on Violence Against Women and Children. She recently wrote *Discourses of Denial: Mediations of Race, Gender and Violence* (2006) and co-edited *Girlhood: Redefining the Limits* (2006). Her articles have been published in the *International Journal of Violence Against Women, Critical Middle Eastern Studies, Social Justice,* and the *Canadian Journal of Communications.*

PARVATHY KANTHASAMY, PhD, is a community mental health advocate at Community Resource Connections of Toronto. She has also been an instructor at the South Asia Studies Program at the University of Toronto; a research associate at the Centre for Refugee Studies at York University; and a Senior Fulbright Fellow at Stanford University. As a community activist, she has worked extensively with abused and other high-risk women. Her research interests include gender and class construction in the Sri Lankan community. Parvathy is a founding member of Vasantham, a Tamil seniors' wellness centre. She has won various awards including the City of Toronto's Status of Women award, recognizing contributions toward equitable treatment for women.

ROBIN A. MASON, M.Ed., PhD, is a research scientist in the Violence and Health Research Program at the Women's College Research Institute and an assistant professor with the Department of Public Health Sciences at the University of Toronto. Her research focuses on the health effects of intimate partner violence (IPV) and the experience of IPV in ethnocultural communities. She also trains and educates health care professionals on these issues. Robin has been involved in developing policies and curricula on IPV locally, provincially and nationally.

FARAH N. MAWANI, M.Sc., PhD Candidate, is completing her thesis in Public Health Sciences at the University of Toronto. Farah is committed to qualitative and quantitative research focused on improving immigrant mental health by influencing policy and program change. She is currently a fellow of the Statistics Canada Tom Symons Research Stipend Program and the Research in Addictions and Mental Health Policy & Services (RAMHPS) CIHR Strategic Training Program. She is past chair of the board of directors for Access Alliance Multicultural Community Health Centre and a member of the Expert Review and Advisory Committee of the Canadian Women's Health Network.

JAIRO ORTIZ, MSW, RSW, is a social work practice leader in the Community Mental Health Program at Toronto Western Hospital. In 1998, he participated as a research associate in the Canadian Incidence Study of Child Abuse and Neglect, directed by Dr. Nico Trocme. Jairo is an adjunct practice professor at the Faculty of Social Work at the University of Toronto, where he did his master's degree. He grew up in Colombia, where he did a degree in clinical psychology prior to immigrating to Canada in 1979.

STELLA RAHMAN, MB, BS, works as a clinical services consultant at the Centre for Addiction and Mental Health where she co-ordinates the Cultural Interpretation Services. She is also a physician from Bangladesh and an accredited Bengali freelance interpreter with the Ministry of the Attorney General. Stella addresses interpreters' requests and helps clinicians work effectively and efficiently with interpreters. She believes that not bridging the language barrier can have tragic consequences, especially in a health care setting, where good communication is essential. Stella sits on many internal and external committees with the goal of establishing best practices in medical interpretation.

LORI E. ROSS, PhD, is a research scientist at the Centre for Addiction and Mental Health and Women's College Hospital in Toronto. Her main research interests are women's mental health, pregnancy and the postpartum period, particularly among marginalized populations. Lori is also a lead investigator on research projects examining mental health problems in immigrant mothers and in co-parenting lesbian and bisexual women.

EDWARD JASON SANTOS, BScN, has completed a bachelor of science in nursing at Ryerson University and is interested continuing his studies at the graduate and post-graduate level. Edward has a particular interest in psychosocial and mental health nursing, with a focus in palliative care research for the geriatric population and in working with immigrant women. Edward has been involved in various research projects on intimate partner violence in the immigrant women community.

YOGENDRA B. SHAKYA, PhD, is the research and evaluation co-ordinator at Access Alliance Multicultural Community Health Centre. His research interests include social determinants of newcomer health, racialization of poverty and international development. Yogendra currently leads a number of community-based participatory research projects at Access Alliance focused on the health impacts of racism and racialized inequalities, refugee mental health and newcomer youth issues.

LAURA SIMICH, PhD, is a cultural anthropologist, an assistant professor of psychiatry at the University of Toronto and a scientist at the Centre for Addiction and Mental Health. Laura specializes in qualitative, community-based and policy-oriented research on social determinants of mental health among newcomers, particularly during refugee resettlement. Her research interests include community mental health and cultural diversity, immigrant family adaptation and contributions to children's mental health, and experiences of social exclusion and mental well-being among non-status immigrants.

EVA SAPHIR, MA, DTATI, has worked in the field of trauma since 1980, when she co-founded and co-coordinated Hospice Wellington for the terminally ill and their families. In 1988, she created the counselling program at Casey House Hospice in Toronto for people with HIV/AIDS. As an original member of Toronto Western Hospital's team of Spanish-speaking therapists, she then spent 15 years working with refugees and immigrants from Latin America as a mental health clinician in their Community Mental Health Program. She also created and co-facilitated an art therapy group at the hospital for Latin people living with HIV. Eva was born in Argentina and is now in private practice in Toronto.